Telephone Numbers & Information

Emergency Medical Service (EMS): _____

Fire: _____ Police: _____ Poison Control Center: 800.222.1222

Local Poison Control: _____ National Suicide Prevention Lifeline: 800.273.8255

Health Care Providers

Name	Specialty	Telephone Number

Pharmacy: _____ Phone Number: _____

Hospital: _____ Phone Number: _____

Employee Assistance Program (EAP): _____

Health Insurance Information

Company: _____ Phone Number: _____

Address: _____

Policyholder's Name: _____ Policy Number: _____

What to Tell Your Doctor or Provider

(Make copies as needed.)

Use this summary when you call or visit a doctor or provider. See pages 13, 14, 36 and 37 for more information.

Symptoms

☐ Pain   ☐ Nausea/vomiting   ☐ Skin problems   ☐ Eye, ear, nose, throat problems

☐ Fever/chills ☐ Breathing problems ☐ Stomach problems   ☐ Muscle or joint problems

Other problems: _____

Specific questions I have now: _____

What I need to do: _____

Medications

	Name/Dose	Name/Dose
Current medications:		
Medication allergies:		

1

Healthier at Home®

Your Guide to Self-Care & Wise Health Consumerism

Written by
Don R. Powell, Ph.D.
and the
American Institute for Preventive Medicine

Note: This book is not meant to be a complete guide to health care. The information is given to help you make informed choices about your health. You should not replace this information for expert medical advice or treatment. Follow your doctor's advice if it differs from what is given in this book. Also, if the problem you are reading about doesn't go away after a reasonable amount of time, you should see or call your doctor.

Please know that many of the designations used by manufacturers and sellers to distinguish their products are claimed as trademarks. Where those designations appear in this book and the American Institute for Preventive Medicine was aware of a trademark claim, the designations have been printed in initial capital letters (e.g., Tums).

This guide is one of many self-care books and programs offered by the American Institute for Preventive Medicine. The goal of all of these products is to help individuals reduce health care costs and improve the quality of their lives.

For more information, call or write:
American Institute for Preventive Medicine
30445 Northwestern Hwy., Suite 350
Farmington Hills, MI 48334
248.539.1800 / Fax 248.539.1808
E-mail: aipm@healthylife.com

For free health information:
Go to: www.HealthyLearn.com. At this site, type a topic in the box for "Search MedlinePlus."

Online instructional video:
An online video shows you how to get the maximum benefit from this book.
Go to: www.HealthyLearn.com and click on "Self-Care and You Instructional Video."

{*Note*: "Life Art Image. Williams and Wilkins. All rights reserved." applies to many illustrations in this book.}

ISBN-13: 978-0-9765048-0-1
ISBN-10: 0-9765048-0-4

Acknowledgements

Susan Schooley, M.D., Medical Director, Detroit Region and Chair, Department of Family Medicine, Henry Ford Medical Group, Detroit, MI; Medical Director, American Institute for Preventive Medicine, Farmington Hills, MI

Edward Adler, M.D., S.A.C.P., Attending Physician, Division of Geriatric Medicine, William Beaumont Hospital, Royal Oak, MI

Richard Aghababian, M.D., Past President, American College of Emergency Physicians, Washington, DC

Sara D. Atkinson, M.D., Child & Adolescent Psychiatry; General Psychiatry, Menninger Clinic, Topeka, KS

Jeffrey D. Band, M.D., Corporate Epidemiologist, Chief of Infectious Diseases and Medical Director, InterHealth: Health Care for International Travelers, William Beaumont Hospital, Royal Oak, MI

Mark H. Beers, M.D., Senior Director of Geriatrics and Associate Editor, Merck Manual, West Point, PA

Joseph Berenholz, M.D., F.A.C.O.G., Diplomate, American College of Obstetrics and Gynecology, Clinical Instructor, Detroit Medical Center, Detroit, MI

Dwight L. Blackburn, M.D., Former Medical Director, Anthem Blue Cross/Blue Shield, Louisville, KY

Douglas D. Blevins, M.D., Departments of Infectious Disease, Internal Medicine, Lewis-Gale Clinic, Salem, VA

Frances B. DeHart, R.N., B.S.N., Former Health Management Specialist, HealthFirst, Greenville, SC

Peter Fass, M.D., Former Medical Director, KeyCorp, Cleveland, OH

Steve Feldman, M.D., Internal Medicine, William Beaumont Hospital, Royal Oak, MI

Elaine Frank, M.Ed., R.D., Vice President, American Institute for Preventive Medicine, Farmington Hills, MI

Barry A. Franklin, Ph.D., Director, Cardiac Rehabilitation and Exercise Laboratories, William Beaumont Hospital, Royal Oak, MI

Gerald Freidman, M.D., Medical Director, Physicians Health Plan, Kalamazoo, MI

Abe Gershonowicz, D.D.S., Family Dentistry, Sterling Heights, MI

Lary Goldman, M.D., FACC, Cardiovascular Specialists, P.C., Farmington Hills, MI; Cardiologist, William Beaumont Hospital, Royal Oak, MI

Gary P. Gross, M.D., Dermatologist, Lewis-Gale Clinic, Salem, VA

Bruce Gursky, D.D.S., Complete Dental Care, Madison Heights, MI

J. Bruce Hagadorn, M.D., Otolaryngologist, Lewis-Gale Clinic, Salem, VA

Donald Hayes, M.D., Former Medical Director, Sara Lee Corporation, Winston-Salem, NC

William Hettler, M.D., Director, University Health Service, University of Wisconsin, Stevens Point, WI

Ronald Holmes, M.D., Former Director, Division of General Pediatrics, Professor, Department of Pediatrics, University of Michigan Medical Center, Ann Arbor, MI

William J. Kagey, M.D., Pediatrician, Lewis-Gale Clinic, Salem, VA

Jeanette Karwan, R.D., Director, Product Development, American Institute for Preventive Medicine, Farmington Hills, MI

Steven N. Klein, M.D., FACS, FASCRS, Chairman, Department of Colon and Rectal Surgery and of the Credentials and Qualifications Committee, William Beaumont Hospital, Royal Oak, MI

James Kohlenberg, M.D., Internal Medicine, John R Medical Clinic, Madison Heights, MI and William Beaumont Hospital, Royal Oak, MI

Richard S. Lang, M.D., M.P.H., Head, Section of Preventive Medicine, Department of Internal Medicine, Cleveland Clinic Foundation, OH

Table of Contents

Section I
Wise Health Care Choices

Chapter 1. Medical Care

Chapter 2. Medical Exams & Tests

Chapter 3. Medications

Chapter 4. Complementary & Alternative Medicine

Chapter 5. Medical Decisions

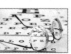

Chapter 11. Respiratory Conditions

Chapter 12. Skin Conditions

Chapter 13. Digestive & Urinary Problems

Chapter 14. Muscle & Bone Problems

Chapter 15. General Health Conditions

Chapter 16. Mental Health Conditions

Chapter 17.
Men's Health Issues

Chapter 18.
Women's Health Issues

Chapter 19. Children's
Health Problems

Chapter 20. Dental &
Mouth Concerns

Section IV
Emergencies & First Aid

Chapter 21.
Emergency Procedures

Chapter 22. Emergency
Conditions / First Aid

Index

Section 1

Wise Health Care Choices

There is a lot to know about health care. This section will help you make wise choices. It gives information, such as: How to choose a doctor; when to have medical exams and tests; and how to use medicines safely. These and other topics can help you take charge of your health. They can help you take care of your family's health needs, too.

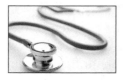

Chapter 1
Medical Care

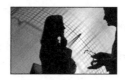

Chapter 2
Medical Exams
& Tests

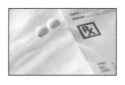

Chapter 3
Medications

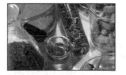

Chapter 4
Complementary &
Alternative
Medicine

Chapter 5
Medical
Decisions

Chapter 1

Medical Care

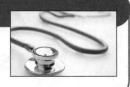

Choosing a Doctor or Health Care Provider

Finding the right doctor or health care provider for you is a big part of your medical care. Don't wait until you get sick to find one. When you look for or change doctors, follow these tips:

- Look for one who accepts your health plan. Check with the plan. Ask the person at work who handles employee benefits.

- If you belong to a managed care plan, get a list of providers who work with the plan. Health Maintenance Organizations (HMOs) and Preferred Provider Organizations (PPOs) are two types of managed care plans. The doctor(s) you see now may be on your HMO or PPO list.

- Ask relatives and friends for doctors they trust and have given them good medical care.

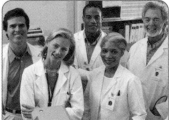

Make a list of things you want in a doctor or provider, such as close location, certain gender, age, etc.

- Find out if a doctor is taking new patients. Check with your health plan. Call the doctor's office.

- Look for a doctor you can relate to. How do you want medical decisions to be made? The doctor alone? You and the doctor together? Find one that meets your needs.

- Ask about office hours and staffing. Ask how many patients are scheduled to be seen in an hour and how long they usually wait to see the doctor.

- Ask how payment is handled. Must you pay at the time of your visit or can you be billed?

- Find out what other providers serve as backups when the doctor is away. Ask what you should do at non-office hour times.

- Find out which hospital(s) the doctor or provider sends patients to.

- Look for a doctor who is competent and can care for all your general health needs. Ask if and who the doctor will refer you to for any special health needs.

Find out about doctors, hospitals, and healthcare services from:

HealthyLearn® • www.HealthyLearn.com
Click on "Medline Plus®" and then on "Directories."

American Board of Medical Specialties (ABMS)
866.ASK.ABMS (275.2267)
www.abms.org

Federation of State Medical Boards
888.ASK.FCVS (275.3287)
www.fsmb.org

Health Grades
www.healthgrades.com

U.S. Department of Health & Human Services
www.healthfinder.gov

See Your "Primary" Doctor Before You See a Specialist

Primary care doctors manage your medical care. If you are a member of a Health Maintenance Organization (HMO), your primary care doctor is the doctor you select from the HMO plan to coordinate your medical care. This person could be a family doctor, internist, obstetrician/gynecologist, etc. Whether or not you belong to an HMO, call or see your primary care doctor before you see a specialist. If your primary care doctor cannot take care of your needs, he or she will refer you to a specialist.

Tell & Ask the Doctor/Provider Checklists

(Make copies as needed. Use the lines to fill in the information.)

Checklist 1 – Before You Call or See Your Doctor/Provider

Your signs and symptoms (in the order they occurred and what makes them better or worse): _____

Results of home testing, such as your temperature: _____

Medicines you take (prescribed, over-the-counter, herbal products, vitamins, etc.): _____

Allergies to medicines, food, etc.: _____

Family and personal medical history: _____

Your lifestyle: Eating, drinking, sleeping, exercising habits, sexual functioning, etc.: _____

Concerns you have about your health and/or what you think the problem may be due to:_____

What you would like the doctor to do for you: _____

Your pharmacist's phone number and fax number: _____

{*Note:* If needed, have your medical records, results of lab tests and X-rays, etc. from other health care providers sent to your doctor before your visit.}

Checklist 2 – During the Doctor/Provider Visit or Call

Tell the doctor what you wrote down in Checklist 1. (Take the list with you.) _____

_____

Ask your doctor these questions:

What do you think the problem or diagnosis is? _____

_____

What, if any, tests are needed to rule out or confirm your diagnosis? _____

_____

What do I need to do to treat the problem? Do I need to take medicine? How can I prevent the

problem in the future? _____

_____

When do I need to call or see you again? _____

_____

How are costs handled for this visit and for tests? _____

_____

Checklist 3 – After the Doctor/Provider Visit or Call

Follow your doctor's advice.

Call the doctor's office if you don't understand his or her instructions.

Tell your doctor if you feel worse, have other problems or side effects from the medicines, etc.

Keep return visit appointments.

Choosing a Health Plan

Know Your Options

- If you get health insurance through work, find out what health plan choices are offered. Get information from the employee benefits office and/or from the insurance companies. Find out the time of year when you can join or change health plans. Even if an employer gives only one health plan choice, find out what the health plan provides. Find out what you need to do to get the health care that you and family members need.

- If you do not get health insurance through work, find out about health insurance from:
  - An insurance broker. This person can assess your needs and recommend a health plan to purchase on your own.
  - Professional organizations and social or civic groups that offer health plans to members.

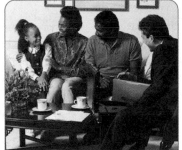

An insurance broker can recommend health plan options.

  - Your state's Health Department, Department of Community Health, or State Medicaid Office (for some low-income and disabled people).

- Find out if you are eligible for Medicare. Contact 800.MEDICARE (633.4227), your local Social Security Administration, or access www.medicare.gov on the Internet.

Comparing Health Plans

Different Types of Health Plans

- *Health Savings Account (HSA).* Money set aside by you or your employer (on a tax-free basis) to pay for current and future medical expenses.

- *High-deductible Health Plan.* A plan that gives comprehensive coverage for high cost medical events. It includes a high-deductible and a limit on annual out-of-pocket costs. A health savings account or health spending account is usually coupled with this type of plan.

- *Indemnity Plan.* This type of health plan is also called fee-for-service. You can use any medical provider. The provider bills for each service given. You and the insurance plan each pay part of the bill as stated by the plan.

- *Managed Care Plans.* These kinds of plans provide services and handle payment for them. You have less paperwork with these plans compared to an indemnity plan. Managed care plans use certain doctors, hospitals, and health care providers. There are three basic types of managed care plans.
  - *Health Maintenance Organization (HMO).* With this, you pick a primary doctor who manages all of the medical services you receive.

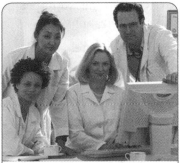

Managed care plans have many doctors to choose from.

  HMOs offer a range of health benefits. This includes preventive care.

- *Preferred Provider Organization (PPO).* With this, a network of providers gives medical services at a discount to its members. With a PPO, you can choose one or more providers from a list of those who participate with the health plan.

- *Point-of-Service (POS).* With this, you have the option to go to providers outside of the plan's network of providers. Some of the cost is still paid for by the plan.

Plans vary; so do costs and what is covered. With any plan, a basic premium is paid by you and/or your employer. After that, you pay extra costs (deductibles, co-pays, etc.). These costs vary. They depend on the plan. Compare costs and how each plan handles services. These include:

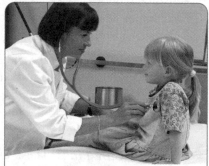

Find out if a health plan covers checkups and immunizations.

- Routine checkups, health screenings, and immunizations.

- Hospital care.

- Emergency and urgent care.

- Care by specialists.

- Maternity care.

- Preventive services, such as programs for weight loss.

- Prescription drugs.

- Vision care.

- Dental care.

- Mental health care.

- Substance abuse services.

- Physical therapy.

- Alternative health care.

- Home health care.

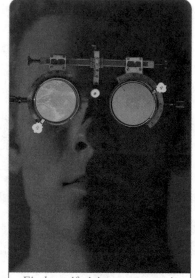

Find out if vision coverage is part of the plan.

Compare what different plans cover. Decide what is important to you and your family. Choose the plan that best meets your needs. Look at the quality of care, too.

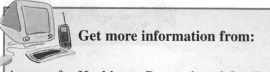

Get more information from:

Agency for Healthcare Research and Quality
www.ahrq.gov

Health Insurance Checklist

(Make copies of this form. Fill one out every year.)

Check off insurances that you have.

Types of Insurance	Name of Plan	Who to Contact
☐ Employer Insurance	_____	_____
☐ Individual Policy	_____	_____
☐ Medicare 　 Medicare Choices Helpline 　 Date called to apply for: _____ 　{*Note:* Call 3 months before, or no later than 3 months after you turn age 65.}		www.medicare.gov 800.MEDICARE (633.4227)
☐ Prescription Drug and 　 Other Assistance Programs	_____	www.medicare.gov 800.MEDICARE (633.4227)
☐ Local Social Security 　 Administration Number: _____		_____
☐ Medicaid Information:	_____ _____	www.cms.hhs.gov
☐ Medigap or Supplemental 　 Insurance	_____	_____
☐ Disability Insurance	_____	
☐ Long-Term Care Insurance	_____	http://longtermcareinsurance.org 800.587.3279
☐ Other	_____	_____

Using Your Health Plan

Know Your Health Plan

- Find out what the plan covers. Ask your employer, insurance company, or use the Web site you are given to get information.

- Read your health plan's policy and member handbook or Web site information. If you don't understand something, talk to your health benefits staff at work. Ask someone at the health plan's member services.

- Find out how services are paid for. What is your role to cover payment?

- If you belong to a managed care plan, find out how to get a list of the plan's providers. Ask how you find out about changes in covered services or in providers.

- Find out if the health plan has an advice hotline. Often, this is a toll-free number you can call 24 hours a day.

- Find out if services are covered when you are out of your home state or in another country.

- Find out if and how prescription drugs are covered. Find out if you have a co-pay for medicines and how much it is for generic and brand name drugs. Does the plan have a preferred list of medications (formulary)? If so, get a copy from the health plan. Take it to each doctor visit.

- Do you have to use the plan's mail order pharmacy? A mail order pharmacy may charge you the same co-pay amount for 90 days that you would pay for 30 days at a drug store.

- Find out how to file a complaint and an appeal if you and your doctor do not agree with the health plan's decision to provide care.

Be Involved in Your Health Care

- Discuss your needs with your doctor or health care provider.

- Ask questions. Ask for clear answers. Make sure you understand what you are told to do. Take notes. Ask another person to go with you, if necessary.

- Follow your doctor's advice. If you can't, let the doctor know.

- Learn about your condition from your doctor. (See, also, **Gather Facts** on page 35.)

- Keep track of medical needs for each family member. (See **Family Medical Record** on page 25.)

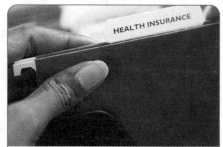

Keep copies of medical claim statements and payment receipts.

- If you are not satisfied with the service you get, discuss your concerns with the doctor or health care provider. If you are still not satisfied, consider using another provider.

Get more information from:

Agency for Healthcare Research and Quality (AHRQ)
www.ahrq.gov

Consumer Reports Best Buy Drugs
www.CRBestBuyDrugs.org

Preventing Medical Errors

Medical errors are a leading cause of death and injury. It has been reported that as many as 195,000 people a year die in U.S. hospitals due to medical errors.

Medical errors occur when a planned part of medical care doesn't work out or when the wrong plan was used. This can happen in hospitals, nursing homes, etc. and in your home. Examples of medical errors are:

- A wrong medicine is prescribed or taken.

- Too much medicine is taken.

- Mistakes are made before, during, or after surgery.

- The wrong problem is treated.

To help prevent medical errors, be your own watch dog. Take an active role in every decision about your health care.

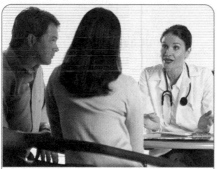

A family member or friend can be another 'set of ears.'

If necessary, have a family member or friend oversee your care.

General Tips

- Learn about your health problem and its treatments. Talk with your doctor and/or nurse. Use other trusted sources. (See **Gather Facts** on page 35.)

- Speak up if you have questions or concerns. You have a right to question anyone who is involved with your care.

- Make sure that someone, such as your personal doctor, is in charge of your care. This is very important if you have many health problems or are in a hospital.

- Make sure that all doctors, etc. involved in your care have your health information. Do not assume that they know everything they need to.

- Ask a family member or friend to be with you at office visits, etc. He or she can help get things done and speak up for you if you can't.

- Know that "more" is not always better. Find out why a test or treatment is needed. Ask how it can help you. You could be better off without it.

- If you have a test, don't assume that no news is good news. Find out the results.

- If you are having surgery, make sure that you, your doctor, and your surgeon all agree and are clear on what will be done. Before you are taken into surgery, mark the body part to be operated on. (Use the marker, etc. the doctor gives you to do this.)

Medication Tips

- Make sure that all of your doctors, etc. know the medicines you take. This includes prescribed and over-the-counter (OTC) ones. It also includes vitamin and herbal supplements. Bring a list of your medicines and/or your medication bottles to your doctor visits.

- Make sure your doctor and pharmacist know about any allergies and adverse reactions you have had to medicines.

- When your doctor writes a prescription, make sure you can read it. If you can't read it, the pharmacist might not be able to read it either!

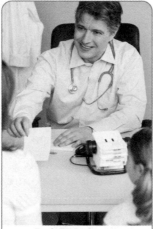

- Let your doctor know if you have problems swallowing pills. Some prescribed medicines do not work the right way when they are crushed.

Before a doctor prescribes a medicine, tell him or her about any allergies you have.

- Ask for information about your medicines in words you can understand. Do this when medicines are prescribed and when you receive them.

- When you receive your medicine, check the label. Make sure it has your name on it. If you have any questions, ask the pharmacist.

- Ask your pharmacist for the best device to measure liquid medicines. Also, ask questions if you're not sure how to use it.

- If you get medicines from a mail order pharmacy, call their customer service number for questions and concerns.

Hospital Stay Tips

- If you have a choice, choose a hospital with a good rating and a lot of experience in the procedure or surgery you need.

- Ask all health care workers who have direct contact with you if they have washed their hands. If not, request that they do.

- Tell the doctors, nurses, surgeon, and anesthetist any allergies you have. Make sure that things you are allergic to are written on your chart.

- If you are having surgery, make sure that you, your doctor, and your surgeon all agree and are clear on exactly what will be done.

- Follow pre-surgery instructions. Mark or sign your initials on the limb or area to be operated on.

- When you are discharged from the hospital, ask your doctor to explain the treatment plan you will use at home. Get written instructions for diet, activity, medicines, reasons to call your doctor, and when you need to be seen again.

- Ask for written information about the side effects your medicine could cause. Ask which ones you should contact your doctor for.

Get more information from:

Agency for Healthcare Research and Quality (AHRQ)
www.ahrq.gov

Chapter 2

Medical Exams & Tests

A Routine Checkup

A routine checkup from a doctor or health care provider is a way to find out your health status. It allows you to ask questions, too. It also helps you find out if you have a health problem you don't know about. Some diseases, such as high blood pressure and some cancers, may not have symptoms in the early stages. Tests and exams can help detect these. (See **Health Tests & When to Have Them** on page 22.)

The Basic Parts of a Checkup

- A complete medical history. This includes family health history, past illnesses, and current problems.

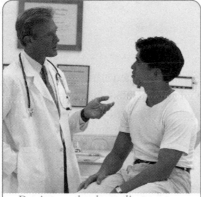
During a checkup, discuss your health concerns with your doctor.

- A check on how well your eyes, ears, heart, bowels, etc. function.

- A check of your blood pressure, pulse, temperature, etc.

- A medical exam.

- Routine tests. These include blood tests and a chest X-ray.

- A check of specific health concerns.

- Vaccinations, as needed.

Tests & What They Are For

Abdominal Aortic Anuerysm. This checks for problems with the aorta (the main artery in the body) and other structures in the upper abdomen.

Blood Pressure Test. This checks the force of blood against the walls of the arteries. The top number (systolic pressure) measures the force as the heart beats. The bottom number (diastolic pressure) measures the force between heartbeats when the heart is being refilled. High blood pressure may have no symptoms. It can lead to a heart attack and/or stroke.

Chlamydia Screening. This checks for chlamydia bacteria, which is transmitted sexually.

Cholesterol Blood Test. This checks the levels of fatty deposits (cholesterol) in the blood. High LDL-cholesterol levels are linked to heart disease.

Colorectal Cancer Screening. This checks for early signs of colorectal problems, including cancer.

Diabetes Screening. This checks for normal and abnormal blood sugar levels.

Mammogram. This X-ray detects breast problems.

Osteoporosis Screening. This measures bone density to predict the risk for fractures.

Pap Test. This checks for early signs of cervical cancer.

Professional Breast Exam. A health care provider examines the breasts for problems.

Prostate Cancer Screening. Two screening tools are a digital rectal exam and a PSA blood test. Men should talk to their doctors about the benefits and risks of these tests.

Health Tests & When to Have Them*

Health Test	Ages 18–29	Ages 30–39	Ages 40–49	Age 50 and older
Regular Dental Checkup	Every 6-12 months			
Physical Exam	Every 5 years	Every 2-4 years		Every 1-2 years
Blood Pressure	At every office visit or at least every 2 years			
Vision Exam	Every 5 years	Every 2-4 years		Every 1-2 years age 65+
Cholesterol Blood Test	Starting at age 35 (men); 45 (women at increased risk for coronary heart disease) or as advised			
Pap Test — W O M E N	At least every 3 years ages 20-65. As advised after age 65.			
Chlamydia Screening	All sexually active women ages 24 and younger; ages 25+ if at an increased risk			
Professional Breast Exam[1]			Discuss with doctor	
Mammogram[1]			Every 2 years ages 50-74 or as advised	
Osteoporosis Screening	Starting at age 65 (60 for women at increased risk for fractures) as often as advised			
Prostate Cancer Screening[2] — M E N			By age 50, discuss with doctor	
Abdominal Aortic Aneurysm Screening				One-time screening for men ages 65-75 who have ever smoked
Colorectal Cancer Screening[3]				Ages 50 to 75

Note: These are general guidelines. Adults should also be screened for alcohol misuse, depression, obesity, and tobacco use. If you are at an increased risk for an illness, tests may need to be done sooner or more often. Extra tests (e.g., screening for diabetes, glaucoma) may also need to be done. Persons with high blood pressure or high cholesterol should be screened for diabetes. Follow your doctor's advice. Check with your health plan to see if and when tests are covered. Get updates and more information on tests and exams from the Agency for Healthcare Research and Quality's "Guide to Clinical Preventive Services" at www.ahrq.gov/clinic/pocketgd.htm.

1. Breast cancer screening guidelines vary with different health groups. For ages 40-49 and 74+, discuss your breast cancer risk and the pros and cons of these screening tests with your doctor or health care provider. Women at a high risk for breast cancer should seek expert medical advice about breast cancer screening and prevention.
2. African American men and men with a brother or father diagnosed with prostate cancer should discuss the pros and cons of screening for prostate cancer with their doctors by age 45; by age 40 for men with multiple family members diagnosed with prostate cancer before age 65.
3. Follow your doctor's advice. Screening test options include a high-sensitivity stool blood test, sigmoidoscopy, and colonoscopy. How often testing is needed depends on the test(s) given and on your personal risk factors.

Immunization Schedule

Age ▶ Vaccine[1] ▼	Birth	1 mon	2 mos	4 mos	6 mos	12 mos	15 mos	18 mos	19 mos-3 yrs	4–6 yrs	7–12 yrs	13–18 yrs
Hepatitis B	HepB-1	HepB-2		*HepB (if needed)*	HepB-3 or 4						HepB Series[2]	
Rotavirus			RV-1	RV-2	RV-3 *(if needed)*							
Diphtheria Tetanus Pertussis			DTaP-1	DTaP-2	DTaP-3	DTaP-4				DTaP-5	Tdap (11-12 yrs)	Tdap[2]
Haemophilus Influenzae type b			Hib-1	Hib-2	*Hib (if needed)*	Hib-3 or 4						
Pneumo-coccal[3]			PCV-1	PCV-2	PCV-3	PCV-4			PCV[3] *(if needed)*			
Inactivated Poliovirus			IPV-1	IPV-2	IPV-3					IPV-4	IPV Series[2]	
Influenza[4]					Seasonal flu vaccine (yearly)							
Varicella						Varicella-1				Varicella-2	Varicella Series[2]	
Measles, Mumps, Rubella						MMR-1				MMR-2	MMR Series[2]	
Hepatitis A						HepA (2 doses)						
Meningo-coccal[5]											MCV 11-12 yrs[5]	MCV[2]
Human Papilloma-virus[6]											HPV[2,6] (3 doses) for girls aged 11-12 years (or from 9-26 years)	

1. For updates, contact CDC Immunization Program at 800.CDC.INFO (232.4636) or www.cdc.gov/vaccines. Ask your child's doctor what vaccines, health screenings, and checkups your child needs.
2. **Catch-up (make-up)** vaccines should be given to children and teenagers who have not already had them.
3. PCV vaccine protects against meningitis and some pneumonias. One dose is needed for all healthy children aged 24-59 months who are not completely vaccinated for their age. Some high-risk children age 2 years and older may also need a vaccine called PPV.
4. Starting at age 6 months, get H1N1 flu vaccine(s) as advised.
5. The MCV vaccine and booster vaccines are also advised for persons aged 2-55 years at increased risk for meningococcal disease. Follow your doctor's advice.
6. Males aged 9-26 years may be advised by their doctors to get 3 doses of HPV vaccine.
7. Adults may also need vaccines for: Varicella; Measles, Mumps, Rubella; Hepatitis A and/or B; and/or Human Papillomavirus. Follow your doctor's advice.

Adult Immunizations[7]			
Td (Tetanus Diphtheria)	Seasonal Flu Vaccine[4]	Zoster (Shingles) Vaccine	Pneumococcal Vaccine
Every 10 years	Yearly at age 50 and older or as advised	Once at age 60+	Once at 65 years or as advised

Vaccines for Traveling Abroad

Before you travel to other countries, find out if you need certain vaccines. Get information from the CDC Travelers' Information Line. Call 800.CDC.INFO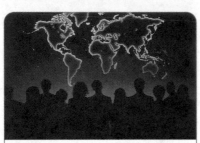

Before you travel abroad, find out if certain vaccines are required.

(232.4636) or use the www.cdc.gov/travel Web site. Discuss your needs with your doctor.

Home Medical Tests

Home medical tests let you check for and monitor health conditions at home.

Self-Testing Kits
- Diagnose when conditions are or are not present. These include kits that test for blood cholesterol level and blood in the stool.

- Monitor a chronic condition. These include kits that test for blood sugar levels and blood pressure readings.

The U.S. Public Health Service and the Food and Drug Administration (FDA) give tips for safe and proper use of self-testing kits. (Each of these does not apply to all tests.)

- Don't buy or use a test kit after the expiration date.

- Follow storage directions on the label.

- Note special precautions, such as not eating certain foods before testing.

- Study the package insert. First, read it through to get a general idea of how to perform the test. Then, go back and review the instructions and diagrams until you fully understand each step.

- Know what the test is meant to do and what it doesn't do. Tests are not always 100% accurate.

- Some test results rely on comparing colors. If you're colorblind, ask someone who is not colorblind to help you read the results.

- Follow instructions exactly. Don't skip a step.

- When you collect a urine sample, use a sterile or clean container.

- Some steps need to be timed. Use a watch or clock with a second hand.

- Note what you should do if the results are positive, negative, or unclear.

- If something is not clear, don't guess. Call the "800" number on the package or call a pharmacist for information.

- Keep test kits that have chemicals out of the reach of children. Throw away used test materials as directed.

Report any malfunction of a self-test to the manufacturer or to the:

U.S. Pharmacopoeia Practitioner's Reporting Network
12601 Twinbrook Parkway
Rockville, MD 20852
800.227.8772 or www.usp.org

Family Medical Record

A. Medical Conditions in Your Family (Father, mother, grandparents, brothers, sisters, aunts, uncles)

Condition	Relative	Age of Onset	Age and Cause of Death
Alcohol / Drug Abuse			
Allergies / Asthma			
Arthritis			
Bowel Disorder (Crohn's Disease, Colitis)			
Cancer & Type			
Cataracts / Glaucoma			
Depression			
Diabetes			
Hearing Problems			
Heart Disease / Stroke			
High Blood Pressure			
Migraine Headaches			
Pneumonia			
Smoker			
Thrombosis (Blood Clots)			
Thyroid Problems			

Other

B. Medical Log (Keep one for each family member.)

Condition/Surgery	Date Diagnosed	Doctor/Treatment/Comments
_____	_____	_____
_____	_____	_____
_____	_____	_____
_____	_____	_____

Blood Type _____

Allergies _____Drug Sensitivities _____

Chapter 3

Medications

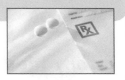

Safe Use of Medications

- Things to tell your doctor:
  - Things you have had an allergic reaction to.
  - If you are pregnant or breast-feeding.
  - If another doctor is also treating you.
  - If you have diabetes or kidney or liver disease.
  - If you use alcohol, tobacco, or drugs.

- See that your doctor has an up-to-date list of all the medicines you take. This includes prescribed and over-the-counter (OTC) ones, vitamins, and herbal supplements. Keep an up-to-date list in your wallet.

- Ask your doctor these questions: What is the medicine for? When should I take it? How long do I need to take it? Should I take it with or without food? Can I crush the pill or open up the capsule if I can't swallow it whole? Write these things down so you don't forget what was said.

- Tell your local and mail order pharmacist what medicines and supplements you take. List these on the form the health plan sends you. Harmful mixtures with other drugs and with foods can be identified.

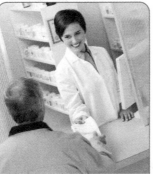

Your local or mail order pharmacist can answer questions about medications.

- Keep medicines in their original containers or in ones with sections for daily doses.

- Let your doctor know about your past reactions to certain medicines. As some people age, they may be more sensitive to some medications, such as painkillers or sedatives.

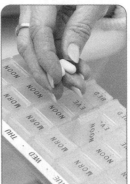

Containers with sections for daily doses and times can remind you when to take medicines.

- Ask about the possible side effects of a medication. Find out what you should do if you have any.

- Ask if you can drink alcohol while taking the medication(s). Alcohol can lessen the effects of some medicines. Other medicines, such as sedatives, can be deadly when used with alcohol.

- Don't take someone else's medication.

- Throw away medications that have expired. Crush pills and dissolve them in water. Mix this with used coffee grounds or kitty litter and put it in the garbage in a sealed bag.

- Try to reduce the need for some medications, such as sleeping pills or laxatives. A hot bath and a glass of milk might help you fall asleep. Having more fiber in your diet can reduce or replace the need for a laxative. Check with your doctor on ways other than medicines to help treat your problem.

- Even if you feel better, don't stop taking a prescribed medicine unless your doctor tells you to. Also, don't skip doses.

Over-the-Counter (OTC) Medications

Over-the-counter (OTC) medications are ones that you can get without a prescription. Often, they are less potent than prescribed ones. When taken in large amounts, though, an OTC medicine might equal or exceed the dose of a prescribed

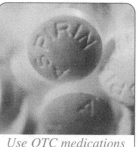

Use OTC medications as directed.

medicine. Read the information on the label. To learn more about OTC medicine labels, access www.fda.gov. Search for "over-the-counter medicine label." An example is in the next column.

Use OTC Medicines Wisely

- Ask your doctor or health care provider what OTC products are safe for you to use and what you should take for pain and fever.

- To prevent harmful side effects and interactions, review all of the OTC medicines, supplements, and herbal remedies that you take with your doctor.

- Do not take OTC medicines on a regular basis unless your doctor tells you to.

- Read the package labels. Heed the warnings listed. If you are unsure whether or not an OTC medication will help or harm you, check with your doctor or pharmacist.

- Store medicines in a dry place and out of children's reach. Do not call medicine "candy."

- Before you take a medicine, check the expiration date. Discard expired medicines. Crush pills. Dissolve them in water. Mix this with used coffee grounds or kitty litter and put it in the garbage in a sealed bag.

- If you have an allergy to a medicine, check the list of ingredients on OTC medicine labels. Find out if what you are allergic to is in them. Some labels will warn persons with certain allergies to avoid taking that medicine.

- Do not take any OTC product if you are pregnant or nursing a baby unless your doctor or health care provider says it is okay.

- Before taking herbal remedies and supplements, check with your doctor.

Drug Facts (Sample OTC label from www.fda.gov.)

Active ingredient (in each tablet)	Purpose
Chlorpheniramine maleate 2 mg	Antihistamine

Uses temporarily relieves these symptoms due to hay fever or other upper respiratory allergies:
- sneezing ■ runny nose ■ itchy, watery eyes ■ itchy throat

Warnings
Ask a doctor before use if you have
- glaucoma ■ a breathing problem such as emphysema or chronic bronchitis
- trouble urinating due to an enlarged prostate gland

Ask a doctor or pharmacist before use if you are taking tranquilizers or sedatives

When using this product
- You may get drowsy ■ avoid alcoholic drinks
- alcohol, sedatives, and tranquilizers may increase drowsiness
- be careful when driving a motor vehicle or operating machinery
- excitability may occur, especially in children

If pregnant or breast-feeding, ask a health professional before use.
Keep out of reach of children. In case of overdose, get medical help or contact a Poison Control Center right away.

Directions

adults and children 12 years and over	take 2 tablets every 4 to 6 hours; not more than 12 tablets in 24 hours
children 6 years to under 12 years	take 1 tablet every 4 to 6 hours; not more than 6 tablets in 24 hours
children under 6 years	ask a doctor

Other information: store at 20-25ºC (68-77ºF). Protect from excessive moisture.
Inactive ingredients: D&C yellow no. 10, lactose, magnesium stearate, microcrystalline cellulose, pregelatinized starch

Your Home Pharmacy

Basic Over-the-Counter (OTC) Medications that Can Help with Self-Care

Medicines	Common Uses	Side Effects/Warnings/Interactions
Antacids (e.g., Tums, Rolaids, Mylanta).	Stomach upset. Heartburn.	Don't use for more than 2 weeks without your doctor's advice. Don't use high-sodium ones if on a low-salt diet. Don't use if you have chronic kidney failure.
Antidiarrheal medicine (e.g., Kaopectate, Imodium A-D, Pepto-Bismol♦).	Diarrhea.	Don't give Pepto-Bismol that has salicylates to anyone under 19 years of age due to its link to Reye's Syndrome. Also, Pepto-Bismol can cause black stools.
☆**Antihistamines** (e.g., Chlor-Trimeton, Benadryl).	Allergies. Cold symptom relief. Relieves itching.	May make you drowsy or agitated. Can cause dry mouth and/or problems with urinating. Don't use with alcohol, when operating machines, or when driving. Don't use if you have problems passing urine, glaucoma, or an enlarged prostate.
☆**Cough suppressant** (e.g., Robitussin-DM or others with dextromethorphan).	Dry cough without mucus.	May make you drowsy. People with glaucoma or problems passing urine should avoid ones with diphenhydramine.
☆**Decongestant** (e.g., Sudafed, Dimetapp).	Stuffy and runny nose. Postnasal drip. Allergies. Fluid in the ears.	Don't use if you have high blood pressure, diabetes, glaucoma, heart disease, a history of stroke, or an enlarged prostate.
☆**Expectorant** (e.g., Robitussin or others with guaifenesin).	Cough with mucus.	Don't give with an antihistamine.
Laxatives (e.g., Ex-Lax, Correctol [stimulant-types], Metamucil [bulk-forming type].	Constipation.	Long-term use of stimulant-type can lead to dependence and to muscle weakness due to potassium loss.
Throat anesthetic (e.g., Sucrets, Chloraseptic spray).	Minor sore throat.	Don't give throat lozenges to children under age 5.
Toothache anesthetic (e.g., Anbesol).	Toothache. Teething.	Call doctor before giving to babies under 4 months old.

♦ Do not give aspirin or any medication with salicylates, such as Pepto-Bismol to anyone under 19 years of age due to its link to Reye's Syndrome.

☆ Do not give OTC medicines for colds, coughs and/or the flu to children under 6 years old.
For children 6 years old and older, follow their doctor's advice.

Chart continued on next page

Medicines	Common Uses	Side Effects/Warnings/Interactions
Pain Relievers		
Acetaminophen (e.g., Tylenol, Anacin-3, Datril, Liquiprin, Panadol, Tempra).	Gives pain relief. Lowers fever. Does not reduce swelling.	More gentle on stomach than other OTC pain relievers. Can result in liver problems in heavy alcohol users. Large doses or long-term use can cause liver or kidney damage.
Aspirin♦* (e.g., Bayer, Bufferin).	Gives pain relief. Lowers fever and swelling.	Can cause stomach upset (which is made worse with alcohol use). May cause stomach ulcers and bleeding. Avoid if you: Have an ulcer, have asthma, are under 19 years of age (due to its link to Reye's Syndrome), and/or are having surgery within 2 weeks. High doses or prolonged use can cause ringing in the ears.
Ibuprofen* (e.g., Advil, Motrin, Adult and Children's Advil). **Ketoprofen*** for adults (e.g., Actron, Orudis KT). **Naproxen Sodium*** for adults (e.g., Aleve).	Gives pain relief. Lowers fever and swelling.	Can cause stomach upset and peptic ulcers. Take with milk or food. Can make you more sensitive to the effects of the sun. Don't use if you are allergic to aspirin. Don't use if you have a peptic ulcer, blood clotting problems, or kidney disease.

♦ Do not give aspirin or any medication with salicylates, such as Pepto-Bismol, to anyone under 19 years of age due to its link to Reye's Syndrome.

* These medicines are examples of nonsteroidal anti-inflammatory drugs (NSAIDs).

Medication Interactions

Talk to your doctor or pharmacist about all of the medications you take. These include prescribed and OTC medicines and dietary supplements (vitamins, minerals, herbal products). Heed warnings on labels, too.

■ *Drug-drug interactions.* These can make a drug work less, increase the action of a drug, or cause side effects, even harmful ones. For example, unless told to by a doctor, do not take an antihistamine if you take medicine for high blood pressure or a sedative or tranquilizer.

■ *Drug-condition interactions.* Some medical conditions make taking certain drugs harmful. One example is taking a nasal decongestant if you have high blood pressure.

■ *Drug and food/beverage interactions.* Alcohol should not be mixed with certain drugs. Grapefruit juice should not be taken with certain medicines for high blood pressure and high blood cholesterol.

The "Side Effects/Warnings/Interactions" columns on page 28 and this page point out common medication interactions for OTC medicines.

Common Drug Interactions

Drug	Harmful or Less Effective With*
Acid reducers (for heartburn).	Asthma drug – theophylline. Blood thinner – warfarin. Tricyclic antidepressants, such as Elavil and Pamelor.
Antibiotics.	Some birth control pills.
Asthma drug – theophylline.	Beta-blockers. Caffeine. Cimetidine (in acid reducers).
Blood thinner – warfarin. Get a copy of "Blood Thinner Pills: Your Guide to Using Them Safely" from www.ahrq.gov/consumer/btpills.pdf.	Antacids. Aspirin. High doses (400 IU or more) of vitamin E. Vitamin K and/or foods high in it (liver, broccoli, brussels sprouts, kale, spinach, etc.). Grapefruit juice. Grapefruit.
Some statin drugs to lower cholesterol.	Grapefruit juice. Grapefruit.
Nitrates to dilate blood vessels.	Cialis. Levitra. Viagra.

* This does not include all medicines and foods that can cause harmful reactions with these drugs. Ask your doctor or pharmacist for more information.

Overhauling Your Medicine Cabinet

- Take everything out of the medicine cabinet.

- Check expiration dates. Throw out all outdated medicines. If you're not sure about a certain item, call your pharmacist. Ask what the shelf life is.

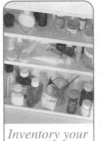

Inventory your medicine cabinet at least once a year.

- Discard old tubes of cream that are hardened or cracked. Throw out any liquid medicines that look cloudy or filmy.

- If medications are not in original containers and clearly labeled, throw them away. Some medicines come in tinted glass, for example, because exposure to light may cause them to deteriorate.

- **Every medication is a potential poison.** If there are children in the house, keep all medicines and vitamins locked in a high cabinet, well out of their reach.

- Activated charcoal and syrup of ipecac are not advised for home use for swallowed poisons. Call the Poison Control Center at 800.222.1222 for advice.

Basic Supplies to Help with Self-Care
▪ Adhesive bandages, sterile gauze, first aid tape, and scissors.
▪ Antibiotic ointment.
▪ Antiseptic ointment or wipes.
▪ Eye dropper.
▪ Heating pad/hot water bottle. Heat pack.
▪ Humidifier or vaporizer (cool-mist).
▪ Ice pack.
▪ Tweezers.
▪ Petroleum jelly.
▪ Rubbing alcohol.
▪ Sunscreen with a sun protection factor (SPF) of 15 or more.
▪ Thermometer (digital or ear).
▪ Tongue depressor and flashlight.

Chapter 4
Complementary & Alternative Medicine

Complementary and alternative medicine (**CAM**) is a group of many different health care systems, practices, and products. These are not yet a part of mainstream medicine. In general, they are not used in hospitals. They are not taught widely in medical schools. They are not usually paid for by health insurance plans.

Complementary medicine is used *with* mainstream medicine. **Alternative** medicine is used *in place of* it. A survey done by the National Center for Complementary and Alternative medicine (NCCAM) found that 36% of adults in the U.S. use some form of CAM. This figure did not include the use of prayer and megavitamin therapy for health reasons. When it did, 62% of adults said they used CAM. Doctors may advise the use of some forms of CAM for patients.

Types

The National Center for Complementary and Alternative Medicine (NCCAM) puts common CAM practices into 5 groups.

1. *Alternative medical systems.* These are complete systems of theory and practice. Often, these systems have been used in other countries for centuries. They can be very different from mainstream medicine used in the U.S.

   - *Ayurveda* ("ah-yur-VAY-dah"). This system of diagnosis and treatment has been used in India for more than 5,000 years. It includes yoga, meditation, herbs, massage, specific diets, and controlled breathing.

   - *Homeopathy.* This method is based on the idea that "like cures like." Things that cause certain symptoms in a healthy person can also cure those symptoms in someone who is sick. They must be given in small, highly diluted amounts.

   - *Naturopathy.* This uses methods to allow the body to heal itself rather than treat disease. It uses diet, herbal medicine, acupuncture, homeopathy, body manipulation, etc.

2. *Biological-based methods.* These use substances found in nature, such as herbs, foods, and vitamins. Other "natural," but unproven therapies are in this group, too. An example is using shark cartilage to treat cancer.

   - *Aromatherapy.* This uses essential oils from plants for relaxation and for symptom relief.

   - *Herbal therapies.* These use chemicals from herbs, plants, or plant parts that act upon the body in a therapeutic way.

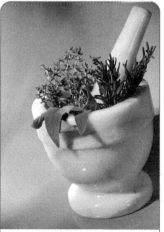

Check with your doctor before using herbal therapies.

- *Dietary supplements.* These include vitamins, minerals, herbs or other botanicals, amino acids, enzymes, organ tissues, and metabolites. Forms they come in include extracts, concentrates, tablets, capsules, gel caps, liquids, and powders. Dietary supplements are called foods, not drugs. They do not need FDA approval before they are sold. The company that makes them is required to give honest label information that does not mislead the public. For more information on dietary supplements, access the Center for Food Safety and Applied Nutrition at www.cfsan.fda.gov.

3. *Energy therapies.* These focus on energy fields that start within the body (biofields) or ones from other sources (electromagnetic fields).

   - *Electromagnetic fields.* These are used to manage pain and migraine headaches and to treat asthma or cancer.

   - *Qi gong* ("chee-GUNG"). This is part of traditional Chinese medicine. It uses movement, meditation, and controlled breathing to enhance the flow of "qi" in the body. (Qi is an ancient term for vital energy.)

   - *Reiki* ("RAY-kee"). This Japanese word stands for Universal Life Energy. With Reiki, spiritual energy is channeled through a Reiki practitioner to heal a patient's spirit. Healing the spirit heals the physical body.

   - *Therapeutic touch.* This comes from an ancient technique called laying-on of hands. It believes that the healing force of the therapist affects the patient's recovery. Healing is promoted when the body's energies are in balance. By passing their hands over the patient, healers can identify energy imbalances.

4. *Manipulative and body-based methods.* These are based on manipulation and/or movement of one or more body parts. Examples are:

   - *Acupressure.* This applies pressure to certain places (acupoints) on the body by pressing on them with fingers or hands.

   - *Acupuncture.* This uses needles that are inserted into the skin at certain sites (acupoints).

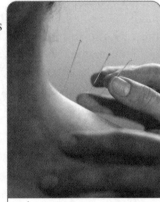

Acupuncture uses very thin needles.

   - *Chiropractic.* This seeks to put the body into balance through manual realignment of the spine and other joints and muscles.

   - *Massage.* This uses touching and rubbing techniques mostly on the muscles.

5. *Mind-body medicine methods.* These enhance the mind's ability to affect symptoms and how the body functions. These include meditation, prayer, mental healing, yoga, tai chi, and therapies that use creative outlets, such as art, music, or dance.

Safe Use

Products and services of Complementary and Alternative Medicine (CAM) may be safe and effective. A lack of scientific research to prove this, though, is one reason they are not part of mainstream medicine. Things that are CAM methods today, could become a part of mainstream medicine in the future.

How can you tell if a CAM product or service is one you should use? Follow these tips:
- Use credible sources for information:
  - "CAM on PubMed." Contact the National Center for Complementary and Alternative Medicine (NCCAM) Clearinghouse at 888.644.6226 or www.nccam.nih.gov. An "Alerts and Advisories" section is also listed on the Web site.
  - PDR for Herbal Medicines. Look for this book at your local library or bookstore.
  - Your doctor, health care provider, or pharmacist. Discuss conventional and alternative treatments you use now and ones you are thinking about trying. Find out if an herbal product, megadose of a vitamin, etc. could be harmful with other medicines you take or conditions you have. Ask for a referral or list of practitioners who are trained and certified in the alternative medicine you want to explore.
  - Local and state medical boards, other health regulatory agencies or boards, and consumer affairs departments. These give information on a provider's credentials and about reported problems with products and services.

- Avoid products and services that claim to have "secret formulas" or "miraculous breakthroughs." Just because a product is labeled "natural," doesn't mean it's safe.

- Females who are planning to get pregnant, are pregnant, or who breast-feed should not use herbal products unless directed by a doctor. They should also take vitamin supplements as advised. For a list of herbs to avoid during pregnancy, access The American Pregnancy Association's Web site at www.americanpregnancy.org.

- Give nutritional supplements to children as advised by their doctors.

Follow the directions on the product label. Report unwanted side effects to your doctor or health care provider.

Consider costs, too. Health plans do not usually pay for CAM methods. Some therapies, such as chiropractic, may be covered. Find out if a chiropractor (or other CAM provider) accepts your health insurance. Ask, too, if you need a referral from your doctor for any or all of the costs to be covered.

Herbs

Herbs and other nutritional supplements can act in the same way as drugs. Check with your doctor before you take them.

Health problems using herbs can result from:
- The contents of a product. Some have harmful metals, organisms, etc.

- Taking too much.

- Interactions with medications.

- Effects on existing medical conditions.

Herb Alert Chart		
Herb	**Proposed Uses**	**Warnings**
Echinacea.	To prevent colds & flu, fight infections, and boost the immune system.	Could cause liver damage if taken with antifungal medicines (e.g., Nizoral). Since it boosts the immune system, it should not be taken by persons with autoimmune conditions (e.g., AIDS, lupus, multiple sclerosis) or who take medicines (e.g., cyclosporine) to suppress the immune system.
Ginko.	To improve mental function and promote circulation to the limbs.	Do not use if you take blood-thinners (e.g., aspirin, warfarin) or have a bleeding disorder.
Ginseng.	To increase energy.	Don't use if you take medicines for high blood pressure, diabetes, or heart disease. Don't use if you take MAOI medicines for depression (e.g., Nardil, Parnate). Ginseng can cause irritability when mixed with caffeine.
Kava.	To treat anxiety, insomnia, premenstrual syndrome, and stress.	FDA advisory links products with Kava to severe liver damage. Don't use if you take anti-anxiety and antidepressant medicines. Don't use with alcohol.
Saw Palmetto.	To treat symptoms of an enlarged prostate.	Don't self-diagnose. See a doctor. Follow his or her advice. Don't take with medicine prescribed for an enlarged prostate.
St. John's Wort.	To treat mild to moderate depression.	Should not be used with prescribed antidepressants, such as SSRIs (e.g., Zoloft, Paxil) and MAOIs (e.g., Nardil, Parnate). Makes birth control pills and some medicines for asthma, HIV, and heart disease less effective.

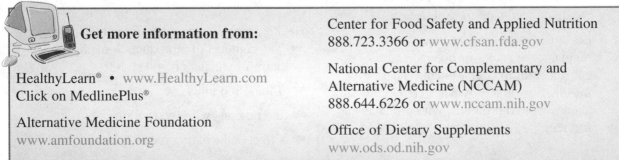

Get more information from:

HealthyLearn® • www.HealthyLearn.com
Click on MedlinePlus®

Alternative Medicine Foundation
www.amfoundation.org

Center for Food Safety and Applied Nutrition
888.723.3366 or www.cfsan.fda.gov

National Center for Complementary and Alternative Medicine (NCCAM)
888.644.6226 or www.nccam.nih.gov

Office of Dietary Supplements
www.ods.od.nih.gov

Chapter 5

Medical Decisions

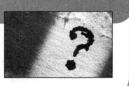

Gather Facts

Decisions you make about your health can affect the length and quality of your life. Choose wisely. To do this, you need to gather facts. Use these sources:

- You. You know more about you than anyone else. Be in touch with how you feel, physically and emotionally. Keep track of past and present health concerns.

- Your doctor. Ask for his or her advice. Your doctor may also have written materials on your condition.

- Medical resources. These include:

  - The Internet's world wide web. Look for credible sites, such as www.medlineplus.gov, www.healthfinder.gov, and other Web sites which end in .gov. Other credible sites are ones from hospitals, medical centers, and medical associations. Most often, these sites end in .edu and .org. Web sites for certain health concerns are listed in many topics in Section III of this book. Beware of Web sites that promote health fraud and quackery. Access www.quackwatch.org for information. Also, check with your doctor before you follow advice from a Web site. The advice may not be right for your needs.

- Not-for-profit groups. These include the American Cancer Society, the American Heart Association, and the American Diabetes Association. To get information, call their toll-free numbers or access their Web sites. These are listed in the topics **Cancer**, **Diabetes**, and **Heart Disease** in Section III.

- Government agencies. One is the National Heart, Lung, and Blood Institute (NHLBI). Access www.nhlbi.nih.gov.

- Support groups for conditions, such as breast cancer. Check local hospitals for lists of support groups near you. Also, contact the National Self-Help Clearinghouse at 212.817.1822 or access www.selfhelpgroups.org.

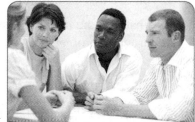

Support groups can be a source of practical information on medical conditions.

Your job is to gather facts. Use the **Key Questions Checklist** and **Medical Decision Comparison Chart** on the next pages to help you know what facts to look for. Once you have the facts, you and your doctor can make the medical decision(s) best suited to your needs.

Key Questions Checklist

1. **Diagnosis**
   - What is my diagnosis?
   - Is my condition chronic or acute?
   - Is there anything I can do to cure, treat, and/or prevent it from getting worse?
   - Is my condition contagious or genetic?
   - How certain are you about this diagnosis?

2. **Treatment**
   - What is the recommended treatment?
   - Is there a support group for my condition?

   If you are discussing medications:
   - What will the medicine do for my particular problem?
   - When, how often, and for how long should I take the medicine?
   - How long before the medicine starts working?
   - Will there be side effects?
   - Will there be interactions with other medications I am taking?

   If you are discussing a test:
   - What is the test called and how will it help identify the problem? Will it give specific or general information?
   - Will more tests be necessary?
   - How accurate and reliable is the test?
   - How should I prepare for the test?
   - Where do I go for the test?
   - How and when will I get the test's results?

   If you are discussing surgery:
   - What are my options for surgery? Which one do you advise?
   - How many of these surgeries have you done and what were the results?
   - Can I get a step-by-step account of the procedure, including anesthesia and recovery?

3. **Benefits vs. Risks**
   - What are the benefits if I go ahead with the treatment?
   - What are the possible risks and complications?
   - Do the benefits outweigh the risks?

4. **Success**
   - What is the success rate for the treatment?
   - Are there any personal factors that will affect my odds either way?
   - How long will the results of treatment last?

5. **Timing**
   - When is the best time to begin the treatment?
   - When can I expect to see results?

6. **Alternatives**
   - What will happen if I decide to do nothing?
   - What are my other options?

7. **Cost**
   - What is the cost for the treatment?
   - What related costs should I consider (e.g., time off work, travel, etc.).

8. **Decision**
   - You can now make an informed decision.
   - You have the right to choose or refuse treatment.

Medical Decision Comparison Chart

(Make copies as needed.) Use this chart to help you compare medical options that are available to you.

Diagnosis _____

	Option One	Option Two	Option Three
Treatment			
Benefits			
Risks			
Success			
Timing			
Alternatives			
Cost			
Decision	☐ Yes ☐ No	☐ Yes ☐ No	☐ Yes ☐ No

Patient Rights

According to the American Hospital Association (AHA), all hospital patients are entitled to certain standards of care. The AHA developed a voluntary code called The Patient's Bill of Rights. This gives guidelines for both staff and patients. It gives you these rights:

- To considerate and respectful care.

- To obtain from your doctor complete, current information about your diagnosis, treatment, and prognosis. These should be given in terms you can understand.

- To receive from your doctor information necessary to give informed consent before the start of any procedure and/or treatment.

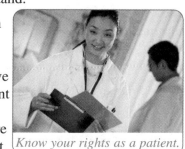

Know your rights as a patient.

- To expect reasonable continuity of care.

- To refuse treatment to the extent the law permits. To be informed of the medical effects of your action.

- To privacy for your medical care. This includes all communications and records about your care.

- To expect that, within its capacity, a hospital must make a reasonable response to your request for services.

- To get information about any connection between your hospital and other health care and educational institutions, as it relates to your care.

- To be advised if the hospital proposes to take part in or perform human experiments that could affect your care or treatment.

- To examine and receive an explanation of your bill no matter how it is paid.

- To know what hospital rules and regulations apply to your conduct as a patient.

- To obtain a copy of your written medical records.

Informed Consent

Informed consent means that you agree to treatment only after it has been explained to you and that you understand it. You should know the nature of the treatment, its benefits and risks, and the likelihood of its success. You should also be told if your treatment is an experimental one.

The doctor should review any alternatives to surgery or other procedures. There are no guaranteed outcomes in medicine, but informed consent enables YOU to make a rational and educated decision about your treatment.

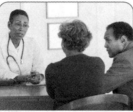

The doctor should review any alternatives to surgery or other procedures.

With Informed Consent

- You cannot demand services that go beyond what are considered "acceptable" practices of medicine or that violate professional ethics.

- You must recognize that you may be faced with some uncertainties or unpleasantness.

- You should, if competent, be responsible for your choices. Don't have others make decisions for you.

Advance Directives

Hospitals and nursing homes are required to give you information about your rights as a patient under their care. Advance directives are a legal way for you to declare your wishes to choose or refuse medical treatment.

{Note: If you live in or get medical care in more than one state, have advance directives for all states involved.}

Two Types of Advance Directives

- *Living Will.* This written document states what medical treatment you would want or not want if you were unable to state it yourself. A living will applies when you can't express your wishes on your own **and** you have a terminal illness or condition from which you aren't expected to survive.

In writing, you may choose or refuse:

- *Measures to Support Life,* such as a respirator (a machine to breathe for you).

- *Measures to Sustain Life,* such as tube feedings and kidney dialysis (a machine that does the work of your kidneys).

- *Measures to Enhance Life.* These keep you comfortable, but don't prolong life. Examples are pain medications and hospice care.

- *Durable Power of Attorney for Health Care.* This written document names a **person** who would make treatment decisions for you if you are not able to make them yourself. This person would state your wishes. Your condition does not have to be terminal or irreversible to have someone speak on your behalf.

Each state has its own laws on advance directives. Get forms for them from your lawyer, local hospital or library, or from your state's Web site. Other places you can get forms and information are:

- Put It in Writing
  www.putitinwriting.org

- U.S. Living Will Registry
  www.uslivingwillregistry.com

After you complete advance directives, discuss them with your family and close friend(s). Give your doctor a copy, too.

Health & Safety Guidelines

This section gives information you can use every day to help keep you healthy and safe. Guidelines given can help you prevent health problems, too.

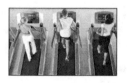

Chapter 6
Staying Well

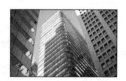

Chapter 7
Workplace Health
& Safety

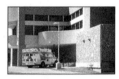

Chapter 8
Be Prepared for
Disasters & Threats

Ten Basic Tips to Stay Healthy & Safe

Make health and wellness a priority in your life.

- Get at least 6 to 8 hours of sleep each night.

- Don't smoke. If you smoke, quit. (See page 50.)

- Balance work and play.

- Eat healthy foods. (See pages 44 to 46.)

- Maintain a healthy weight. (See page 48.)

- Get regular exercise. (See pages 42 to 43.)

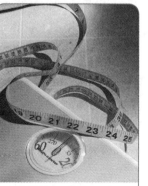

Get to and stay at a healthy weight.

- Have regular screening tests and exams. (See **Health Tests & When to Have Them** on page 22.)

- Wash your hands often to lessen the chance of picking up cold and flu viruses and other germs.

- Protect yourself from injuries. (See **Home Safety Checklist** on page 54, **Personal Safety Checklist** on page 55, and **Workplace Health & Safety** on pages 57 to 60.)

- Keep informed of health updates. Listen to the news. Read the newspaper. Access the Web sites in this book. Beware of sites that promote health fraud and quackery. Access www.quackwatch.org for information.

Chapter 6

Staying Well

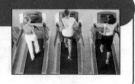

HealthyLife® Risk Appraisal

Step 1. In the Healthy Habits™ Test that follows, write the number of years gained or lost for each health habit. Total this number. Write it in BOX A on the bottom of this page.

Years

A. Physical Fitness. *If you exercise:*

At least 3 times a week or are physically active at work, add 3 years. _____

Rarely and work at a sedentary job, subtract 2 years. _____

B. Cigarette Smoking

If you smoke daily or ever have, subtract 14 years. _____

If you stopped smoking at about:

• Age 60 add back 3 years. _____

• Age 50, add back 6 years. _____

• Age 40, add back 9 years. _____

C. Weight Control. *If you are:*

Within 5 pounds of your healthy weight, add 1 year. _____

Overweight by 11-30 pounds, subtract 1 year. _____

Overweight by 31 or more pounds, subtract 2 years. _____

D. Alcohol.

If you drink moderate amounts of alcohol daily, add 3 years. _____

If you drink heavily, subtract 8 years. _____

E. Blood Pressure. *If the lower number is:*

Under 90, add 4 years. _____

Between 90-104, subtract 2 years. _____

Above 104, subtract 4 years. _____

F. Stress

If you are relaxed most of the time, and have a positive attitude, add 4 years. _____

If you have a high degree of stress in your life, subtract 2 years. _____

G. Auto Safety. *If you wear a seatbelt:*

100% of the time, add 3 years. _____

None of the time, subtract 3 years. _____

H. Cholesterol. *If your cholesterol is:*

200 or lower, add 2 years. _____

Between 201 and 239, subtract 1 year. _____

240 or above, subtract 2 years. _____

BOX A: Healthy Habits™ Years
Total from A-H in Step 1 _____

Step 2. Find your gender, race, and age in the following Life Expectancy Table. Note the average age you can expect to live in the "Life Span" column for your gender and race. Write this number in Box B in the next column.

Life Expectancy Table							
Females				Males			
White		Black		White		Black	
Age	Life Span	Age	Life Span	Age	Life Span	Age	Life Span
20	81.5	20	77.7	20	76.6	20	71.2
21	81.5	21	77.7	21	76.7	21	71.3
22	81.5	22	77.7	22	76.8	22	71.4
23	81.6	23	77.8	23	76.8	23	71.5
24	81.6	24	77.8	24	76.9	24	71.6
25	81.6	25	77.8	25	77.0	25	71.7
26	81.7	26	77.9	26	77.1	26	71.8
27	81.7	27	77.9	27	77.1	27	71.0
28	81.7	28	78.0	28	77.2	28	72.0
29	81.7	29	78.0	29	77.2	29	72.2
30	81.8	30	78.1	30	77.3	30	72.3
31	81.8	31	78.1	31	77.3	31	72.4
32	81.8	32	78.2	32	77.4	32	72.5
33	81.8	33	78.3	33	77.5	33	72.6
34	81.9	34	78.3	34	77.5	34	72.7
35	81.9	35	78.4	35	77.6	35	72.8
36	82.0	36	78.4	36	77.6	36	72.9
37	82.0	37	78.5	37	77.7	37	73.0
38	82.0	38	78.6	38	77.8	38	73.1
39	82.1	39	78.7	39	77.9	39	73.2
40	82.1	40	78.8	40	77.9	40	73.4
41	82.2	41	78.9	41	78.0	41	73.5
42	82.2	42	79.0	42	78.1	42	73.6
43	82.3	43	79.1	43	78.2	43	73.8
44	82.4	44	79.2	44	78.3	44	73.9
45	82.4	45	79.3	45	78.4	45	74.1
46	82.5	46	79.5	46	78.5	46	74.3
47	82.6	47	79.6	47	78.7	47	74.5
48	82.7	48	79.8	48	78.8	48	74.7
49	82.8	49	79.9	49	78.9	49	74.9

Life Expectancy Table							
Females				Males			
White		Black		White		Black	
Age	Life Span	Age	Life Span	Age	Life Span	Age	Life Span
50	82.9	50	80.1	50	79.1	50	75.1
51	83.0	51	80.3	51	79.2	51	75.4
52	83.1	52	80.5	52	79.4	52	75.6
53	83.2	53	80.6	53	79.5	53	75.9
54	83.3	54	80.8	54	79.7	54	76.2
55	83.4	55	81.0	55	79.9	55	76.5
56	83.5	56	81.3	56	80.1	56	76.8
57	83.6	57	81.5	57	80.3	57	77.1
58	83.8	58	81.7	58	80.5	58	77.5
59	83.9	59	81.9	59	80.7	59	77.8
60	84.1	60	82.2	60	80.9	60	78.2
61	84.2	61	82.4	61	81.1	61	78.5
62	84.4	62	82.7	62	81.3	62	78.9
63	84.6	63	83.0	63	81.6	63	79.3
64	84.8	64	83.3	64	81.9	64	79.7
65	85.0	65	83.6	65	82.2	65	80.2
66	85.2	66	83.9	66	82.4	66	80.6
67	85.5	67	84.2	67	82.5	67	81.0
68	85.7	68	84.6	68	83.1	68	81.5
69	86.0	69	84.9	69	83.4	69	81.9
70	86.2	70	85.3	70	83.7	70	82.4

Source: National Vital Statistics Report, Vol. 56, No. 9, December 28, 2007

BOX B: Life Span from Step 2 _____

Box C: Healthy Habits™ Life Span
Add Box A _____ (from page 40)
  + Box B _____
  = Total _____

This total estimates how long you may live based upon your health habits. As you make changes listed in this chapter, retake the test to see if you've added years to your life span.

Be Physically Active

Physical activity increases fitness. It helps build and maintain healthy bones, muscles, and joints. It helps manage weight and control blood pressure. It helps you look and feel better. It also lowers the risk for heart disease, colon cancer, and type 2 diabetes.

- Each week, adults should do at least 2 hours and 30 minutes of moderate-intensity (or 1 hour and 15 minutes of vigorous-intensity) physical activity. Additional physical activity may be needed to lose weight and prevent weight gain.

- Children and teens should do at least 60 minutes of physical activity every day.

Types of Exercise

- *Aerobic Exercise.* This type speeds your heart rate and breathing. It promotes cardiovascular fitness. Examples are walking briskly, swimming, jumping rope, and jogging.

Three Steps of Aerobic Exercises

1. *Warm Up.* Spend 5 to 10 minutes stretching or doing the aerobic activity at a slower pace.

2. *Aerobic Activity.* To be aerobic, the activity you choose should:

   - Be steady and nonstop

   - Last a minimum of 20 minutes. You can start out for shorter periods of time, many times a day. For example, start

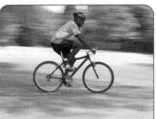
Aerobic exercise uses large muscles of the lower body (legs, buttocks).

   with 5 minutes, 4 times a day. Try to do more minutes each time.

- Allow you to speak without gasping for breath.

- Result in your target heart rate. This is 60 to 80% of your maximum heart rate. (See "Target Heart Rate Zone" below.)

Target Heart Rate Zone		
Age	Beats Per Minute	Approximate Beats Per 10 Seconds
20	120 to 160	20 to 27
25	117 to 156	19 to 26
30	114 to 152	19 to 25
35	111 to 148	18 to 25
40	108 to 144	18 to 24
45	105 to 140	17 to 23
50	102 to 136	17 to 23
55	99 to 132	16 to 22
60	96 to 128	16 to 21
65+	93 to 124	15 to 20

3. *Cool Down.* Cool down slowly. Choose a slower pace of the activity you were doing. For example, if you were walking briskly, walk slowly. Or, stretch for about 5 minutes.

Strengthening Exercises

Do muscle-strengthening activities that involve all major muscle groups. Adults need to do these on 2 or more days a week; children and teens should do these at least 3 days a week.

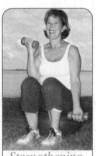
Strengthening exercises help build muscle.

Benefits of Strengthening Exercises

- They let your muscles work longer before they get tired. This is called endurance.

- They improve your bone density. This helps prevent osteoporosis and fractures.

Strengthening Exercise Guidelines

- Use weights or a stretch band. Try out different ones to find what's right for you. For strengthening, you should be able to do at least 2 sets and repeat these 8 times. The weight is too heavy if you can't. If you can easily do more than 3 sets, 12 times, use a heavier weight.

- Give muscles a day to rest in between workouts. If you work out every day, do the upper body one day; the lower body the next.

- Move slowly. Don't jerk the weights up. Don't drop them too fast.

- Keep your knees and elbows slightly bent.

- Breathe out when you are at the hardest part of the exercise. Breathe in when you return to the starting position. Don't hold your breath.

- Work opposing muscles. For example, after you work the front of the arm (biceps), work the back of the arm (triceps).

- Talk to your doctor or a fitness consultant for a complete exercise program.

Do stretching exercises before and after every strengthening or aerobic workout.

Stretching Exercises
These make your body more flexible. This helps to prevent injury during sports, exercise, and everyday activities.

Stretching Exercise Guidelines

- Try slow, relaxing stretches like those in yoga or tai chi.

- Try swimming. It builds flexibility.

- Stretch after exercise when muscles are warmed up. Stretch gradually.

- Don't bounce. Don't hold your breath. Exhale as stretching continues.

- Stretch every day, even if you don't exercise.

- Don't stretch areas where pain is felt.

Other Ways to Be Physically Active
- Recreation. Swim, golf, dance, etc.

- Active hobbies, such as working in the garden.

- Chores, such as washing windows, etc.

Physical Activity Advice
- Check with your doctor before starting any new vigorous exercise if you have a chronic health problem or if you are over age 40 (men) or 50 (women).

- Get physically active. Maintain or increase physical activity if you are already active. Stay active throughout your life.

- Choose activities that fit in with your daily routine.

- If muscles or joints start to hurt while you exercise, ease up.

Get more information from:

HealthyLearn®
www.HealthyLearn.com • Click on MedlinePlus®

U.S. Department of Health & Human Services
www.health.gov/paguidelines

Eat for Good Health

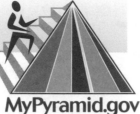

MyPyramid.gov
STEPS TO A HEALTHIER YOU

Use **My Pyramid – Steps to a Healthier You**. To find out about this, call 888.7.PYRAMID (779.7264) or go to www.mypyramid.gov. In the "MyPyramid Plan" box, fill in your age, sex, and physical activity level. See what you will learn in the next column.

- How many calories you should eat each day.
- How much to eat from basic food groups, subgroups, and oils, to meet your calorie needs. Serving sizes are given in cups, $1/2$ cups, etc.
- How to plan a healthy menu.
- How to keep track of the foods and beverages you eat and drink and the activities you do.
- Information about foods from MyFoodapedia.
- Tips for physical activity, eating out, a sample menu, and more.

Here is a sample of a "MyPyramid" plan for a 40 year old female who exercises less than 30 minutes a day.

Grains 6 ounces / day	**Vegetables** 2 cups / day	**Fruits** $1^1/2$ cups / day	**Milk** 3 cups / day	**Meat & Beans** 5 ounces / day
■ Make half your grains whole ■ Aim for at least **3 ounces** of whole grains a day	■ Vary your veggies ■ Aim for these amounts each week: **Dark green veggies** = 2 cups **Orange veggies** = $1^1/2$ cups **Dry beans & peas** = $2^1/2$ cups **Starchy veggies** = $2^1/2$ cups **Other veggies** = $5^1/2$ cups	■ Focus on fruits ■ Eat a variety of fruits ■ Go easy on fruit juices	■ Get your calcium-rich foods ■ Go low-fat or fat-free when you choose milk, yogurt, or cheese	■ Go lean with protein ■ Choose low-fat or lean meats and poultry ■ Vary your protein routine – choose more fish, beans, peas, nuts, and seeds

Find your balance between food and physical activity. Be physically active for at least 30 minutes most days of the week.

Know your limits on fats, sugars, and sodium. Your allowance for oils is **5 teaspoons a day**. Limit extras – solid fats and sugars – to **195 calories a day.**

Your results are based on a 1800 calorie pattern. This calorie level is only an estimate of your needs. Monitor your body weight to see if you need to adjust your calorie intake.

Healthy Eating Tips

- *Choose whole-grain products and fruits and vegetables daily.* These give vitamins and minerals, fiber, and other substances that are important for good health. Have 20 to 35 grams of dietary fiber per day.

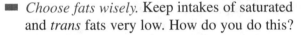

- *Choose fats wisely.* Keep intakes of saturated and *trans* fats very low. How do you do this?

  - Limit animal fats. This means meat fat and full-fat dairy products.

  - Strictly limit *trans* fats which come from hydrogenated oils. These are in stick margarine, cookies, snack crackers, vegetable shortening (and foods fried in this).

Read food labels to find out the grams of saturated fat and *trans* fat an item has per serving. Aim to have less than 2 grams of *trans* fat a day.

Use only monounsaturated and polyunsaturated fat for added fats.

Monounsaturated Fats – Preferred
(These are mostly liquid at room temperature.)
Canola, olive, and peanut oils.
Natural fat in avocado.
Fat in almonds, peanuts, pecans.

Polyunsaturated Fats – Use in Moderation
(These are mostly liquid at room temperature.)
Safflower, corn, sunflower, soybean, and sesame seed oils.
Soft tub margarine.
Fat in walnuts, sunflower and pumpkin seeds.
Mayonnaise.

- *Reduce salt (sodium) and increase potassium.* Having less than 2,300 milligrams of sodium (about 1 teaspoon of salt) per day may reduce the risk of high blood pressure. This is from all sources: Salt added in cooking and at the table; salt in processed food; and sodium that occurs naturally in foods. Read the Nutrition Facts on food labels for sodium content.

Getting more potassium also helps lower blood pressure. Potassium is in many foods, such as fruits and vegetables, milk products, and meats. Processed foods add salt, but not potassium.

- *If you drink alcoholic beverages, do so in moderation.* The topic, **Use Alcohol Wisely** on page 51, explains this.

- *Keep foods safe to eat.* (See **Food Poisoning** on pages 158 and 159.) Read how to avoid getting food poisoning in the **Prevention** column.

Another guide for healthy eating is the **DASH Eating Plan**. This is listed on page 46. DASH stands for Dietary Approaches to Stop Hypertension. For more information,

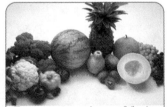

Eat more servings of fruits and vegetables a day.

including menus and recipes for different DASH Eating Plans, access www.nhlbi.nih.gov. Search for "DASH Eating Plan."

The DASH Eating Plan for 2,000 and 1,600 Calories/Day					
Food Group	Daily Servings: 2000	1600	Serving Sizes	What Each Food Group Gives	Examples and Notes
Grains & grain products.	7–8	6	1 slice bread. 1 ounce dry cereal. ½ cup cooked rice, pasta, or cereal.	Major source of energy & fiber.	Whole wheat breads and cereals. Bagels. Low-fat crackers. Unsalted pretzels & popcorn.
Vegetables.	4–5	3–4	1 cup raw leafy vegetable. ½ cup cooked vegetable. 6 ounces vegetable juice.	Rich sources of potassium, fiber, and magnesium.	Tomatoes. Potatoes. Carrots. Green beans & peas. Squash. Broccoli. Collards. Kale. Spinach. Lima beans.
Fruits.	4–5	4	1 medium fruit. ¼ cup dried fruit. ½ cup fresh, frozen, or canned fruit. 6 ounces fruit juice.	Important sources of potassium, fiber & magnesium.	Apricots. Bananas. Dates. Oranges & grapefruits (and their juices). Melons. Peaches. Pineapples. Prunes. Raisins. Strawberries.
Low-fat or fat-free dairy foods.	2–3	2–3	8 ounces milk. 1 cup yogurt. 1½ ounces cheese.	Major sources of calcium & protein.	Buttermilk. Fat-free or low-fat milks and yogurts. Low-fat & fat-free cheeses.
Lean meats, poultry & fish.	2 or less	1–2	3 ounces cooked lean meat, skinless poultry, or fish.	Rich sources of protein & magnesium.	Lean meats (trim visible fats). Broil, roast, or boil. Choose fish often.
Nuts, seeds, & dry beans.	4–5 per wk.	3 per wk.	⅓ cup or 1½ ounces nuts. 2 Tbsp. or ½ ounce seeds. ½ cup cooked dry beans or peas.	Rich sources of energy, protein, magnesium, fiber, & potassium.	Almonds. Peanuts. Walnuts. Sunflower seeds. Kidney beans. Lentils. Dried peas.
Fats & oils.	2–3	2	1 teaspoon vegetable oil or soft margarine. 1 Tbsp. low-fat margarine or mayonnaise. 2 Tbsp. light dressing.	DASH has 27% of calories as fat (low in saturated fat). This includes fat in or added to foods.	Soft margarine. Low-fat mayonnaise. Light salad dressing. Vegetable oil (such as olive, corn, canola).
Sweets.	5 per wk.	0	1 Tbsp. sugar, jelly, or jam. ½ ounce jelly beans. 8 ounces lemonade.	Sweets should be low in fat.	Maple syrup. Sugar. Jelly. Hard candy. Fruit punch. Sorbet.

Nutrition for Children

Guidelines for Healthy Eating
Birth to 2 Years Old

- Breast-feed your baby from birth to 6 months of age. Breast-feed for the first year, if you can. If you can't breast-feed or don't want to, give iron-enriched formula (not cow's milk) for the first 12 months. After that and up to age 2, use whole cow's milk to replace formula or breast milk. Don't limit fat for the first 2 years of life.

- Follow your child's doctor's advice on breast-feeding and what formula and vitamins to give your baby. Breast-fed babies who do not get regular exposure to sunlight may need vitamin D supplements.

- Start solid foods as advised by your baby's doctor. It is common to do this at 4 to 6 months of age. Iron-enriched infant rice cereal is usually the first food given.

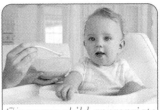

Give your child appropriate foods for his or her age.

- Start new foods one at a time. Wait 1 week before adding each new cereal, vegetable, or other food. Doing this makes it easier to find out which foods your baby has a problem with.

- Use iron-rich foods, such as grains, iron-enriched cereals, and meats.

- Do not give honey to infants during the first 12 months of life.

- Don't let a baby fall asleep with a bottle that has formula, juice, or milk. The sugars in these can cause tooth decay.

- Don't give foods that can lead to choking, such as hard candies and bits of hot dogs.

Two Years and Older

- Give a variety of healthy foods for meals and snacks. Follow guidelines from the MyPyramid for Kids Web site listed below. Let your child choose which healthy foods and how much to eat to satisfy his or her hunger.

- Help your child maintain a healthy weight. Give proper foods. Promote regular exercise. Lead by example. Children learn from what they see parents do, as well as, from what parents say. Eat with your children. Be a role model for good eating. Exercise, too.

- Let your child help plan meals and snacks, shop for food, and prepare foods.

- Don't force your child to eat certain foods. Don't use food to reward or punish behavior.

- Teach healthy behaviors in a fun way. For ideas to help get children to eat well and be more active, access the Web sites with a ☆ sign in the box below.

Get more information from:

☆Food & Nutrition Service
Eat Smart, Play Hard
www.fns.usda.gov/eatsmartplayhard

Healthier US.GOV
www.healthierus.gov / dietaryguidelines

☆MyPyramid.gov for kids and preschoolers
www.mypyramid.gov/kids
www.mypyramid.gov/preschoolers

☆Team Nutrition
www.fns.usda.gov/tn/default.htm

☆We Can!
http://wecan.nhlbi.nih.gov

Control Your Weight

Being overweight increases your risk for high blood pressure, high blood cholesterol, heart disease, stroke, diabetes, certain types of cancer, arthritis, and breathing problems.

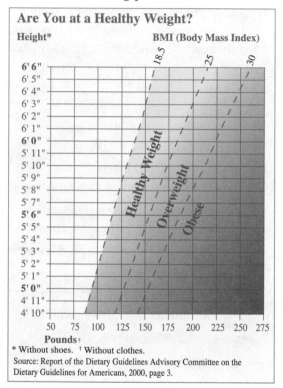

Are You at a Healthy Weight?

Height*   BMI (Body Mass Index)

Heights listed: 6'6", 6'5", 6'4", 6'3", 6'2", 6'1", 6'0", 5'11", 5'10", 5'9", 5'8", 5'7", 5'6", 5'5", 5'4", 5'3", 5'2", 5'1", 5'0", 4'11", 4'10"

BMI lines: 18.5, 25, 30

Regions: Healthy Weight, Overweight, Obese

Pounds†: 50 75 100 125 150 175 200 225 250 275

* Without shoes. † Without clothes.
Source: Report of the Dietary Guidelines Advisory Committee on the Dietary Guidelines for Americans, 2000, page 3.

Check Off Your Weight Group

☐ Healthy Weight = BMI from 18.5 to 24.9.

☐ Overweight = BMI from 25 to 29.9.

☐ Obese = BMI of 30 or higher.

If you are in the overweight or obese group, contact your doctor.

A BMI above the healthy range may be fine if you have lots of muscle and little fat. In general, though, if your BMI is above the healthy range, you may benefit from weight loss.

Ways to Control Your Weight

- Get regular physical activity to balance calories from the foods you eat.

- Eat 5 to 9 servings of vegetables and fruits a day. Eat whole grains with little added fat or sugar.

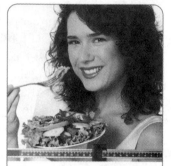

Eat a variety of fruits and vegetables.

- Eat at regular times.

- Choose sensible portion sizes. Limit high calorie foods (e.g., cookies, cakes, french fries, fats, oils, and spreads). Don't buy high calorie snack foods. Limit second helpings.

- Don't drink sweetened beverages.

- Eat when you are truly hungry, not as a response to emotions.

- Reduce total calories. Choose low-fat foods.

- When you eat out, avoid all-you-can-eat restaurants. Choose ones with low-fat foods.

- Eat slowly. Take at least 20 minutes to eat.

- Don't follow crash diets. Don't use ones with excessive protein (from foods or supplements) unless supervised by your doctor.

- Only take over-the-counter medicines and weight loss aids with your doctor's okay.

Get more information from:

HealthyLearn® • www.HealthyLearn.com
Click on MedlinePlus®

Weight-control Information Network (WIN) www.niddk.nih.gov. Click on "Weight Loss & Control" under "Health Information."

Control Your Cholesterol & Triglycerides

Cholesterol is a fat-like substance made in the body (mostly in the liver) and is in animal foods (dietary cholesterol), such as: Organ meats like liver; egg yolks, meats, poultry, and fish; and dairy products with fat. Plant foods have no cholesterol.

Total Blood Cholesterol Goal
Less than 200 mg/dL

{*Note:* Goals for LDL-cholesterol are based on your risk factors for heart disease. Ask your doctor what your heart disease risk level is.}

LDL ("bad") Cholesterol Goals Deposits cholesterol in the artery walls.	
Less than 70 mg/dL	If at "very high-risk."
Less than 100 mg/dL	If at "high-risk."
Less than 70 mg/dL	Optional goal for this risk level.
Less than 130 mg/dL	If at "moderate high-risk."
Less than 100 mg/dL	Optional goal for this risk level.
Less than 160 mg/dL	If at "lower/moderate risk."

HDL ("good") Cholesterol Goals Helps remove cholesterol from the blood
40 mg/dL or higher for men
50 mg/dL or higher for women

Triglycerides are fat-like substances carried through the bloodstream to the tissues which store it for later use as energy. Triglycerides come from the fat in both animal and plant foods.

Triglycerides Goal
Less than 150 mg/dL

{*Note:* High-risk blood cholesterol levels are only one risk factor for heart disease. Learn about other risk factors in **Heart Disease** on pages 232 and 233.

Ways to Reduce Cholesterol
- Take medications, if prescribed.
- Limit foods with saturated fats. Strictly limit *trans* fats. These are hydrogenated oils in foods, such as stick margarine and snack foods.
- Use salad dressings and margarines made with plant sterols and stanols (e.g., Benecol and Take Control brands.)
- Choose lean beef, pork, lamb, chicken, and turkey. Limit serving sizes.
- Eat a variety of fruits and vegetables (5 to 7 or more servings/day) and whole-grain products (6 or more servings/day).
- Get 20 to 35 grams of dietary fiber a day.
- Eat fish 2 to 3 times a week (especially ones high in omega-3 fatty acids, such as salmon).
- Use nonfat and low-fat dairy products.
- Limit dietary cholesterol to 300 mg. per day (200 mg. if your cholesterol is elevated).
- If you drink alcohol, do so in moderation. (See "**Use Alcohol Wisely**" on page 51.)
- Be physically active. (See pages 42 to 43.)

Ways to Reduce Triglycerides
- Lose weight if you are overweight. Follow a low-fat diet. Limit alcohol, sugar, and foods with sugar.
- Get regular exercise.
- Take medications, if prescribed.

Get more information from:
HealthyLearn® • www.HealthyLearn.com
Click on MedlinePlus®

National Heart, Lung, and Blood Institute
www.nhlbi.nih.gov

Be Tobacco-Free

Not using tobacco (smoking, chewing, etc.) is one of the best things you can do for your health. Why? Using tobacco products is linked to many serious illnesses:

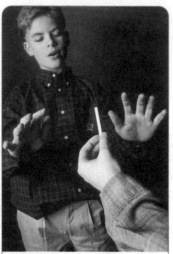

Quitting smoking sets a good example for children.

- Cancers of the lungs, mouth, throat, bladder, cervix, kidney, and stomach, as well as, a certain type of leukemia.

- Heart disease, emphysema, pneumonia, and abdominal aortic aneurysm.

- Cataracts, gum disease, and tooth decay.

Ways to Quit Using Tobacco
- Use an OTC nicotine replacement product, such as a patch, gum, or lozenges. Use as directed.

- Talk to your doctor about prescribed medicines. Some contain nicotine. Others do not contain nicotine, but alter brain chemistry to help reduce cravings.

To increase your chances of success, take part in a stop smoking class and/or use the behavior change techniques that follow.

- Throw away all your cigarettes, cigars, etc. Hide all smoking items like matches, lighters, ashtrays, etc.

- Whenever you have an urge to smoke, dip, or chew, take a deep breath through your mouth. Slowly exhale through pursed lips. Repeat 5 to 10 times.

- Get rid of familiar tobacco triggers. Change your daily routine. Do things you don't associate with tobacco use.

- In place of cigarettes, snuff, etc., use other things that will give oral gratification (e.g., sugarless gum, mints, and toothpicks).

- Create a "ciggy bank." Put the money you used to spend on cigarettes, cigars, etc. in a jar. Buy yourself a reward.

- Place a rubber band on your wrist. Snap it when you get an urge to smoke, dip, or chew.

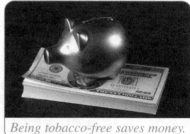

Being tobacco-free saves money.

- Talk to a nonsmoking friend for support.

- Make a list of good things you've noticed since you quit.

- Each day, renew your commitment to not use tobacco products.

Get more information from:

American Lung Association
800.586.4872 • www.lungusa.org/tobacco

National Cancer Institute's Smoking Quitline
877.44U.QUIT (448.7848)

Smokefree.Gov
800.QUITNOW (784.8669)
www.smokefree.gov

Use Alcohol Wisely

- If you drink, do so in moderation. This means no more than 2 drinks a day for males; 1 drink if you are female or age 65 or older. One drink has one half of an ounce of pure alcohol (e.g., 12 oz. of regular beer, 4 to 5 oz. of wine, 1½ oz. of 80-proof liquor).

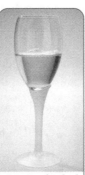

Limit alcohol to 1 to 2 drinks per day.

- Ask your doctor how much, if any, alcohol you can have with conditions you have and/or medications you take. Heed warnings on over-the-counter medicine labels, too.

- Drink slowly. You are apt to drink less.

- After you have 1 or 2 drinks with alcohol, have drinks without alcohol.

- Eat when you drink. Food helps to slow alcohol absorption.

- Don't drink and drive. Designate a driver who will not be drinking.

- Coffee or fresh air cannot make you sober. To get sober, stop drinking.

- Know your limit and stick to it. You may decide it is better not to drink at all.

Persons Who Should Not Drink

- Children and teenagers.

- Women who may become pregnant or who are pregnant or breast-feeding.

- Persons who can't restrict drinking to moderate levels.

- Persons who plan to drive or take part in other activities that require attention, skill, or coordination.

Questions to Detect an Alcohol Problem

Answer the questions that follow. A key word in each of these 4 questions spells CAGE.

- Have you ever felt you should Cut down on your drinking?

- Have people Annoyed you by criticizing your drinking?

- Have you ever felt bad or Guilty about your drinking?

- Have you ever had a drink to steady your nerves or to get rid of a hangover (Eye opener)?

One "Yes" answer means there might be an alcohol problem. Two or more "Yes" answers means it is highly likely that you may have an alcohol problem. In either case, contact your doctor or other health care provider to discuss your responses to these questions. You may have answered "No" to all four CAGE questions, but there could still be a problem. Some men say, "But I only drink beer." This doesn't mean they don't have an alcohol problem.

{*Note:* Most alcoholics deny or don't see that they have a disease. Alcoholism is a serious condition that is treatable. If you suspect a drinking problem in you, a family member, or a friend, seek advice.}

 Get more information from:

Center for Substance Abuse Treatment (CSAT)
800.662.HELP (662.4357)
www.findtreatment.samhsa.gov

Your Mind + Your Body = You

Your mind and your body are one unit. They define who you are.

How you think and feel plays a role in your mental and physical health. These, in turn, affect your state of mind. Your brain makes chemicals that control pain. These are called **endorphins**. It also makes **gamma globulin**. This helps your immune system. Another chemical it makes is called **interferon**. This helps your body fight viruses. How much of these chemicals your brain makes depends on your physical health, attitude, and emotions. Aerobic exercise increases endorphin levels. Having a positive attitude may do this, too. Positive thinkers tend to deal with pain better than negative thinkers do.

Taking care of your body and mending your "mind" can help prevent and treat health conditions. Ways to do this include:

- Meditation and yoga. **Yoga** uses body postures, movements, and breathing exercises. These unite the body, mind, and spirit. Yoga improves blood pressure and circulation. It increases flexibility and mental fitness.

- Relaxation exercises.

- **Biofeedback**. Biofeedback devices help you learn to control your body's automatic responses to stress. Then you learn to control stress without these devices.

- Humor. Laughter can reduce stress, lower blood pressure, and elevate mood.

- Spirituality. Connecting to a higher power, praying, etc. can provide hope, help you deal with things you cannot change, and help you cope with illness. Reaching out to help others and attending a place of worship can provide a sense of community and shared purpose.

- Mental imagery. Imagining soothing pictures in the mind can relax the body and reduce stress. Practice the exercise in the box below.

Personal Mental Imagery
Choose a scene that relaxes you, such as watching a sunset. Imagine being there using these 10 steps:
1. Find a comfortable sitting or other position.
2. Gently close your eyes.
3. Focus only on a gentle breathing pattern.
4. Think about the relaxing scene you chose. Picture being there and what you do when your mind and body are so very, very relaxed. Create and capture the image of your quiet place.
5. Pretend that you are really there. Picture all the colors...Hear the sounds...Smell the aromas...Taste...Touch your surroundings as if you are really there...Enjoy...Relax...
6. Feel the calm and peace...Allow yourself to feel good...Let your whole body relax and enjoy the moment.
7. Pause for 5 to 10 minutes and become filled with relaxation.
8. Allow the relaxation to re-energize your body and mind.
9. As you feel comfortable, slowly open your eyes, feeling totally refreshed.
10. Escape to your special place anytime you wish to relax, if even for a moment.

Get more information from:

Center for Mind-Body Medicine
www.cmbm.org

Manage Stress

Stress is the way you react to any changes (good, bad, real, or even imagined). Any change in daily habits causes stress. Some stress is productive and gives you the edge needed to achieve things. Other stress can be harmful and can lead to or worsen some health problems.

Ways to Manage Stress

- Maintain a regular program of healthy eating, good health habits, and adequate sleep.

- Exercise regularly. This promotes physical fitness and emotional well-being.

- Don't let your emotions get "bottled up" inside. Share your feelings with others.

- Learn to manage your time efficiently.

- Avoid unnecessary arguments or quarrels.

- Do a "stress rehearsal." Prepare for stressful events by imagining yourself feeling calm and handling the situation well.

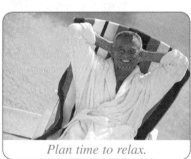

Plan time to relax.

- Minimize your exposure to things that cause distress.

- Practice a relaxation technique daily.

- Spend time helping others.

- Balance work and family or personal life.

- Engage in activities you enjoy and look forward to. Discover the "elf" in yourself. Learn to have fun and laugh.

- Accept the things you cannot change in yourself or others.

- Forgive yourself for mistakes.

- Take satisfaction in your accomplishments. Don't dwell on your shortcomings.

- Develop and maintain a positive attitude.

- Surround yourself with cheerful people. Avoid stress-carriers.

- Set realistic goals for yourself.

- Seek professional help if you have one or more of these problems caused by stress:

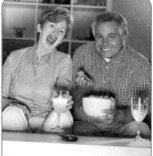

Do things that make you laugh.

- Excessive worry, anxiety, or nervousness

- Crying spells or feeling of hopelessness

- Insomnia or loss of appetite

- Withdrawal from friends, coworkers, and relatives or getting angry at everyone

Get more information from:

HealthyLearn®
www.HealthyLearn.com
Click on MedlinePlus®

The National Institute for Occupational Safety and Health (NIOSH)
800.CDC.INFO (232.4636)
www.cdc.gov/niosh/jobstress.html

Home Safety Checklist

☐ Keep your doors locked.

☐ Use a peephole in the front door.

☐ If you live alone, arrange for daily contact with a neighbor, relative, etc.

☐ Clearly post emergency numbers. Teach children how to call **9-1-1**, etc. for help.

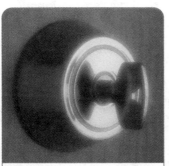

After calling 9-1-1, unlock the door so EMS personnel can get in quickly.

☐ Stock first aid supplies. In case of accidental poisoning, call the Poison Control Center (800.222.1222) for advice.

☐ Install smoke alarms and a carbon monoxide detector. Check them every 6 months. Keep a fire extinguisher handy.

☐ Never smoke in bed or when you feel drowsy. Better yet, don't smoke at all!

☐ If you use a space heater, make sure it has an emergency shut off.

☐ Plan an escape route in case of fire. Practice it with all household members every couple of months.

☐ Keep flashlights handy.

☐ Use night lights.

☐ Keep stair areas well lit.

☐ Have snow and icy patches cleared from the sidewalk and steps.

☐ Be careful or stay home if it is icy or slippery outside.

☐ Monitor your medication use. Let your doctor know if medicine(s) affect your vision, balance, etc. If prescribed sedatives or tranquilizers, be careful when you take them. They can increase the risk of falls.

☐ Don't get up too quickly after lying down, resting, or eating a meal. Low blood pressure can cause dizziness.

☐ Wear nonslip, snug-fitting shoes and slippers.

☐ Use safety mats or nonskid tape in your tub and shower. Install grab bars in the shower and tub, too.

☐ If you use a shower bench, use one with rubber tips on its legs.

☐ Before getting in the tub, test the bath water. Make sure it is not too hot.

☐ Never lock the bathroom door.

☐ Use a cane or walker, if necessary.

☐ Install handrails on both sides of the stairs. Keep clutter off stairs.

☐ Don't use loose area rugs. See that carpet on stairs is nailed down securely.

☐ Arrange furniture so there is a clear path for walking. Test if furniture is sturdy enough to lean on.

☐ Clear away phone or electrical wires from walk paths.

☐ Use a step stool with a safety rail.

☐ Be alert to spills or wet floors.

☐ To pick up things, bend at your knees and keep your back straight. Don't stoop.

To Keep Children Safe

- Never leave a young child alone in the bathtub or on a bed or table.

- Never give a young child toys or items with small parts. He or she may choke on them.

- Keep medicines and vitamins in "child-safe" bottles and where children can't reach them.

- Never put your baby in a crib with bars that are spaced more than 2 inches apart.

- Make sure the mattress fits the crib so your baby can't get stuck in the spaces.

- Never tie anything around your baby's neck. He or she could choke. Take strings and ties off baby clothes. They can get caught on things and choke your baby. Cut and tie off window blind cords and keep them out of your child's reach.

- Keep cleaners, chemicals, etc. out of your child's reach. Don't grow poisonous plants.

- Keep electric cords out of the way so your child doesn't trip on them.

- Keep guard rails around space heaters.

- Lock guns in one place and bullets in another. Don't let your child get the keys.

- Don't allow diving into water that is less than 9 feet deep. Put a life-preserver on your child when near the water.

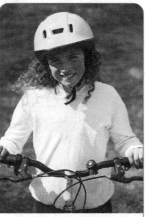

Make sure your child wears a helmet when he or she rollerblades, rides a bike, etc.

Personal Safety Checklist

- ☐ Ask your pharmacist or doctor if the medicines you take might make you unsteady or make it unsafe for you to drive.

- ☐ Wear a medical alert tag to identify health concerns. Get one from a drug store or from: MedicAlert Foundation International. Contact 800.344.3226 or www.medicalert.org.

- ☐ Walk with a companion.

- ☐ Use a cane or walker if you feel more secure walking with one.

- ☐ Wear a helmet when you ride a bike, rollerblade, etc.

- ☐ Have eye exams on a regular basis.

- ☐ Don't carry large amounts of cash. Carry credit cards or money in an inside pocket.

- ☐ Don't give your name or phone number to strangers.

- ☐ Always wear a seat belt when in a vehicle.

- ☐ Focus when you are driving. Don't do things, such as talking on a cell phone, that could distract you.

- ☐ Don't drink and drive. Don't drive at night if you have limited night vision.

- ☐ Keep emergency supplies (e.g., flares, blankets, water) in your car.

Get more information from:

HealthyLearn®
www.HealthyLearn.com
Click on MedlinePlus®

National Safety Council
www.nsc.org

Healthy Travel Checklist

Before You Go

☐ Find out about health concerns where you are going and if immunizations are needed. (See **Vaccines for Traveling Abroad** on page 24.)

☐ Carry all needed prescriptions (in their original containers) and supplies with you. Get a letter from your doctor, for taking a controlled substance, injectable medicines, notice for having a pacemaker, artificial joint, etc.

☐ Find out what your health insurance plan covers and if you need extra insurance.

☐ Talk to your doctor. Find out if you need to adjust medicine dosages and activity schedules. Arrange for special needs (e.g., wheelchair, special meals, etc.) with the airline, etc.

For Motion Sickness

☐ Get plenty of rest before the trip.

☐ Take an OTC medication (i.e., Dramamine®) 30 minutes before travel begins.

☐ If traveling by airplane, request a seat over the wings. Open the overhead vents and direct air at your face.

☐ On a cruise ship, get a cabin near the middle and close to the waterline. Spend as much time as you can on deck in the fresh air.

☐ When traveling by car or train, gaze straight ahead, not to the side. Sit by an open window for fresh air except in a polluted area.

☐ If you feel sick, breathe slowly and deeply. Avoid smoke and food odors. Eat crackers.

To Help Prevent Jet Lag

☐ Three nights before you leave, change your bedtime. If traveling to a different time zone and going east, go to bed 1 hour earlier for each time zone you cross; if traveling west, go to bed 1 hour later for each time zone.

☐ Once on the plane, change your watch and activity to match the time where you are going. If it is daytime there, stay awake; if nighttime, sleep on the plane.

Other Tips for Air Travel

☐ To reduce the risk for blood clots in the legs, extend your feet and flex your ankles several times while sitting. Get up and walk every hour or so.

☐ To avoid ear pain, chew gum, suck on hard candy, or yawn during take-offs and landings.

☐ Drink water, not alcoholic or caffeinated beverages, before and during the flight.

To Stay Safe While You Are Away

☐ Do not look like a tourist. Wear plain clothes and little, if any, jewelry.

☐ Avoid first floor rooms and those with doors facing outside. Lock your door using the safety chain. Make sure that windows and connecting doors are locked.

☐ Study the emergency exit map to prepare for an escape.

☐ Walk at night with others and in well-lit, safe areas. Ask hotel staff for advice.

Get more information from:

International Association for Medical Assistance to Travellers (IAMAT) 716.754.4883 or www.iamat.org

Chapter 7

Workplace Health & Safety

General Guidelines

The health of the U.S. economy depends on healthy and productive workers. Workers' health depends on what they do (or don't do) on and off the job.

General Guidelines

- Practice good health habits. This helps you be healthy and alert at work.

- Follow your doctor's treatment plan for conditions you have. Exercise. Take medications as directed, etc.

- Manage stress. (See **Manage Stress** on page 53.)

- Prevent and manage back pain. (See **Back Pain** on pages 184 to 187.)

- Set realistic goals. Budget your time. Rank order tasks.

- Don't commit to doing too much.

- Balance work, personal, and family life.

- Don't drink alcohol or use illegal drugs before or during work. Don't use medicines that cause drowsiness, especially if you operate machines. Ask your doctor if and how medicines you take can affect you on the job. Follow his or her advice. Alcohol and drug use and abuse affect the person using the substance, as well as co-workers. (See also, **Alcohol & Drug Problems** on page 263.) If you or a co-worker have an alcohol or drug problem, talk in confidence to the contact person in your Employee Assistance Program (EAP).

- Learn how to respond to accidents.

  - Know where the closest fire extinguisher is. Learn how to use it the right way.

  - Know your closest fire escape route. Plan a fire drill with your co-workers.

  - Post emergency phone numbers (EMS, fire, police, Poison Control Center) near phones.

  - Take first aid courses for CPR, for choking, and how to treat injuries.

  - Find out if your workplace has an Automated External Defibrillator (AED) to use if someone has a heart attack. Find out where it is. (Find out about AEDs on pages 354 and 355.)

Prevent Injuries

Most workplace injuries can be prevented. What you need to do depends on the job you do and the hazards you are exposed to. Your place of work may have certain standards and safety measures. Some are set by the Occupational Safety and Health Administration (OSHA). Know and follow your workplace's safety rules. Ask questions if you don't understand them.

General Safety Tips

- Help prevent slip and falls.

  - Keep walk areas free from clutter. Secure telephone and electrical cords to prevent tripping.

  - Wear nonskid shoes or footwear with a tread pattern to prevent slips, if needed.

  - Keep walking surfaces dry and free of water, grease, etc.

- Use proper lighting. Look where you are going. Don't carry things that block your vision.

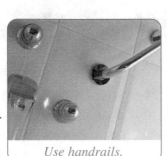

Use handrails.

- Don't lean back in your chair.

- Don't climb on chairs or boxes. Use a ladder that lets you safely reach items.

- Don't pile items on stairs or against doors.

- Report injuries and "near misses" of injuries to your supervisor or to security. Follow your company's rules for this.

Safety for High Risk Occupations
Certain jobs may require workers to:

- Use Material Safety Data Sheets (MSDSs). These tell you how to use chemicals safely. They can be on printed pages and in a computer. Know where this data is. Use the information given.

- Wear protective headgear (e.g., hard hats, hair covers, etc.).

- Wear safety glasses with side shields, goggles, face shields, tinted glasses to reduce glare, etc. Keep eyewear clean and in good condition. Replace it if it is broken or has a defect.

- Wear ear plugs or special ear muffs. These protect hearing from damage.

- Wear steel-toe shoes or boots.

- Protect your lungs from dust, fumes, gases, vapors, etc. If needed, use the right type of mask or respirator for the material you are working with. Not all masks filter all particles or gases. Have your respirator "fit tested" to assure safe use.

Prevent Musculoskeletal Disorders

Musculoskeletal Disorders (MSDs) affect muscles, tendons, nerves, joints, ligaments, cartilage, and discs in the spine. They do not result from slips, falls, or similar accidents. Common Work-Related Musculoskeletal Disorders (WMSDs) are low back pain, carpal tunnel syndrome, and tendonitis. These are caused by:

- Repeating the same motion. This can result in **Repetitive Motion Injuries**. (See page 202.)

- Awkward or static postures

- Using a great deal of force to do a job

- Vibration

WMSDs can be prevented or reduced using **ergonomics**. This is the science of fitting the job to the worker.

One way to prevent and deal with WMSDs is to use proper workstation positions. (See **Proper Position and Support for Computer Users** on page 59.)

Other Workstation Proper Positions

- Keep your head upright and your ears, shoulders, and hips in a straight line.

- Keep your work within reach without having to stretch or strain your arms, shoulders, or back. Don't stretch to reach items on an assembly line. Wait for the items to reach you.

- Change positions or tasks often. This avoids repeated stress on a single body part.

- Use the proper tools for the job. Use tools made to reduce vibration and/or pressure, if needed.

Proper Position and Support for Computer Users

Computer screen should be about 2 feet away from eyes.

Use a wrist rest, if needed. Keep wrists straight. Also, put the mouse next to and on the same level as the keyboard.

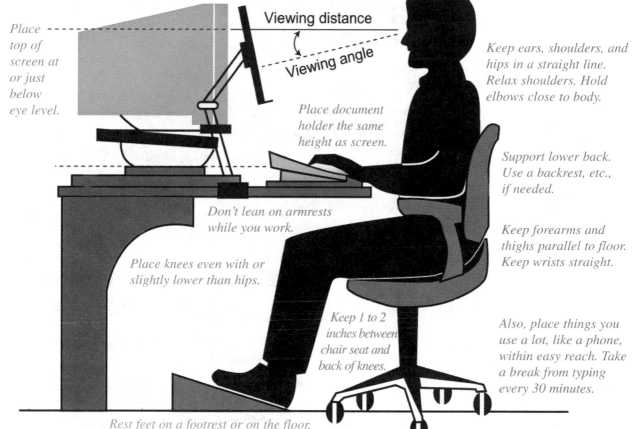

Place top of screen at or just below eye level.

Viewing distance

Viewing angle

Place document holder the same height as screen.

Keep ears, shoulders, and hips in a straight line. Relax shoulders. Hold elbows close to body.

Support lower back. Use a backrest, etc., if needed.

Don't lean on armrests while you work.

Place knees even with or slightly lower than hips.

Keep forearms and thighs parallel to floor. Keep wrists straight.

Keep 1 to 2 inches between chair seat and back of knees.

Also, place things you use a lot, like a phone, within easy reach. Take a break from typing every 30 minutes.

Rest feet on a footrest or on the floor.

Workstation Exercises

A. Shoulder Stretch

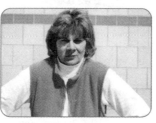

Push your shoulders backwards, then up towards your ears, then forward to make circles. Repeat 3 to 5 times. Do it again in the other direction.

B. Neck Rolls

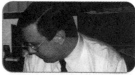

Touch your chin to chest. Slide your chin from shoulder to shoulder until you feel looser.

C. Finger Fan

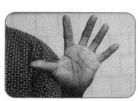

Spread the fingers of both hands wide. Hold for 5 seconds, then relax. Repeat 3 times.

D. **Tall Stretch**

Reach up as high as you can 3 times, first with one hand and then with the other or do both hands at the same time.

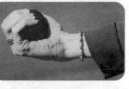

E. **Squeeze a Ball**

Squeeze a foam ball 5 to 10 times. Put the ball down and stretch your fingers.

F. **Arm Circles**

Extend your arms straight out and move them slowly around in smaller to larger circles, forward then backward. Do this several times.

Manage Job Stress

Job stress causes a worker to feel overly taxed both mentally and physically. It affects both workers and employers.

What Causes Job Stress?
- Too much work to do. Conflicting expectations.

- Lack of support from co-workers and bosses.

- Crowded, noisy, unsafe work conditions. Infrequent rest breaks.

- Rapid changes for which workers are not prepared. Job insecurity.

If not dealt with, job stress can lead to health problems.

Signs & Symptoms of Job Stress
- Hard time concentrating. Headache.

- Sleep problems. Stomach problems.

- Short temper.

- Job dissatisfaction. Low morale.

- Increase in being late for work or not going to work.

Ways to Manage Job Stress
- Schedule your time and tasks to be done. Use a calendar, planner, "TO DO" lists, etc. Rank order tasks. Break tasks down into steps. Check off items that are done.

- Organize your work space to make it easier to find things. Get rid of items and e-mails that you don't need.

- Ask for help from your boss and co-workers, as needed. Ask your boss for the order in which your job tasks need to be done.

- Take breaks. Get enough sleep.

- Leave work at work. Try not to take work home. If this is not possible, take as little work home as you need to.

- Plan for and take vacations that give you a rest from work.

- Relax as much as you can. (See also, **Manage Stress** on page 53 and **Self-Care / Prevention** for **Stress & Posttraumatic Stress Disorder** on pages 285 and 286.)

Get more information from:

National Institute for Occupational Safety and Health (NIOSH)
800.CDC.INFO (232.4636) or www.cdc.gov/niosh

Occupational Safety and Health Administration (OSHA)
202.693.1999 or www.osha.gov
For emergency situations: 800.321.OSHA (6742)

Chapter 8

Be Prepared for Disasters & Threats

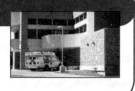

For persons in the U.S., the chances of being the victim of a terrorist act or other life-threatening event is very slim compared to the many risky lifestyle behaviors they take part in. These include cigarette smoking, drinking too much alcohol, and reckless driving.

Even so, the fear of public health disasters and threats causes concern and alarm.

No one can promise absolute safety, but steps can be taken to be more prepared than scared of possible crises. The National Weather Service operates the most advanced weather and flood warning and forecast system in the world. This helps protect lives and property. The U.S. Government has increased measures to prevent attacks of terror. Airports, employers, schools, retailers, etc. are taking steps to prevent and be prepared for disasters of many kinds.

Plans to Make Before a Disaster

By acting on the items that follow, you and your family can be prepared for many types of disasters that can occur quickly and with little or no warning.

- Write down, ahead of time, the steps to take for different disasters (e.g., house fires, floods, etc.). Go through drills for each plan with the whole family. Make sure the car always has gas in case you have to leave an area.

- Know your place of work's emergency plans. Find out about them from your supervisor, Employee Assistance Program (EAP), etc.

- Take a course in first aid from the Red Cross, your police or fire department, etc.

- Give each family member a prepaid phone card with about a ten dollar value. Instruct children how to use the card and a pay phone. Some cell phone services may be overwhelmed in a crisis.

- Set up a "check-in" plan. Choose someone for family members to call or e-mail to check on each other. Pick someone far enough away who would not likely be part of the same event. Of course, call each other on cell, regular, or pay phones.

- Choose two places to meet. One is at home or near your home. Choose another place farther away in case you can't get home. Make plans for the safety of your children.

- If you have children in school, find out the school's crisis plan. Know the school's policy for sending children home. See that the school has current phone numbers for you and other caregivers (in case you can't be reached). Find out what the school needs to have to release your child to assigned caregivers.

- If you have a pet, plan for its safety.

- When you enter a building, find emergency exits and stairways. Plan ahead how to get out quickly from buildings, vehicles, crowded public places, etc.

■ Make an emergency supply kit. Put these things in backpacks or containers that one or more family members can easily carry:

• Three days' supply of bottled water (one gallon a day per person, if possible). Put these next to, not in, your backpack, etc.

• Food that won't spoil. A hand can opener.

• Flashlight and extra batteries.

• A battery powered radio or TV and extra batteries.

• First-aid kits for the home and the car.

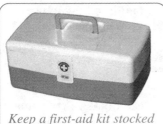

Keep a first-aid kit stocked and ready-to-go.

• Sleeping bags or blankets.

• A change of clothing for each person.

• Items for family members with special needs, such as baby supplies, medicines, etc.

• Duct tape and dry towels that you can make wet to make a room airtight.

• One small bottle of regular bleach (not scented). This may be needed to purify water. Use 2 drops of bleach per quart of water.

• Cash, credit cards, and important documents (or photocopies of them).

Web sites that give information on being ready for disasters are www.disasterrelief.org and www.redcross.org. {*Note:* Access these and other Web sites listed in this chapter as soon as you can. Don't wait until a crisis occurs. You may not have time to do it then. You may not have electricity to run your home computer.}

Be Prepared for Certain Disasters

Knowledge is power! Be aware of warning signs for certain disasters. Learn actions to take to increase the chance for your safety and the safety of others.

For Weather Disasters

■ Find out and be prepared for disasters that are likely to occur in your area (e.g., floods, hurricanes, tornadoes, earthquakes, etc.).

■ Tune in, daily, to weather forecasts. The Emergency Alert System (EAS) uses radio and TV stations to issue a WATCH (for an expected emergency) or a WARNING (for an emergency in progress or one that is about to occur). Contact The National Weather Service at www.nws.noaa.gov.

■ Heed the warnings given. Emergency sirens may also sound. Know when your area does a practice drill for sirens. Then you won't confuse this with a real emergency.

■ Watch for fallen power lines. Avoid them.

For Bomb Threats

■ Don't touch strange packages.

■ Be suspicious if packages have a ticking sound or have wires or aluminum foil sticking out from them.

■ Leave the building as fast as you can.

■ Call local police and the building manager.

■ When leaving a building, try not to walk by windows.

For Biological Terrorism

Biological terrorism includes anthrax, smallpox, and other biological agents. If a biological attack occurs, the public will be informed and told what to do. Stay calm and listen for instructions on the radio or television.

{*Note:* For up-to-date information on biological agents, contact The Centers for Disease Control and Prevention at 888.246.2675 or www.bt.cdc.gov.}

For Smallpox

Smallpox is caused by a specific virus. It was wiped out as a disease in 1977, but may exist in labs in some foreign countries. This makes it possible for use in germ warfare. Smallpox is very contagious.

What Can You Do?

- Listen to the news on a regular basis. If a confirmed case of smallpox occurs, the public will be told what to do.

- For people exposed to smallpox, a vaccine (from an emergency supply) can be given to lessen the severity of the illness or even prevent it. The vaccine needs to be given within 4 days after exposure, though.

For Explosions and Fires

- Follow fire prevention measures. Install and maintain smoke alarms. Plan escape routes from both your home and your place of work. {*Note:* For a more complete list of fire prevention tips, contact the National Fire Protection Association at www.nfpa.org or contact www.firesafetytips.com.}

- Know the building's emergency plan.

- Know where fire exits are.

- Keep fire extinguishers handy. Make sure they work.

- Learn first aid.

- Keep a battery-operated radio, flashlights, and extra batteries, a first-aid kit, and bright tape to mark off unsafe areas on each floor.

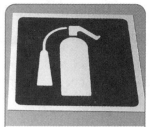

Know where fire extinguishers are and how to use them.

- Stay calm. Exit the building quickly.

- If things fall from above, get under a strong table or desk. Exit as soon as you can.

When Inside a Building Where a Fire Occurs

- Get out! Stay low (crawl). Cover your nose and mouth with a wet cloth. Exit the building as fast as you can.

- Feel the top, middle, and bottom of a closed door for heat. If the door is not warm, brace yourself against the door and open it slowly. If the door is warm, find another way out.

- Always stay below the smoke. After you are out, **call 9-1-1!**

When Trapped in a Collapsed Building

- Use a flashlight, if you have one.

- Don't move more than necessary so you won't kick up dust. Cover your nose and mouth with clothing.

- To help someone find you, tap a pipe or wall or whistle. Don't yell. Yelling can cause you to breathe in dangerous amounts of dust. Shout only as a last resort.

- Wait for emergency workers. (Untrained people should not try to go inside a collapsed building for any reason.)

For Harmful Chemical Exposures

Once in awhile, you hear about chemical leaks from industrial sites. The threat of chemical warfare is also on the minds of Americans. Of utmost concern is to keep your home safe.

What Can You Do?

- Install carbon monoxide detectors in your home and garage. Follow instructions given.

- If the alarm sounds, open windows and doors. Leave the building right away. **Call 9-1-1** if persons are dizzy, weak, short of breath, confused, etc. If not, turn off all appliances that use fuel. Have a qualified person inspect your home.

- Don't run cars and lawn mowers in the garage. Don't use gas ranges for heat.

- Have your home furnace, chimney, and flue checked by a qualified person every year. If you think there is a gas leak, open a window and leave the house. Then, call the local gas company. Follow their advice.

- Use common sense. Biohazard suits and expensive gas masks are a waste of money.

- If you work at a company where a harmful chemical leak or exposure could occur, follow your workplace safety guidelines. Follow instructions on Material Safety Data Sheets (MSDSs). These tell you how to use chemicals safely.

- In the event of a chemical leak or exposure, follow the advice of local officials. You may be told to "evacuate" or "shelter in place."

Evacuate

- If told to leave the area, do so right away.

- Take your emergency supply kit, if available.

- Wear pants, long-sleeves, and sturdy shoes.

- Take pets.

- Lock your home.

- Travel on routes approved by local officials. Shortcuts could be dangerous or closed.

- Watch for fallen power lines and avoid them.

Shelter in Place

If told to "shelter in place," stay in your home or workplace.

- Close and lock windows and outside doors.

- Turn off heating and cooling units and fans.

- Close the fireplace flue.

- Get your emergency supply kit, if available.

- Turn on the radio and listen for what to do.

- If you can, go to an inside room above ground level. Choose a room with no or few windows.

- Seal vents and cracks around doors with duct tape and wet towels. Tape all the faucets and drains, too.

Contact with chemicals can kill. For this reason, do not leave the shelter to help victims. Persons trained to deal with harmful chemicals should treat victims.

 Get information on other types of disasters, such as shootings, arson, hijackings, and kidnappings, from:

www.fbi.gov and www.cia.gov

Section III

Common Health Problems

Knowledge is power. Knowing what to do to prevent common health problems can help keep you from getting sick. When you do get sick, you should know what to do, too.

- Should you get medical help fast?
- Should you call your doctor?
- Should you wait and see if the problem gets better?
- Can you take care of the problem yourself?
- What things should you do?

This section can help you answer these questions. It tells what you can do to help prevent getting common health problems and what to do when you have one of them.

Sometimes you can treat these problems with self-care. Sometimes you need medical help. This section can help you ask the right questions and find the answers to take care of your health.

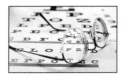
Chapter 9
Eye Conditions

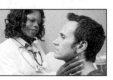
Chapter 10
Ear, Nose &
Throat Problems

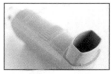
Chapter 11
Respiratory
Conditions

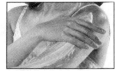
Chapter 12
Skin Conditions

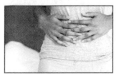
Chapter 13
Digestive &
Urinary Problems

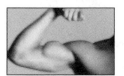
Chapter 14
Muscle & Bone
Problems

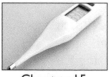
Chapter 15
General Health
Conditions

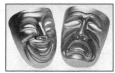
Chapter 16
Mental Health
Conditions

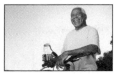
Chapter 17
Men's Health
Issues

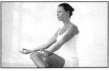
Chapter 18
Women's Health
Issues

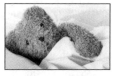
Chapter 19
Children's Health
Problems

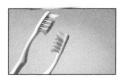
Chapter 20
Dental & Mouth
Concerns

How to Use This Section

- Find the health condition in the index or in the Table of Contents. Go to that page. The problems are listed in chapters. Each chapter covers certain conditions, such as **Eye Conditions**, and **Ear, Nose & Throat Problems**, etc. The topics in each chapter are listed in order from A to Z.

- Read about the problem, what causes it (if known), its symptoms, and treatments.

- Read the "Questions to Ask." Start at the top of the flow chart and answer YES or NO to each question. Follow the arrows until you get to one of these answers:
  - Get Medical Care Fast.
  - See Doctor.
  - See Counselor or Call Counselor.
  - Call Doctor.
  - Use Self-Care.

What the Instructions Mean

Get Medical Care Fast
If your symptoms are listed under this heading, get medical care without delay. See **Recognizing Emergencies** on page 351 for warning signs of a medical emergency. For one or more of these signs, go to a hospital emergency department if you can do so safely. If not, call **9-1-1**, your local rescue squad, or an ambulance. Don't call **9-1-1** or use a hospital emergency department if symptoms do not threaten life. Call your doctor right away or go to an "urgent care" center. Some hospital emergency departments have a "Prompt Care" area to treat problems, such as a sprained ankle.

Ask your doctor ahead of time where you should go for a sprained ankle or similar problem that needs prompt care, but not emergency care.

Find out, now, how your health insurance covers medical emergencies, so you'll know what to do.

Know phone numbers for emergency medical help. Write them down near your phone and on the **Telephone Numbers & Information** list on page 1 of this book. Call **9-1-1** where the service is available. If your HMO prefers that you use a certain ambulance service, find out their number and write it on page 1.

See Doctor
If your symptoms are listed under this heading, you should be seen by your doctor for medical advice. Contact your doctor or health care provider to find out how soon you should be seen.

The term "doctor" can be used for a number of health care providers:
- Your doctor.
- Your Health Maintenance Organization (HMO) clinic, primary doctor, or other health care provider.
- Walk-in clinic.
- Physician's assistants (P.A.s), nurse practitioners (N.P.s), or certified nurses (C.N.s) who work with your doctor. This includes your "Nurse Call" Information Service.
- Home health care provider.
- Your psychiatrist.
- Your dentist.

Write down phone numbers for your health care providers on page 1 of this book.

See Counselor or Call Counselor

If your symptoms are listed under this heading, call your mental health counselor, if you have one. If not, call your doctor for a referral. You will get advice on what to do.

The term "counselor" can be used for a number of mental health care providers:

- Your counselor or therapist, if you already have one.

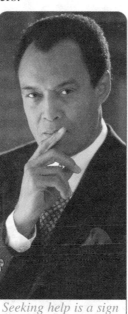

- A mental health professional provided by your Employee Assistance Program (EAP) at work.

- A mental health center.

- A clinical psychologist.

- A social worker with a master's degree (M.S.W.).

- Another health care provider in the mental health field, such as a psychiatric nurse.

Seeking help is a sign of strength, not weakness.

{*Note:* Your primary care doctor may be able to provide some counseling, too, or help you by making a referral to another mental health care provider. If you belong to a Health Maintenance Organization (HMO) or other managed health care plan, you may need a referral from your primary care doctor for services to be covered. Also, a counselor may have you join a self-help/support group.}

Call Doctor

Call your doctor or health care provider and state the problem. He or she can decide what you should do. He or she may:

- Tell you to make an appointment to be seen.

- Send you to a laboratory for tests.

- Prescribe medicine or treatment over the phone.

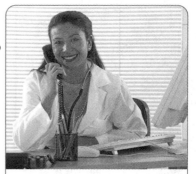

Your doctor or a staff member will respond to your call.

- Tell you specific things to do to treat the problem.

Use Self-Care

You can probably take care of the problem yourself if you answered NO to all the questions. Use the "Self-Care" measures that are listed. Call your doctor if you don't feel better soon, though. You may have some other problem.

Online Instructional Video

An online video shows you how to get the maximun benefit from this book.

Go to: www.HealthyLearn.com and click on "Self-Care and You Instructional Video."

To learn more about topics covered in this Guide and other health issues, access www.HealthyLearn.com. At this site, type a topic in the box for "Search MedlinePlus."

Chapter 9

Eye Conditions

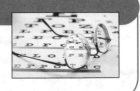

Cataract

A **cataract** is a cloudy area in the lens or lens capsule of the eye. A cataract blocks or distorts light entering the eye. Vision gradually becomes dull and fuzzy, even in daylight. Most of the time, cataracts occur in both eyes, but only one eye may be affected. If they form in both eyes, one eye can be worse than the other, because each cataract develops at a different rate.

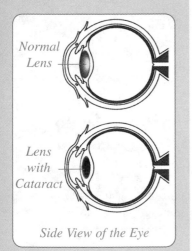

Normal Lens

Lens with Cataract

Side View of the Eye

Signs & Symptoms

- Cloudy, fuzzy, foggy, or filmy vision.
- Pupils (normally black) appear milky white.
- Frequent changes in eyeglass prescriptions. Better near vision for a while, but only in far-sighted people.
- Sensitivity to light and glazed nighttime vision. This can cause problems when driving at night.
- Blurred or double vision. Changes in the way you see colors.
- Seeing glare from lamps or the sun. Halos may appear around lights.

Vision with cataracts

Causes

- The most common form of cataracts come with aging due to changes in the chemical state of lens proteins. More than half of Americans age 65 and older have a cataract.
- Cataracts can also result from damage to the lens capsule due to trauma; from ionizing radiation or infrared rays; from taking corticosteroid medicines for a long time; and from chemical toxins. Smokers have an increased risk for cataracts. So do persons with diabetes and glaucoma.

Treatment

Treatment includes eye exams, corrective lenses, cataract glasses, and cataract surgery, when needed.

A person who has cataract surgery usually gets an artificial lens at the same time. A plastic disc called an intraocular lens (IOL) is placed in the lens capsule inside the eye.

Cataract, Continued

It takes a couple of months for an eye to heal after cataract surgery. Experts say it is best to wait until your first eye heals before you have surgery on the second eye if it, too, has a cataract.

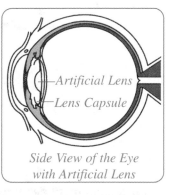

Side View of the Eye with Artificial Lens

—Artificial Lens
—Lens Capsule

Questions to Ask

Do you have any of the **signs and symptoms of cataracts** listed on page 68?

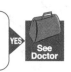
YES → See Doctor

NO
Use Self-Care

Self-Care / Prevention

To Help Prevent Cataracts

- Limit exposing your eyes to X-rays, microwaves, and infrared radiation.

- Avoid overexposure to sunlight. While outdoors, wear sunglasses with UV block and wear a hat with a brim.

- Wear glasses or goggles that protect your eyes whenever you use strong chemicals, power tools, or other instruments that could result in eye injury.

- Don't smoke. Avoid heavy drinking.

- Keep other illnesses, such as diabetes, under control.

- Eat foods high in beta-carotene and/or vitamin C, which may help to prevent or delay cataracts. Examples are carrots, cantaloupes, oranges, and broccoli.

To Treat Cataracts

- Be careful about driving at night. Let someone else drive if you can't see well.

- Wear sunglasses with UV block.

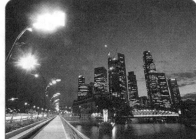

Night vision can be one of the first things affected by cataracts.

- When indoors, don't have lighting too bright or pointed directly at you. Install dimmer switches so you can lower the light level. Use table lamps, not ceiling fixtures.

- Use soft, white (not clear) light bulbs.

- Arrange to have light reflect off walls and ceilings.

- Read large print items. Use magnifying glasses, if needed.

- Schedule eye exams as advised by your doctor.

- Wear your prescribed glasses.

Get more information from:

HealthyLearn® • www.HealthyLearn.com
Click on MedlinePlus®

National Eye Institute (NEI)
www.nei.nih.gov

Eyestrain from Computer Use

Persons who use computer video display terminals (VDTs) at work and/or at home may notice eyestrain.

Signs & Symptoms

- Eye discomfort or irritation. This includes dry, red, and/or watery eyes.
- Eye fatigue.
- Having a hard time focusing.
- Back pain, shoulder pain, and headaches may also occur.

Treatment

Self-care measures prevent and treat eyestrain when using VDTs.

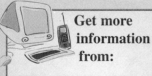

Get more information from:

HealthyLearn®
www.HealthyLearn.com
Click on MedlinePlus®

Prevent Blindness America
www.preventblindness.org

Causes

The cause of eyestrain is most likely from conditions that surround the VDT, not the VDT itself. These include improper positioning of the VDT and supplies, poor lighting, and/or poor posture.

A pre-existing eye problem may also be the cause.

Questions to Ask

Do you still have **signs and symptoms of eye strain** despite using self-care measures? **YES** Call Doctor

NO Use Self-Care

Self-Care / Prevention

- Place the screen so that your line of sight is 10 to 15 degrees (about one-third of a 45-degree angle) below horizontal.
- Position the VDT screen about 2 feet away from your eyes. This is a little farther away than normal reading distance.
- Dust the screen often.
- Reduce glare. Place the VDT at right angles to a window. Turn off or shield overhead lights. Wear a visor to block them, if needed.
- Place your paperwork close enough that you don't have to keep refocusing when switching from the screen to the paper. Use a paper document holder placed at the same height as the VDT screen.
- Blink often to keep your eyes from getting dry. Use "artificial tear" eyedrops, if needed.
- Tell your eye specialist that you use a VDT. Glasses and contacts worn for other activities may not be good for VDT work. With bifocals, the near-vision part of the lens is good for looking down, as when you read, but not for looking straight ahead, as when you look at a video display screen. You may need single-vision lenses for VDT work.
- If the image on the VDT screen is blurred, dull, or flickers, have it serviced right away.

Floaters & Flashes

Signs & Symptoms

- **Floaters** are specks, dots, cobwebs, or wavy lines that seem to fall within the line of sight. They rarely affect eyesight. They are more visible against a plain or dark background.

- **Flashes** are streaks of light that "flash" across the field of vision. They can occur when the eyes are closed or in extreme darkness.

Causes

With aging, the middle portion of the eye, called the vitreous, becomes less solid and more liquid. This allows particles (floaters), which have always been in the eye, to begin to move around. Flashes can occur when the vitreous shrinks and pulls on the retina of the eye. This is common. On rare occasions, when the vitreous detaches from the retina, it can rip or tear the retina. This may lead to a **detached retina**. The retina peels away from the eye wall causing sight loss.

Risk Factors for Floaters and Flashes
- Eye diseases or injuries.

- A tear in the retina. Aging and cataract surgery increase the risk for this.

- High blood pressure.

- Migraine headaches.

- Nearsightedness.

Treatment

Self-care is enough to treat floaters and flashes unless they are due to another medical condition.

Questions to Ask

> Do you have any of these **signs of a detached retina**?
> - A floater appears suddenly.
> - A large red floater disturbs vision.
> - It looks like a curtain is over your field of vision.
> - The number of floaters and/or light flashes keep increasing.

YES → Get Medical Care Fast

NO ↓

> With floaters or flashes, do you have any of these problems?
> - A loss of side vision.
> - Bleeding in the eye.
> - The floaters don't move as you look at them.

YES → Get Medical Care Fast

NO ↓

> With floaters or flashes, do you have a history of migraine headaches or high blood pressure? Or, do the floaters or flashes last 10 to 20 minutes in both eyes?

YES → See Doctor

NO ↓

Use Self-Care

Self-Care / Prevention

- Move your eyes up and down (not side to side) several times.

- Don't focus on or stare at plain, light backgrounds, such as a blank pastel wall or the light blue sky.

- You may notice flashes less if you avoid moving suddenly, don't bend over, and don't get up quickly from sitting or lying down.

Glaucoma

Glaucoma is a group of eye diseases that damages the optic nerve and causes vision loss.

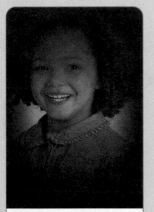

Vision with glaucoma

Signs & Symptoms

For Chronic (Open-Angle) Glaucoma

This type takes place gradually, and causes no symptoms early on. Loss of side (peripheral) vision and blurred vision are the first signs.

Later, symptoms include:
- Vision loss in side and central vision, usually in both eyes.
- Blind spots. Seeing halos around lights.
- Poor night vision.
- Blindness, if not treated early.

For Acute (Angle-Closure) Glaucoma

This type is a medical emergency! These symptoms occur suddenly:
- Severe eye pain and nausea.
- Blurred vision. Seeing halos around lights.
- Redness in the eye. Swollen upper eyelid.
- Severe headache that throbs.

Causes

Glaucoma occurs when the pressure of the liquid in the eye gets too high and causes damage to the optic nerve. Increased eye pressure without damage is not glaucoma, but increases the risk for it. Antihistamines and long-term corticosteroid use can trigger or worsen glaucoma.

Risk Factors for Glaucoma

- Aging, especially being over age 60.
- Being African American over age 40.
- Having a family history of glaucoma.
- Having diabetes.
- Being nearsighted.

Glaucoma, Continued

Treatment

Glaucoma may not be preventable, but the blindness that could result from it is. Get tested for glaucoma when you get regular vision exams. If pressure inside the eyeball is high, an eye doctor will prescribe eye drops. Oral medicines may also be prescribed.

Medicines used for acute glaucoma are prescribed for life. If medicines do not control the pressure, your doctor may advise:

- Ultrasound.
- Laser beam surgery.
- Other surgical procedures.

Questions to Ask

Do you have **signs and symptoms of acute glaucoma** listed on page 72?

YES ▸ Get Medical Care Fast

NO ▾

Do you have any **signs and symptoms of chronic glaucoma** listed on page 72?

YES ▸ See Doctor

NO ▾

Use Self-Care

See Self-Care / Prevention in next column

Self-Care / Prevention

- Don't smoke. If you smoke, quit.

- Do not take any medicine, including over-the-counter ones, without first checking with your doctor or pharmacist. Most cold medications and sleeping pills, for example, can cause the pupil in the eye to dilate. This can lead to increased eye pressure.

- If prescribed eye drops for glaucoma, use them as directed.

- Ask your eye doctor about low vision services and devices.

- Try not to get upset and fatigued. These can increase pressure in the eye.

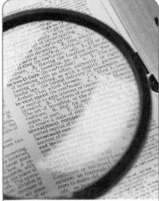

Low vision aids can help you see things better.

Get more information from:

HealthyLearn® • www.HealthyLearn.com
Click on MedlinePlus®

The Glaucoma Foundation
www.glaucoma-foundation.org

National Eye Institute (NEI)
www.nei.nih.gov

Macular Degeneration

Macular degeneration is a progressive eye disorder. Known as **age-related macular degeneration (AMD)**, it is the most common cause of central vision loss in older Americans. The central part of the retina (the macula) deteriorates. This results in the loss of central (straight-ahead) vision. One or both eyes may be affected. The most common type is called the dry form. With this, cells under the retina do not function well, causing subtle to overt blank spots in central vision. Only 1 to 2% of people with the dry form have a lot of vision loss. In the wet form, tiny blood vessels leak blood or fluid around the macula. The wet form is less common than the dry form. It causes more vision loss, though.

Signs & Symptoms

Macular degeneration is painless. It usually develops gradually, especially the dry form. With the wet form, symptoms can occur more rapidly. Symptoms for both forms are:

- Blurred or cloudy vision.
- Seeing a dark or blind spot at the center of vision.
- A hard time reading or doing other close-up work.
- A hard time doing any activity, such as driving, that needs sharp vision.
- Complete loss of central vision. Side vision is not affected.

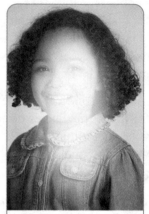

Vision with macular degeneration

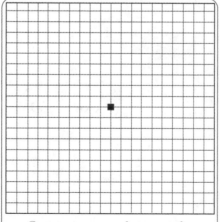

Cover one eye and stare at the center dot in this grid. Seeing blurry, curvy, or distorted lines or empty spots could be a sign of macular degeneration. Repeat, covering the other eye.

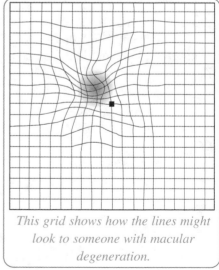

This grid shows how the lines might look to someone with macular degeneration.

Macular Degeneration, Continued

Causes

The exact cause of age-related macular degeneration (AMD) is not known. Risk factors are:

- Advancing age.
- Cigarette smoking. High blood pressure.
- Family history of AMD.
- Having light-colored eyes.
- Exposure to ultraviolet light.
- Poor diet.

Treatment

Treatment for the wet form includes photodynamic therapy and laser therapy. Medicine called "anti-VEGF therapy" can also be given. Most dry form cases are not treatable. Your eye doctor may prescribe special eyeglasses and low vision aids. He or she may also prescribe a specific high dose vitamin and mineral to reduce the risk of advanced AMD.

Questions to Ask

Do you have **signs and symptoms of macular degeneration** listed on page 74, especially if they come on quickly?

YES → See Doctor

NO → Use Self-Care

See Self-Care / Prevention in next column

Self-Care / Prevention

To Reduce the Risk for AMD

- Don't smoke. If you smoke, quit.

- Follow a healthy diet. Include green leafy vegetables and fish.

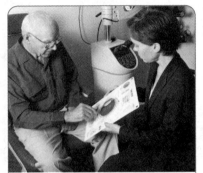

Get your vision checked as often as your doctor advises.

- Protect your eyes from the sun's ultraviolet rays. Wear sunglasses with UV block. Wear a hat with a wide brim.

- Use **Self-Care / Prevention** measures to control **high blood pressure** (see page 239) and **heart disease** (see page 234).

To Treat AMD

- Wear the special eyeglasses and use other vision aids, such as magnifying devices, as advised by your doctor.

- Talk to your doctor before taking vitamin and mineral supplements.

Get more information from:

HealthyLearn® • www.HealthyLearn.com
Click on MedlinePlus®

Macular Degeneration Foundation
www.eyesight.org

National Eye Institute (NEI)
www.nei.nih.gov

Pink Eye (Conjunctivitis)

Pink eye is an inflammation of the conjunctiva. This is the covering of the inside of the eyelids and the whites of the eyes. The medical term for pink eye is **conjunctivitis**.

It is called pink eye when the cause is a bacterial or viral infection. This is because the white part of the eye looks pinkish-red. Conjunctivitis can also be due to an allergic reaction.

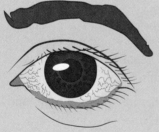

Conjunctivitis

Conjunctivitis Chart		
Signs & Symptoms	Cause	Treatment
Redness of the whites of the eyes. Watery, yellowish-green, or puslike discharge from the eye. Feels like you have something in your eye. May have crusting on the eyelashes, runny nose, and sore throat.	Viral infection (common). Bacterial infection (less common). Both are contagious.	For bacterial infection, prescribed antibiotic eye drops or ointment. Usually starts to clear up in 2 to 3 days. Take eye drops as long as prescribed. Viral infections are self-limiting and resolve without treatment. Antibiotic eye drops or ointment may be prescribed, because it is hard to tell a viral from bacterial infection, since symptoms for both are the same. Can take 14 to 21 days to clear up a viral infection.
Burning, itching, and watery eyes. May feel like you have something in the eye.	Allergic reaction (not contagious). Common irritants are cosmetics, contact lenses, dust, mold, pollen, and smoke.	Avoid the allergen. Use over-the-counter eye drops and/or artificial teardrops. Ask your doctor if it is okay to take an over-the-counter antihistamine.

Questions to Ask

With pink eye, do you have any of these problems?
- A puslike discharge with redness and irritation.
- Your vision is affected and/or your eye(s) hurt a lot.

YES  **See Doctor**

NO

Flowchart continued on the next page

Pink Eye, Continued

Have you tried self-care for a week and symptoms got worse or do you get conjunctivitis often?

YES → **See Doctor**

NO

Use Self-Care

Self-Care / Prevention

For Pink Eye

- Wash your hands often. Don't share towels, washcloths, etc.

- Avoid contact with other people as much as you can until you have used the prescribed antibiotic eye drops, etc. for 24 hours. Follow the rules of your workplace about pink eye. For children, follow the rules of their school.

- With your eyes closed, apply a cotton ball soaked in warm (not hot) water to the affected eye 3 to 4 times a day.

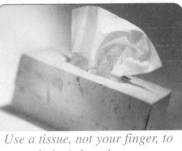

Use a tissue, not your finger, to touch the infected eye area.

Do this for at least 5 minutes at a time. Use a clean cotton ball each time.

- Throw away any makeup that could be contaminated. Don't wear eye makeup until the infection is all cleared up. Don't share makeup with others.

- Don't share eye drops with others.

- Don't put a cover or patch over the eye. This can make the infection grow.

- Don't wear contact lenses while your eyes are infected. Replace contact lenses or disinfect them twice before re-using.

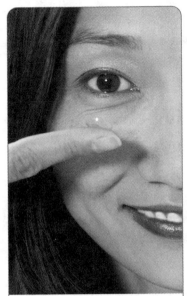

Replace contact lenses or disinfect them before re-using.

For Allergic Conjunctivitis

- Avoid things you know you are allergic to.

- Use over-the-counter eye drops. These soothe irritation and help relieve itching.

- Apply a washcloth rinsed in cold water to the eyes. Do this several times a day.

- Use protective eyewear when you work with chemicals and fumes.

Get more information from:

HealthyLearn® • www.HealthyLearn.com
Click on MedlinePlus®

Stye

A **stye** is an infection in a tiny gland of the eyelid.

Signs & Symptoms

- Red, painful bump or sore on an eyelid.
- Watery or tearing eye that burns and itches.
- The red bump may form a head and appears yellow if it contains pus. This usually drains on its own within days.

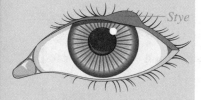

Stye

Causes

Sties form from clogged oil glands at the base of an eyelash.

Treatment

Most sties respond well to self-care and don't need further treatment.

Questions to Ask

With a stye, do you have any of these problems?
- Redness and swelling haven't drained within 1 or 2 days.
- A stye makes it hard for you to see.
- Many sties come at the same time.
- You get one stye right after another.

YES → See Doctor

NO ↓

Use Self-Care

Self-Care / Prevention

- Wash your hands often.
- Don't touch your eyes with your fingers. Use a tissue instead.
- Use clean washcloths and towels each time you wash your face.
- Don't share washcloths, towels, makeup, or eye drops with others.
- Don't expose your eyes to excessive dust or dirt.

To Relieve the Discomfort of a Stye
- Apply warm (not hot), wet compresses to the affected area 3 to 4 times a day for 5 to 10 minutes at a time. Use a clean washcloth each time.
- Don't poke or squeeze the stye. A more serious infection could occur.
- If the stye drains on its own, gently wash the pus away with a clean, wet cloth.

Vision Care

Vision care is taking care of your eyes and general health to prevent or lessen the chances of visual problems.

Vision Care Basics

- Have routine vision tests. (See **Health Tests & When to Have Them** on page 22.) The American Optometric Association gives different guidelines for adults:

Age Group	When to Have Exams
Infants and Children	By 6 months of age; at 3 years of age; before starting first grade, and every 2 years after that.
18 years – 40 years	Every 2–3 years.
41 years – 60 years	Every 2 years.
61 years and older	Every year.

Follow your health care provider's advice for eye exams and treatment for eye and medical conditions. Follow directions for proper use and care of eyeglasses, contact lenses, low vision aids, etc.

- Protect your eyes from the sun. Limit exposure of your eyes to the sun's ultraviolet rays. When outdoors, wear sunglasses with 99 to 100% protection from both UV-A and UV-B rays. Gray lenses are the best choice. Green and brown are okay, too. Wear a wide-brimmed hat. Don't look at the sun during a solar eclipse.

- Protect your eyes from injury. Wear vision protective devices as needed. Examples are safety glasses and protective goggles (for swimming, working with certain machines, etc.).

- Don't smoke. If you smoke, quit.

- Have regular health exams to detect and treat conditions (e.g., diabetes) that can affect your vision or lead to vision loss.

- Get regular exercise for good circulation.

- Maintain a healthy diet. Include foods that are high in antioxidants for eye health (see below). Studies have shown that age-related eye diseases may be slowed by getting these nutrients from foods or when taken in supplement form. Talk to your doctor before you take vitamins, minerals, and/or herbs.

Foods with Antioxidants for Eye Health

- *For Beta-carotene:* Carrots, mangos, sweet potatoes, spinach, cantaloupe, kale, apricots, and broccoli.

- *For Lutein:* Spinach, savoy cabbage, greens, broccoli, peas, and green peppers.

- *For Vitamin C:* Papaya, oranges, grapefruit, strawberries, cantaloupe, green peppers, broccoli, and tomatoes.

- *For Vitamin E:* Almonds, safflower and corn oils, turnip greens, peanuts, and broccoli.

- *For Zeaxanthin:* Orange peppers, corn, collard greens, spinach, kale, and tangerines.

- *For Zinc:* Oysters, fortified breakfast cereals, and meats.

Get more information from:

HealthyLearn® • www.HealthyLearn.com
Click on MedlinePlus®

American Optometric Association
314.991.4100 • www.aoanet.org

National Eye Institute
301.496.5248 • www.nei.nih.gov

Chapter 10

Ear, Nose & Throat Problems

Earaches

Signs & Symptoms

- Mild to severe ear pain.
- Feeling of fullness or discomfort in the ears.
- Tugging at the ear and restlessness in young children.

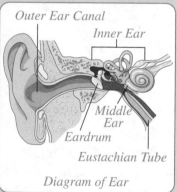

Outer Ear Canal

Inner Ear

Middle Ear

Eardrum

Eustachian Tube

Diagram of Ear

Ruptured Eardrum Signs

- Ear pain.
- Some hearing loss.
- Blood or other discharge from the ear (especially after sticking an object in the ear or exposure to extremely loud noise).

Causes

The most common cause of earaches is plugged Eustachian tubes. These go from the back of the throat to the middle ear. Fluid or pressure in a plugged Eustachian tube causes pain. This is caused by an infection of the middle ear, a cold or sinus infection, or allergies. Other things that can cause ear pain include changes in air pressure in a plane, something stuck in the ear, too much earwax, tooth problems, and ear injuries.

Questions to Ask

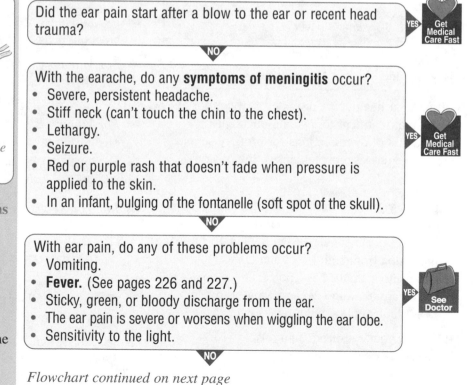

Did the ear pain start after a blow to the ear or recent head trauma?

YES → **Get Medical Care Fast**

NO ↓

With the earache, do any **symptoms of meningitis** occur?
- Severe, persistent headache.
- Stiff neck (can't touch the chin to the chest).
- Lethargy.
- Seizure.
- Red or purple rash that doesn't fade when pressure is applied to the skin.
- In an infant, bulging of the fontanelle (soft spot of the skull).

YES → **Get Medical Care Fast**

NO ↓

With ear pain, do any of these problems occur?
- Vomiting.
- **Fever.** (See pages 226 and 227.)
- Sticky, green, or bloody discharge from the ear.
- The ear pain is severe or worsens when wiggling the ear lobe.
- Sensitivity to the light.

YES → **See Doctor**

NO ↓

Flowchart continued on next page

Earaches, Continued

Does a child show the following signs, especially after a respiratory tract infection, a cold, air travel, or if the child has had ear problems before?
- Constant pulling, touching, or tugging at the ear(s).
- No response to a whistle or a loud clap.
- **Fever.** (See pages 226 and 227.)
- Crying that won't stop.
- Ear(s) that are hot and hurt when touched.
- Acting cranky and restless, especially at night or when lying down.

YES → See Doctor

NO ↓

Does the earache persist, is it more than mild, and does it occur after any of the following?
- A mild ear injury.
- Blowing your nose hard or many times.
- A small object has been stuck in the ear that cannot easily be removed. Or, an insect has gotten in the ear that cannot safely be removed.
- A cold, sinus, or upper respiratory infection.
- Exposure to extremely loud noises, such as rock concerts, heavy machinery, etc.

YES → See Doctor

NO ↓

With the earache, do you also have hearing loss, ringing in the ears, dizziness, or nausea?

YES → See Doctor

NO ↓

Flowchart continued in next column

Does the earache occur with jaw pain, headache, and a clicking sound when you open or close your mouth?

YES → Call Doctor

NO ↓

 Use Self-Care

Self-Care / Prevention

To Help Prevent Ear Pain

- Don't put cotton-tipped swabs, bobby pins, etc., in your ears. This could damage the eardrum.

- Don't blow your nose with too much force.

- If you can, avoid places that have very loud noises (construction sites, etc.). Wear earplugs when exposed to loud noises.

- Keep the volume on low when using stereos, compact discs (CDs), etc. If someone else can hear the music when you are listening to one of these devices with earphones, the volume is too loud.

To Avoid Getting "Swimmer's Ear"

- Wear wax or silicone earplugs.

- Wear a bathing cap.

- Don't swim in dirty water. Swim on the surface not underneath the water.

- Use an over-the-counter product, such as Swim-Ear, as directed.

To Reduce Ear Pain

- Place a warm washcloth next to the ear. Some health professionals recommend putting an ice bag or ice in a wet washcloth over the painful ear for 20 minutes.

- Take an over-the-counter medicine for pain as directed on the label.

Earaches, Continued

Treatment

Treatment includes pain relievers and methods to dry up or clear the blocked ear canal. Self-care can be used to treat many earaches. Severe and/or constant ear pain needs a medical diagnosis. Often, antibiotics *are not* needed for middle ear infections in children. About 8 in 10 children with ear infections get better without antibiotics. Let your child's doctor decide if and when an antibiotic should be prescribed.

To Open Up the Eustachian Tubes and Help Them Drain
- Sit up. Prop your head up when you sleep.
- Yawn. This helps move the muscles that open the Eustachian tubes.
- Chew gum or suck on hard candy. (Do not give to children under age 5.) This tip is especially helpful during pressure changes that take place during air travel, but can also help if you wake up with ear pain.
- When traveling by air, stay awake when the plane takes off and lands. Wear ear plugs.
- Take a steamy shower.
- Use a cool-mist vaporizer, especially at night.
- Drink plenty of cool water.
- Gently, but firmly, blow through your nose while holding both nostrils closed until you hear a pop. This can be done several times a day.
- If okay with your doctor, take a decongestant to help relieve the swelling that causes the pain. (Don't use a nasal spray decongestant for more than 3 days unless directed by your doctor.)
- When you give a baby a bottle, hold the baby in an upright position.

To Treat a Mild Case of "Swimmer's Ear"
The goal is to clean and dry the outer ear canal without doing further damage to the top layer of skin.

- Shake the head to expel trapped water.
- Dry the ear canal. Get a clean facial tissue. Twist each corner into a tip and gently place each tip into the ear canal for 10 seconds. Repeat with the other ear using a new tissue.
- Use an over-the-counter product, such as Swim-Ear. Drop it into the ears to fight infection. Follow package directions.
- Do not remove earwax. This protects the ear canal.

For an Insect in the Ear
- Shine a flashlight into the ear. Doing this may cause the insect to come out. (See, also, **To Remove an Insect from an Ear** on page 396.)

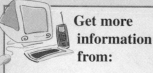

Get more information from:

National Institute on Deafness and Other Communication Disorders (NIDCD)
800.241.1044
www.nidcd.nih.gov

Hay Fever

Hay fever has nothing to do with hay or fever. The medical term for hay fever is **allergic rhinitis**. It is most common in spring and fall when a lot of ragweed is in the air. Some people have hay fever all year, though.

Signs & Symptoms

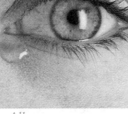

- Itchy or watery eyes.
- Runny, itchy nose.
- Congestion.
- Sneezing.

Allergens can cause itchy or watery eyes.

Causes

Hay fever is a reaction of the upper respiratory tract to allergens.

Treatment

Talk to your doctor if self-care measures do not help. He or she may prescribe:

- Antihistamines. For best results, take the antihistamine 30 minutes before going outside. {*Note:* Some over-the-counter antihistamines can make you more drowsy than prescribed ones. Be careful when driving and operating machinery since some antihistamines can make you drowsy.}

- A decongestant.

{*Note:* Do not give antihistamines, decongestants, and other over-the-counter medicines for colds, coughs, and/or the flu to children less than 2 years old. For children 2 years old and older, follow their doctor's advice.

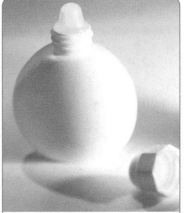

- A corticosteroid nasal spray and eye drops, cromolyn sodium, and oral corticosteroids.

- Skin tests to find out what things you are allergic to.

- Allergy shots.

Your doctor may advise a nasal spray for hay fever symptoms.

It is best to take what your doctor advises instead of testing over-the-counter products on your own.

Questions to Ask

Do you have severe breathing problems or severe wheezing? **YES** → Get Medical Care Fast

NO ↓

Do you have any of these symptoms of an infection?
- **Fever.** (See pages 226 and 227.)
- Green, yellow, or bloody-colored nasal discharge or mucus.
- Throbbing facial pain.

YES → See Doctor

NO ↓

Do you still have hay fever symptoms when you avoid hay fever triggers? Or, do hay fever symptoms keep you from doing daily activities? **YES** → Call Doctor

NO ↓

Use Self-Care

See Self-Care / Prevention on next page

Hay Fever, Continued

Self-Care / Prevention

Avoid Hay Fever Triggers

■ If you are allergic to pollen and molds, let someone else do outside chores. Mowing the lawn or raking leaves can make you very sick.

■ Keep windows and doors shut and stay inside when the pollen count or humidity is high. Early morning is sometimes the worst.

■ Avoid tobacco smoke and other air pollutants.

■ To limit dust, mold, and pollen:
  • Put a plastic cover on your mattress or cover it completely with an allergen-free mattress cover.

  • Sleep with no pillow or with the kind your doctor or health care provider recommends. If you use a pillow, cover it with an allergen-free cover.

  • Don't dry sheets and blankets outside.

  • Try not to have stuffed animals kept in the bedroom. If you must, have only one that can be washed. Wash it in hot water once a week.

  • Use curtains and rugs that can be washed often. Don't use carpeting.

  • Dust and vacuum often. Wear a dust filter mask when you do.

Every week, wash the sheets and blankets on your bed. Wash them in hot water.

  • Put an electronic air filter on your furnace or use portable air purifiers.

  • Shower or bathe and wash your hair after heavy exposure to pollen, dust, etc.

■ Don't have pets. If you have a pet, keep it out of the bedroom. When you can, keep the pet outdoors.

■ Use an air conditioner or air cleaner in your house, especially in the bedroom. Electronic air filters are better than mechanical ones. Clean the filter often. Or, try a doctor-approved air purifier, especially in the bedroom. Devices with HEPA filters can be very effective in cleaning indoor air.

Get more information from:

HealthyLearn®
www.HealthyLearn.com
Click on MedlinePlus®

Asthma and Allergy Foundation of America
800.7.ASTHMA
(727.8462)
www.aafa.org

Hearing Loss

People over age 50 are likely to lose some hearing each year. The decline is usually gradual. About 30% of adults age 65 through 74 and about 50% of those age 85 and older have hearing problems.

Hearing problems can get worse if they are ignored and not treated. People with hearing problems may withdraw from others because they may not be able to understand what others say. Hearing loss can cause an older person to be labeled "confused" or "senile."

Signs & Symptoms

- Words are hard to understand. This worsens when there is background noise.

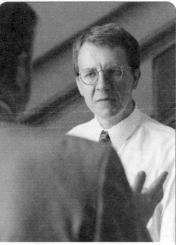

- Certain sounds are overly loud or annoying.

- Hearing a hissing or ringing background noise. This can be constant or it can come and go.

Another person's speech may sound slurred or mumbled.

- Concerts, TV shows, etc. are less enjoyable because much goes unheard.

Causes

- **Presbycusis** (prez-bee-KU-sis). This is a gradual type of hearing loss. It is common with aging. With this, you can have a hard time understanding speech. You may not tolerate loud sounds. You may not hear high pitched sounds. Hearing loss from presbycusis does not cause deafness.

- Ear wax that blocks the ear canal.

- A chronic middle ear infection or an infection of the inner ear.

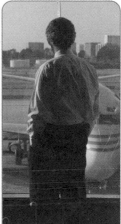

- Medicines (e.g., aspirin).

- Blood vessel disorders, such as high blood pressure.

- Acoustic trauma, such as from a blow to the ear or from excessive noise. **Noise-Induced Hearing Loss (NIHL)** can be from a one-time exposure to an extremely loud sound or to repeated exposure to loud level

Exposure to loud noises increases the risk for hearing loss.

sounds. (See **Decibels of Sound** on page 86.)

- **Ménière's disease.** This is a problem of the inner ear. The hearing loss comes and goes. Dizziness is also a symptom.

- Small tumors on the auditory nerve. Brain tumor (rarely).

Hearing Loss, Continued

Decibels (dB) of Sound

Sound levels are measured in **decibels (dB)**. In general, the louder the sound, the higher the dB.

Type of Sound	dB
Weakest sound heard	0
Whisper	30
Normal talking	60–70
Average radio	75
Busy street	80

Repeated Exposures ≥ 85 can lead to hearing loss

Hair dryer	90
Lawnmower	90
Subway train	95
Rock concert	110–120
Chain saw	120

Ear pain begins at 125 dB

Jet take-off	135

One time exposure >140 dB can cause permanent hearing loss

Siren (at 100 feet)	140
Firearms	140–170
Loudest tone the ear can hear	197

Treatment

- Earwax is removed by a health care provider.
- Hearing aid(s). These make sounds louder.
- Speech reading. This is learning to read lips and facial expressions.
- Auditory training. This helps with specific hearing problems.
- Surgery. This can be done if the problem requires it.

Questions to Ask

When your child is awake, does he or she not respond to any sound, even a whistle or a loud clap? **YES** → See Doctor

NO

With hearing loss, do any of these problems occur?
- A discharge from the ear.
- Ear pain doesn't go away.
- You feel dizzy or it feels like things are spinning around you.
- A recent ear or respiratory infection.
- It feels like your ears are blocked.

YES → See Doctor

NO

Is a nondigital watch not heard when held next to the ear? **YES** → See Doctor

NO

Do you hear a ringing sound in one or both ears all of the time? **YES** → See Doctor

NO

Did you lose your hearing after exposure to loud noises, (e.g., rock concerts, power tools, firearms, etc.) and has this not improved? **YES** → Call Doctor

NO

Use Self-Care

See Self-Care / Prevention on next page

Hearing Loss, Continued

Self-Care / Prevention

For Gradual, Age-Related Hearing Loss

- Ask people to speak clearly, distinctly, and in a normal tone.

- Look at people when they are talking to you. Watch their expressions.

- Try to limit background noise when speaking with someone.

- In a church or theater, sit in the 3rd or 4th row with people sitting around you.

- Install a flasher or amplifier on your phone, door chime, and alarm clock.

To Hear Sounds Better

- Use a hearing aid. There are many kinds. Examples are ones worn:

  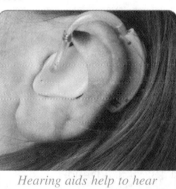

  Hearing aids help to hear sounds better.

  - In-the-Ear (ITE).

  - Behind-the-Ear (BTE).

  - In-the-Canal (ITC).

- To find the hearing aid that works best for you, see an audiologist. Ask him or her about a trial period with different hearing aids to find one you are comfortable with.

- Use devices and listening systems that help you hear better when you use your telephone, mobile phone, TV, stereo, etc.

To Clear Earwax

Use only if the eardrum is not ruptured. (See **Ruptured Eardrum Signs** on page 80.) Check with your doctor if you are not sure.

- Lie on your side. Using a syringe or medicine dropper, carefully squeeze a few drops of lukewarm water into your ear (or have someone else do this). Let the water remain there for 10 to 15 minutes and then shake it out. Now, squeeze a few drops of hydrogen peroxide, mineral oil, or an over-the-counter cleaner, such as Debrox, into the ear. Let the excess fluid flow out of the ear.

- After several minutes, put warm water in the ear again. Let it stay there for 10 to 15 minutes. Tilt the head to allow it to drain out of the ear.

Repeat this entire procedure again in 3 hours if the earwax has not cleared.

Get more information from:

HealthyLearn® • www.HealthyLearn.com
Click on MedlinePlus®

American Speech-Language Hearing Association
800.638.8255
www.asha.org

Better Hearing Institute
Hearing Help-on-Line
www.betterhearing.org

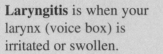

Laryngitis

Laryngitis is when your larynx (voice box) is irritated or swollen.

Signs & Symptoms

- Hoarse, husky, and weak voice or loss of voice.
- Cough.
- Sore throat, fever, and/or trouble swallowing.

Treatment

Self-care treats most cases of laryngitis. If needed, your doctor may prescribe an antibiotic for a bacterial infection.

Get more information from:

HealthyLearn®
www.HealthyLearn.com
Click on MedlinePlus®

American Academy of Otolaryngology - Head and Neck Surgery
www.entnet.org

Causes

Common causes are allergies and irritants like smoke; bacterial or viral infections; and strained vocal cords. Smoking, drinking alcohol, breathing cold air, and using already distressed vocal cords can make the problem worse. Growths on the vocal cords or nerve damage to the vocal cords can also cause hoarseness.

Questions to Ask

Do you have a high fever or are you coughing up yellow, green, or bloody-colored mucus?

NO ↓   YES → See Doctor

Do you have hard, swollen lymph glands in your neck or do you feel like you have a "lump" in your throat that doesn't go away?

NO ↓   YES → See Doctor

Has hoarseness lasted more than a week in a child, more than a month in an adult, or does it become chronic in a smoker?

NO ↓   YES → Call Doctor

Use Self-Care

Self-Care / Prevention

- Don't smoke. Avoid secondhand smoke.
- Don't talk if you don't need to. Write notes, instead.
- Use a cool-mist humidifier in your bedroom.
- Drink a lot of fluids. Drink warm drinks, such as weak tea, with honey and/or lemon juice.
- Gargle every few hours with warm salt water (¼ teaspoon of salt in 1 cup of warm water).
- Run hot water in the shower to make steam. Sit in the bathroom and breathe the moist air.
- Suck on cough drops, throat lozenges, or hard candy. (Don't give to children under age 5.) Take an over-the-counter medicine for pain as directed on the label.

Nosebleeds

Signs & Symptoms

- Bleeding from a nostril.
- Bleeding from the nose and down the back of the throat.

Causes

Nosebleeds are often caused by broken blood vessels just inside the nose. Risk factors include:

- A cold or allergies.
- Frequent nose blowing and picking.
- Dry environment.
- Using too much nasal spray.
- A punch or other blow to the nose.

A nosebleed is serious when heavy bleeding from deep within the nose is hard to stop. This type occurs most often in the elderly. It can be caused by: Hardening of nasal blood vessels; high blood pressure; and medicines that treat blood clots.

Treatment

Self-care treats most nosebleeds. If needed, a doctor can pack the nostril to stop the bleeding or do a treatment that seals the blood vessel that bleeds.

Questions to Ask

Is blood from a nosebleed going down the back of the throat or backward into the mouth? **YES** Get Medical Care Fast

NO

Flowchart continued in next column

Did the nosebleed follow a blow to the head or nose or a severe headache? Or, does the nosebleed occur in a person taking blood-thinning medicine? **YES** 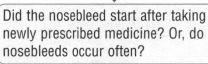 Get Medical Care Fast

NO

In the past 48 hours, did 3 or more nosebleeds occur and did each one take longer than 10 minutes to stop? **YES** See Doctor

NO

Did the nosebleed start after taking newly prescribed medicine? Or, do nosebleeds occur often? **YES** See Doctor

NO

 Use Self-Care

Self-Care / Prevention

- Sit with your head leaning forward. Pinch the nostrils shut. Use your thumb and forefinger to gently squeeze the nose's midsection.

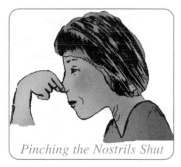

Pinching the Nostrils Shut

- Hold for up to 20 minutes without stopping. Use a clock to time this. Breathe through your mouth while you do this. Repeat a second time, if needed. If a second attempt fails, go to an urgent care center or hospital emergency department. Don't take aspirin or other nonsteroidal anti-inflammatory drugs.

- For the next 24 hours, elevate your head above the level of your heart. Also, try not to blow your nose, lift heavy objects, or exercise hard.

- Use a humidifier or cool-mist vaporizer to add moisture to household air.

Sinus Problems

Signs & Symptoms

Your sinuses are behind your cheekbones and forehead and around your eyes.

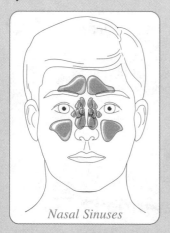

Nasal Sinuses

Healthy sinuses drain almost a quart of mucus every day. They keep the air you breathe wet. Your sinuses can't drain right if they are blocked, infected, or swollen. Sinus problems include:

- A sinus infection. This can be acute or chronic.

- Sinus congestion without an infection.

For a Sinus Infection

- Fever.

- Green, yellow, or bloody-colored nasal discharge.

- Foul-smelling or tasting postnasal drip.

- Severe headache that doesn't get better when you take an over-the-counter pain reliever. The headache is worse in the morning or when bending forward.

- Pain between the nose and lower eyelid. Cheek or upper jaw pain.

- A feeling of pressure inside the head. Stuffy nose.

- Swelling around the eyes, nose, cheeks, and forehead.

- Cough that worsens at night.

- Fatigue.

For sinus congestion without an infection, drainage is clear and there is no fever.

Causes

- Bacterial, viral, or fungal infection. Sneezing hard with your mouth closed or blowing your nose too much with a cold.

- Irritants like tobacco smoke, air pollutants, etc. Hay fever or other allergies.

- A nasal deformity. Sinuses that don't drain well.

Treatment

Sinus congestion without an infection does not need an antibiotic and can be treated with self-care. A decongestant helps break up the congestion.

An acute sinus infection usually clears up in 2 weeks with an antibiotic, a decongestant, and nose drops or a nasal spray. When this is not the case, the problem may be a chronic sinus infection which takes longer to treat and/or may need further investigation to diagnose the cause.

Sinus Problems, *Continued*

An antifungal medicine helps treat a fungal infection in the sinuses. Surgery may be needed to drain the sinuses. Surgery can be done to enlarge a sinus passage that is too narrow to allow proper drainage.

Questions to Ask

With a recent headache, fever, sinus pressure and pain, and yellow, green, or bloody nasal discharge, are all of the following symptoms now present, especially in a child?
- Sudden onset of a fever.
- Redness and swelling of the eyelid(s) or area around the eye(s).
- Protruding eye(s) and pain behind the eye(s).
- Problems moving the eye(s).
- Eye pain and redness.

YES → Get Medical Care Fast

NO ↓

Do you have 2 or more of the following symptoms?
- Fever.
- Green, yellow, or bloody-colored nasal discharge for more than 3 days. This may occur with a foul-smelling or bad-tasting drainage into the back of the throat.
- Headache that gets worse when you bend forward and that may not be relieved with over-the-counter pain relievers.
- Pain (usually throbbing) around the eye(s), cheek(s), upper jaw(s), and/or between the nose and eye socket(s).

YES → See Doctor

NO ↓

Flowchart continued in next column

Have you been treated for a sinus infection and do symptoms not improve after taking the prescribed medicine for 48 hours? Or, do symptoms return after you are done with prescribed treatment?

YES → See Doctor

NO ↓ Use Self-Care

Self-Care / Prevention

- Use a cool-mist humidifier especially in the bedroom. Put a humidifier on the furnace.

- Put a warm washcloth, warm or cold compress over the sinus area of your face. Use the one that helps most for the pain.

- Drink plenty of liquids.

- Take an over-the-counter (OTC) medicine for pain as directed on the label.

- Take an OTC decongestant or an OTC pain reliever with a decongestant (e.g., Tylenol Sinus). {*Note:* Some persons should not take decongestants. See the footnote and **Side Effects/Warnings/Interactions** for **Decongestant** use on page 28.}

- Use nose drops only for the number of days prescribed. Repeated use of them creates a dependency. Don't share nose drops with others. Throw the drops away after treatment.

Get more information from:

HealthyLearn® • www.HealthyLearn.com
Click on MedlinePlus®

National Jewish Health
800.423.8891
www.nationaljewish.org

Sore Throats

Signs & Symptoms

- Dry, irritated throat.

- Soreness or pain in the throat, especially when you talk or swallow. Swollen neck glands.

- The back of the throat and/or the tonsils look bright red or have pus deposits or white spots.

- Enlarged tonsils that feel tender (tonsillitis).

Fatigue, fever, postnasal drip, bad breath, headache, and/or earache can also occur.

Treatment

Self-care treats most sore throats. Your doctor may take a throat culture to see if strep or another type of bacteria is the cause. If so, an antibiotic may be prescribed. Strep throat needs medical care to prevent other health problems. Sore throats caused by viruses **do not** need an antibiotic.

Causes

- Smoking. Dry air. Postnasal drip. Cough. Allergies.

- Viruses, such as with a cold or the flu. (See **Colds & Flu** on page 100.)

- Infection from bacteria, such as strep throat.

Questions to Ask

Do you have severe shortness of breath? Or, can you not swallow your own saliva?

YES → Get Medical Care Fast

NO

With sore throat, do you have a fever higher than 102°F, swollen neck glands, ear pain, bad breath, a skin rash, and/or dark urine? Or, does the back of your throat or tonsils look bright red or have pus?

YES → See Doctor

NO

Have you been in contact with someone who had strep throat in the last 2 weeks, do you get strep throat often, or has a mild sore throat lasted longer than 3 weeks?

YES → Call Doctor

NO

 Use Self-Care

Self-Care / Prevention

- Don't smoke. Avoid secondhand smoke.

- Gargle every few hours with a solution of ¼ teaspoon of salt dissolved in 1 cup of warm water. Don't eat spicy foods.

- Drink plenty of fluids like warm tea. For strep throat, have cold foods and liquids.

- Sit in the bathroom while hot water runs in the shower. Use a cool-mist vaporizer in the room where you spend most of your time.

- Suck on a piece of hard candy or throat lozenge every so often. (Don't give to children under age 5.) Rest your voice, if this helps.

- Take an over-the-counter (OTC) medicine for pain as directed on the label. Take an OTC decongestant for postnasal drip, if okay with your doctor. (See information on **Decongestant** use on page 28.)

Tinnitus (Ringing in the Ears)

Tinnitus is hearing ringing or other noises in the ears when no outside source makes the sounds. Almost everyone gets "ringing in the ears" at one time or another. This may last a minute or so, but then goes away. When hearing these sounds persists, suspect tinnitus. The noises can range in volume from a ring to a roar.

Signs & Symptoms

- Ringing, buzzing, hissing, humming, roaring, or whistling noises in the ears. These problems can persist or come and go.
- Problems sleeping.
- Emotional distress.
- Hearing loss.

Tinnitus can be quite disturbing. It can interfere with normal activities.

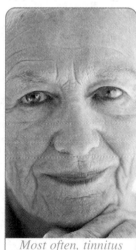

Most often, tinnitus affects older adults.

Causes

Exposure to loud noise which damages nerves in the inner ear is the most common cause. This can be from prolonged exposure or from one extreme incident.

Other Causes

- Ear disorders, such as **labyrinthitis**. This is swelling of canals in the ear that help maintain balance.
- Persistent allergies.
- High blood pressure.
- A reaction to some medications. These include: Aspirin; levodopa (for Parkinson's disease); quinidine (for irregular heartbeats); propranolol (for high blood pressure, etc.); and quinine (for leg cramps).
- **Ménières disease.** With this, dizziness, ringing sounds, and hearing loss occur together. Symptoms come and go.

In some cases, no cause is found.

Treatment

Treatment is aimed at finding and treating the cause of tinnitus. Treatment includes:
- A hearing aid that plays a soothing sound to drown out the tinnitus.
- A tinnitus masker. This is worn behind the ear. It makes a subtle noise to distract the person from tinnitus. The masker does not interfere with hearing and speech.
- Sleeping pills, if needed.
- Counseling or support groups for tinnitus.

Questions to Ask

Did the tinnitus start after taking too much aspirin or other medicines with salicylates, and do you have any of these problems?
- Nausea and/or vomiting.
- Confusion.
- Rapid breathing.

YES → Get Medical Care Fast

NO ↓

Flowchart continued on next page

Tinnitus, Continued

Benign Positional Vertigo (BPV)

Vertigo is a feeling that you or the room around you is spinning or moving. This is due to a problem in the inner ear, the brain's gravity-and-motion detector.

The most common cause of vertigo is **benign positional vertigo (BPV)**. With this, the feeling of spinning occurs quickly when you change the position of your head. (You turn over in bed, bend over, etc.).

With ringing in the ears, do you have any of these problems?
- Severe pain in the ear(s).
- A foreign object is in the ear that cannot be removed.
- A recent ear or head injury.
- You can't hear.

YES → **Get Medical Care Fast**

NO

With ringing in the ears, do you have any of these problems?
- Feeling dizzy or like you are spinning.
- Loss of balance or your walking is unsteady.
- Vomiting or nausea.
- Drainage from the ear(s).
- Sleep habits and/or daily activities are disrupted.

YES → **See Doctor**

NO

Use Self-Care

Self-Care / Prevention

- Wear earplugs or earmuffs when exposed to loud noises. This can prevent noise-induced tinnitus.

- Treat an ear infection right away.

- For mild cases of tinnitus, play the radio or a white noise tape. White noise is a low, constant sound.

- Use biofeedback or other relaxation techniques.

- Limit your intake of caffeine, alcohol, nicotine, and aspirin.

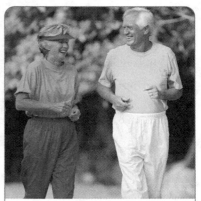

Get regular exercise. This promotes good blood circulation.

- Talk to your doctor if you use the drugs listed in **Causes** on page 93.

- If the noises started during or after traveling in an airplane, pinch your nostrils and blow through your nose. When you fly, chew gum or suck on hard candy to prevent ear popping and ringing sounds in the ear. If possible, avoid flying when you have an upper respiratory or ear infection.

Get more information from:

HealthyLearn®
www.HealthyLearn.com
Click on MedlinePlus®

The American Tinnitus Association
800.634.8978
www.ata.org

Chapter 11

Respiratory Conditions

Asthma

Asthma is a disease that affects the air passages in the lungs. Exposure to "triggers" (see **Asthma Attack Triggers** on this page) causes the airways to narrow. This response is called an "attack" or "episode."

Signs & Symptoms

- A cough lasts more than a week. Coughing may be the only symptom. It may occur during the night or after exercising.

- Prolonged shortness of breath. Breathing gets harder and may hurt. It is harder to breathe out than in.

- Wheezing.

- Chest tightness or pain.

Causes

Genetic factors play a big role. You are more likely to have asthma if you have a family history of it. Being exposed to certain things can set off an immune system response for asthma to develop. Examples are house-dust mites and viral respiratory infections.

Asthma Attack Triggers

- Colds, flu, bronchitis, and sinus infections.

- Breathing an allergen (pollen, dust mites, mold, animal dander) or irritant (tobacco smoke, air pollution, fumes, perfumes).

- Cockroach droppings.

- Sulfites. These are additives in wine, etc.

- Cold air. Temperature and humidity changes.

- Exercise, especially in outdoor cold air.

- Some medicines, such as aspirin.

- Strong feelings (laughing, crying, etc.).

Questions to Ask

Is it so hard for you to breathe that you can't say 4 or 5 words between breaths or you can't eat or sleep? Are you wheezing and do you take corticosteroid medicine or does wheezing not stop after your prescribed treatment?

YES Get Medical Care Fast

NO

Do you have a fever with heavy breathing or is your peak expiratory flow (PEF) reading on your peak flow meter below 50% of your personal best number?

YES Get Medical Care Fast

NO

Is your peak expiratory flow (PEF) 50 to 80% of your personal best number or do you use your bronchodilator more than 2 times a week?

YES See Doctor

NO

Do you have signs of an infection, such as a fever, and/or cough with mucus that is green, yellow, or bloody-colored? Or, are your asthma attacks coming more often or getting worse?

YES  See Doctor

NO

 Use Self-Care

See Self-Care / Prevention on next page

Asthma, Continued

Treatment

Asthma is too complex to treat with over-the-counter products. A doctor should diagnose and monitor asthma. A good way to help manage asthma is to follow a written action management plan that you develop with your doctor. This includes what to do to avoid and deal with asthma triggers, what to do when you have an asthma attack, and what medicines to take. Some kinds are to be taken with an asthma attack. Other kinds are taken daily (or as prescribed) to help prevent asthma attacks.

A yearly flu vaccine is advised. Regular doctor visits are needed to detect any problems and evaluate your use of medicines. It is also important to treat other problems that make it hard to manage asthma. Examples are reflux of stomach acids, being overweight, and sleep apnea.

Self-Care / Prevention

■ Follow your written action management plan. Take medications as prescribed.

■ Avoid your asthma triggers.

■ Don't smoke. Don't let others smoke in your home. Stay away from smoke and air pollution.

■ Drink lots of liquids (2 to 3 quarts a day).

■ Wear a scarf around your mouth and nose when you are outside in cold weather. Doing this warms the air as you breathe it in and prevents cold air from reaching sensitive airways.

■ Stop exercising if you start to wheeze.

■ Try to keep your bedroom allergen-free.

• Sleep with no pillow or the kind your doctor suggests. Use a plastic or "allergen-free" cover on your mattress and pillow (if you use one). Wash mattress pads in hot water every week.

• Use throw rugs, not carpeting. Use curtains or drapes that can be washed often.

• Get someone to dust and vacuum once a week. Use a vacuum with a HEPA filter or double-thickness bags. If you vacuum or dust, wear a dust filter mask.

• Don't use perfumes.

• Put an electronic air filter on your furnace or use portable air purifiers. Change and/or wash furnace and air conditioner filters regularly.

■ Don't eat foods with sulfites, such as wine and some shellfish.

■ Sit up during an asthma attack.

■ Use acetaminophen, not aspirin.

Keep your asthma rescue medicine handy.

Get more information from:

The Asthma and Allergy Foundation of America
800.7.ASTHMA (727.8462) • www.aafa.org

National Heart, Lung, and Blood Institute (NHLBI)
www.nhlbi.nih.gov

Avian Influenza – "Bird Flu"

Avian influenza is called "bird flu," because it naturally occurs in birds. Viruses that cause this do not usually infect humans and other animals, but a growing number of cases have occurred between 1997 and now. There is great concern about outbreaks of "bird flu," because they could lead to widespread infection in humans.

Signs & Symptoms

The viruses cause no or only mild symptoms in wild birds. Certain strains of "bird flu" can cause widespread disease and death in some kinds of wild birds, chickens, and turkeys.

Symptoms in Humans
- Fever.
- Cough.
- Sore throat.
- Muscle aches.
- Eye infections.
- Pneumonia. Severe problems breathing.
- Other serious problems that can threaten life.

Causes

Types of a certain virus cause "bird flu." Infected birds shed the virus in saliva, nasal secretions, and feces. Contact with infected birds or contaminated surfaces can spread the virus to humans. "Bird flu" viruses may be able to change and infect humans directly. This means that the virus could easily pass from one human to another. If this happens, an "influenza pandemic" could occur.

Treatment

When outbreaks occur, sick and exposed animals are killed. This keeps the virus from spreading. Persons who have or might have "bird flu" are isolated. Certain antiviral medicines are given. The Centers for Disease Control and Prevention (CDC) and the World Health Organization (WHO) track and address outbreaks.

Questions to Ask

Do you have symptoms of "bird flu" listed on this page and have you gone to a place with an outbreak of "bird flu" or been in close contact with someone who has?

YES → Call Doctor

NO ↓

Use Self-Care

Self-Care / Prevention

- Before you travel, check the Web sites listed below for current facts on "bird flu." If you will be going to a known site, avoid contact with items and surfaces that may have droppings from an infected bird.

- If you have symptoms of a respiratory infection, cover your nose and mouth with a tissue when you cough or sneeze. Wash your hands often.

Get up-to-date information on "Bird Flu" from:

Centers for Disease Control and Prevention (CDC)
800.CDC.INFO (232.4636)
www.cdc.gov/flu/avian

World Health Organization (WHO)
www.who.int/csr/disease/avian_influenza/en

To Learn More, See Back Cover

Bronchitis

Acute bronchitis is swelling of the air passages of the lung. **Chronic bronchitis** is swelling of the air passages of the lung that persists for a long time or occurs again and again.

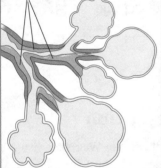

With bronchitis, air passages in the lungs are swollen.

Get more information from:

HealthyLearn®
www.HealthyLearn.com
Click on MedlinePlus®

American Lung Association
800.LUNG.USA
(586.4872)
www.lungusa.org

Signs & Symptoms

For Acute Bronchitis

- A cough starts out dry. Then mucus or phlegm come with the cough. Hoarseness or a sore throat can also occur.
- Chills. Fever less than 102° F.
- Feeling of pressure behind the breastbone or a burning feeling in the chest.

These symptoms can last from 3 days to 3 weeks. They go away when the acute episode is over.

For Chronic Bronchitis

- A cough with mucus or phlegm for 3 or more months at a time. This occurs for more than 2 years in a row.
- Shortness of breath with exertion (in early stages).
- Shortness of breath at rest (in later stages).

Many people, most of them smokers, develop emphysema (destruction of the air sacs) with chronic bronchitis. This is **chronic obstructive pulmonary disease (COPD)**.

Causes

For Acute Bronchitis

- A viral or bacterial infection.
- Pollutants, such as smog.

These attack the mucus membranes within the windpipe or air passages in your respiratory tract leaving them red and inflamed. Acute bronchitis often develops after a cold or other respiratory infection.

For Chronic Bronchitis

- Cigarette smoking. This is the most common cause.
- Air pollution.
- Repeated infections of the air passages in the lungs.

Chronic bronchitis causes permanent damage to the respiratory tract. It can make you more prone to respiratory infections like acute bronchitis and pneumonia. Chronic bronchitis is not contagious.

Bronchitis, Continued

Treatment

For Acute Bronchitis

Most of the time, this type is caused by a virus and goes away without treatment. Sometimes, a doctor may prescribe:

■ Bronchodilators. These medicines open up air passages in the lungs.

■ An antibiotic if you smoke, are older than age 40, or if you have a condition or take medication that makes it hard for you to fight infections.

For Chronic Bronchitis

■ Not smoking. Avoiding secondhand smoke.

■ Avoiding or reducing exposure to air pollution, chemical irritants, and cold, wet weather.

■ Medical treatment as needed, for airway infections and heart problems.

■ Oxygen, as prescribed.

Questions to Ask

With a cough, are you not able to say more than 4 to 5 words between breaths or do you have purple lips? **YES** Get Medical Care Fast

NO

Does a cough persist after an episode of choking on food or a foreign object? **YES** Get Medical Care Fast

NO

Does the cough occur in an infant or young child with rapid breathing and sound like a seal's bark? **YES** See Doctor

NO

Flowchart continued in next column

With a cough, do you have any of these symptoms?
- **Fever.** (See pages 226 and 227.)
- Green, yellow, or bloody-colored mucus.
- Severe or increasing chest pain.
- Shortness of breath at rest and at noncoughing times.
- Vomiting more than once.

YES See Doctor

NO

Have you had a cough longer than 3 weeks and has it not gotten better? **YES** Call Doctor

NO

Use Self-Care

Self-Care / Prevention

■ Don't smoke. Avoid secondhand smoke.

■ Reduce your exposure to air pollution. Use air conditioning, air filters, and a mouth and nose filter mask if you have to. Stay indoors during episodes of heavy air pollution.

■ Rest. Drink plenty of liquids.

■ Breathe air from a cool-mist vaporizer. Bacteria grows in vaporizers, so clean your unit after each use. Breathing in mist with bacteria can make bronchitis worse. Use distilled (not tap) water in the vaporizer.

■ Take an over-the-counter medicine for fever, pain, and/or inflammation as directed.

■ Instead of cough suppressants, use expectorants.

■ Use bronchodilators and/or take antibiotics as prescribed by your doctor. {*Note:* See information "Cough Suppressant" and "Decongestant" use on page 28.}

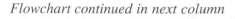

Colds & Flu

Cold & Flu Comparison Chart			
Symptoms*	Cold	Seasonal Flu	H1N1 Flu
Fever.	Rare.	Common. Can be high fever.	Usual. 20% of people may not have a fever.
Chills.	Not common.	Common.	Common.
Headache.	Not common, but can occur due to sinus pressure.	Common.	Very common.
Body Aches.	Slight.	Severe.	Severe.
Fatigue.	Mild.	Moderate to severe.	Moderate to severe.
Itchy/Watery Eyes.	Common.	Not common.	Not common.
Stuffy Nose.	Common.	Runny nose is common.	Not common.
Sneezing.	Common.	Common.	Not common.
Sore Throat.	Common.	Common.	Not common.
Cough.	Cough with mucus.	Often. Dry and hacking cough.**	Usual. Dry cough without mucus.**
Diarrhea / Vomiting.	None.	Not common. More likely to occur in children than adults.	Sometimes.
Chest Pain or Discomfort.	Mild to moderate.	Moderate.**	Often severe.**
Onset of Symptoms.	Develop over a few days. Symptoms mostly affect you above the neck.	Sudden. Symptoms affect the body all over.	Sudden. Symptoms affect the body all over.

* Symptoms can vary from person to person.
** A dry cough that turns into one with mucus and/or chest discomfort that becomes severe could be a sign of a secondary infection.

Cold and flu viruses can be spread through hand shakes and touching objects that has an infected person's mucus on them.

Causes	
Cold	More than 200 different cold viruses.
Seasonal Flu	Different strains of type A and type B viruses for that year's fall and winter months.
H1N1 Flu	H1N1 virus. It was first detected in people in Mexico and in the U.S. in April of 2009. At first, this was called swine flu. In June, 2009, it was declared a **pandemic flu** - one that causes a global outbreak of serious illness that spreads easily from person-to-person.

Colds & Flu, *Continued*

Ways Viruses are Spread

- Breathing air droplets that contain a virus from an infected person's coughs and sneezes.

- Touching an object or surface that has a flu virus on it and then touching your eyes, nose, or mouth. Flu viruses can infect a person for 2 to 8 hours after being left on surfaces like door handles, remote controls, and phones.

You *cannot* get a cold if you sit or sleep in a draft, go outside when your hair is wet, or do not wear a jacket in cold temperatures. You *cannot* get H1N1 flu from eating pork or pork products.

People infected with seasonal flu or H1N1 flu may be able to infect others for up to 7 days after the start of symptoms or until they have been symptom-free for more than 7 days. Children and people with weakened immune systems could be contagious for more than 7 days.

Each year, 36,000 people die from pneumonia and other serious problems from seasonal flu. Get updates on H1N1 flu-related problems and deaths from www.flu.gov.

The risk for serious problems from seasonal and/or H1N1 flu increase with these conditions:

- Asthma, bronchitis, emphysema, or other chronic lung disease.

- Diabetes. Heart disease. Kidney disease.

- Pregnancy.

- A weakened immune system from an illness or medication that lowers the immune response.

- Very severe health conditions, such as cerebral palsy, epilepsy, muscular dystrophy, and sickle cell disease.

Questions to Ask

With a cold, does a child have one or more of these problems?
- Blue color around the lips, fingernails, or skin.
- Quick breathing or a very hard time breathing.
- Grunting sounds with breathing.
- Severe cough or wheezing.
- Fever of 100.4°F or higher in a baby less than 3 months old; 104°F or higher in a child between 3 months and 3 years old.

YES → Get Medical Care Fast

NO ↓

Does an adult have any of these problems?
- Blue color around the lips, fingernails, or skin.
- Severe or increasing shortness of breath.
- Severe wheezing.
- Coughing up true red blood.

YES → Get Medical Care Fast

NO ↓

With or after the flu, do any of these **symptoms of meningitis** occur?
- Stiff neck (can't bend the head forward to touch the chin to the chest).
- Severe headache that persists.
- Red or purple rash that doesn't fade when the skin is pressed.
- Seizure.
- Lethargy.
- In an infant, bulging of the fontanelle (soft spot of the skull).

YES → Get Medical Care Fast

NO ↓

Flowchart continued on next page

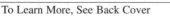

Treatment

Self-care treats colds and most cases of the flu.

Prescribed antiviral medicines can make flu symptoms milder and help you get better sooner if started within 48 hours (36 hours for children) of the start of flu symptoms.

People with a chronic illness should consult their doctors for advice to manage symptoms.

Antibiotics **do not** treat cold and flu viruses.

Antibiotics treat infections from bacteria. Taking them for viruses is a main cause of **antibiotic resistance**. With this, bacteria that were once fought off by antibiotics have become stronger than the medicine. Certain bacteria have become so resistant that it is hard to find an antibiotic that is able to fight off the infection. An example is MRSA – Methicillin-resistant *Staphylococcus aureus*. This can cause an infection that affects the skin or causes pneumonia. MRSA resists treatment from usual antibiotics.

Colds & Flu, Continued

Do flu symptoms improve, but return with a fever and a worse cough? YES **Get Medical Care Fast**

NO

With or after the flu, do these **signs of dehydration** occur?
- Feeling confused.
- Very little or no urine.
- Sunken eyes.
- Dry skin doesn't spring back after being pressed.

 YES **Get Medical Care Fast**

NO

With a cold or the flu, do any of these problems occur?
- Wheezing or trouble breathing.
- Ear pain or swollen, painful neck glands.
- Headache that doesn't go away.
- Sore throat that is very red or has white spots.
- A cough with mucus that is yellow, green, or gray.
- A bad smell from the throat, nose, or ears.
- Fever of 99.5°F and up to 100.4°F in a baby less than 3 months old.
- Fever of 102.2°F and up to 104°F in a child 3 months to 3 years old.
- Fever over 104°F in a person 3 to 64 years old.
- Fever of 102°F or higher in a person age 65 and older.
- Fever and/or other symptoms, like coughing keep getting worse.

YES **See Doctor**

NO

Do you have pain or swelling over your sinuses that gets worse when you bend over or move your head, especially with a fever of 101°F or higher?  YES **See Doctor**

NO

Have you had the flu or a cold for more than a week and not felt better with self-care? Or, do you have new symptoms? YES **See Doctor**

NO

Use Self-Care

See Self-Care / Prevention on next page

Colds & Flu, Continued

Self-Care / Prevention

- Get vaccines† for seasonal flu and H1N1 flu, as advised by your doctor. *Note:* Persons with a severe allergy to eggs should not get flu shots.

  {†Learn up-to-date advice for vaccines from the Centers for Disease Control and Prevention (CDC) at 800.CDC.INFO (232.4636) or www.cdc.gov/vaccines.}

- If you get flu symptoms, call your doctor. Ask if flu testing, an antiviral medicine, or medical care is needed. *Note:* Some antiviral medicines cause mental status changes in older persons and may be worse than flu symptoms.

- Cover your nose and mouth with a tissue when you cough and sneeze. Throw the tissue away after you use it. If you do not have a tissue, cough or sneeze into your elbow or upper sleeve.

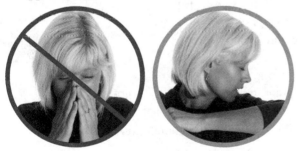

- Wash your hands often with soap and water. Take at least 20 seconds each time. When you can't wash your hands, use alcohol-based wipes or gels to clean your hands. Rub the gel type into your hands until they are dry.

- Avoid touching your eyes, nose, and mouth.

- Try to avoid close contact with people and their things when they have a cold or flu symptoms. If you are sick, avoid contact with others so you do not spread the flu.

- Stay home from work, school, and errands when you are sick. Do not send your children to childcare or school if they are sick.

- Clean and disinfect commonly used objects, such as door handles, phones, railings, light switches, and remote controls.

- Rest and drink plenty of fluids. Eat chicken soup.

- Use over-the-counter (OTC) saline nasal drops or spray, such as Ocean brand. Use as directed.

- Gargle with warm salt water. Mix ¼ teaspoon of salt in 1 cup of warm water.

- Use a cool-mist vaporizer to add moisture to the air.

- If needed, take OTC medicines to reduce fever and pain and to relieve cough and congestion. Take these as directed. *Note:* Do not give aspirin to anyone under 19 years old. Aspirin and other medicines with salicylates have been linked to Reye's syndrome. Do not give OTC medicines for colds, coughs, and flu to children under 6 years old, unless advised by their doctors.

- Eat nutritious foods. Do regular exercise. Manage stress. Get enough sleep.

- For a sore throat, see **Self-Care / Prevention** on page 92.

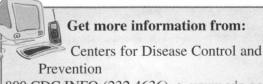

Get more information from:

Centers for Disease Control and Prevention
800.CDC.INFO (232.4636) • www.cdc.gov
www.cdc.gov/flu • www.flu.gov

A **cough** is a reflex action. It clears the lungs and airways of irritants, mucus, a foreign body, etc.

Signs & Symptoms

There are 3 kinds of Coughs

- *Productive.* This cough brings up mucus or phlegm.

- *Nonproductive.* This cough is dry. It doesn't bring up any mucus.

- *Reflex.* This cough is from a problem somewhere else like the ear or stomach.

Treatment

How to treat a cough depends on what kind it is, what caused it, and other symptoms. Treat the cause and soothe the irritation. Self-care can treat most coughs. If the cause is due to a medical condition, treatment for that condition is needed.

Coughs

Causes

- Tobacco smoke. Dry air.

- **Asthma.** (See page 95.)

- An allergy or an infection.

- Acid reflux from the stomach. (See **Heartburn & Indigestion** on page 161.)

- Certain medications, like ACE inhibitors for high blood pressure.

- Something stuck in the windpipe.

- A collapsed lung.

- A growth or tumor in the bronchial tubes or lungs.

Questions to Ask

With a cough, do any of these problems occur?
- A very hard time breathing.
- Chest pain that spreads to the neck, arm, tooth, or jaw.
- Sudden, severe pain in the chest wall followed by a cough and breathlessness without pain.
- Fainting.
- Coughing up true red blood.
- Fever of 100.4°F or higher in a baby less than 3 months old; 104°F or higher in a child between 3 months and 3 years old.
- The cough persists after an episode of choking on food or a foreign object.

YES Get Medical Care Fast

NO

In a child, does the cough occur with one or more of these problems?
- Rapid breathing.
- Fever of 99.5°F and up to 100.4°F in an infant less than 3 months old; between 102.2°F and up to 104°F in a child 3 months to 3 years old; 104°F or higher in a child 3 years old and older.
- The cough sounds like a seal's bark.

YES See Doctor

NO

Flowchart continued on next page

Coughs, Continued

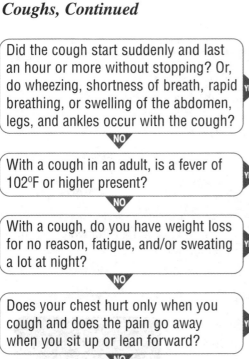

Did the cough start suddenly and last an hour or more without stopping? Or, do wheezing, shortness of breath, rapid breathing, or swelling of the abdomen, legs, and ankles occur with the cough? **YES → See Doctor**

NO

With a cough in an adult, is a fever of 102°F or higher present? **YES → See Doctor**

NO

With a cough, do you have weight loss for no reason, fatigue, and/or sweating a lot at night? **YES → See Doctor**

NO

Does your chest hurt only when you cough and does the pain go away when you sit up or lean forward? **YES → See Doctor**

NO

Do you cough up green, yellow, or bloody-colored mucus, with or without an odor? **YES → See Doctor**

NO

Has the cough lasted more than 2 weeks without getting better? **YES → Call Doctor**

NO

Use Self-Care

Self-Care / Prevention

For Coughs that Bring Up Mucus
- Drink plenty of liquids.
- Don't smoke. Avoid secondhand smoke.
- Use a cool-mist vaporizer, especially in the bedroom. Put a humidifier on the furnace.
- Take a shower. The steam helps thin mucus.

- Use an over-the-counter expectorant medicine, as directed. This helps you spit out phlegm or mucus. Try a decongestant for postnasal drip. {*Note:* See information on "Decongestant" use and "Expectorant" use on page 28.}

For Coughs that Are Dry
- Drink lots of liquids. Hot drinks like tea with lemon and honey soothe the throat.
- Suck on cough drops or hard candy. (Don't give these to children under age 5.)
- Take an over-the-counter cough medicine that has dextromethorphan.{*Note:* See information on "Cough Suppressant" use on page 28.}
- Make your own cough medicine. Mix 1 part lemon juice and 2 parts honey. (Don't give this to children less than 1 year old.)

Other Tips
- Don't smoke. Avoid secondhand smoke. Avoid chemical gases that can hurt your lungs.
- Don't give children under age 5 small objects that can easily get caught in the throat or windpipe. Examples are buttons, balloons, peanuts, and popcorn. Even adults should be careful to chew and swallow foods slowly so they don't "go down the wrong way."
- If you cough and have heartburn symptoms when you lie down, try a liquid antacid. Don't lie down for 2 to 3 hours after you eat.

Get more information from:

HealthyLearn® • www.HealthyLearn.com
Click on MedlinePlus®

American Lung Association
800.LUNG.USA (586.4872) • www.lungusa.org

Emphysema is a chronic lung condition. With emphysema, the air sacs in the lungs are destroyed. The lungs lose their ability to stretch. This makes it harder to get air in and out of the lungs.

When emphysema occurs with **chronic bronchitis** (see page 98), it is called **chronic obstructive pulmonary disease (COPD)**.

Symptoms of COPD are:
- Coughing that produces large amounts of mucus.
- Shortness of breath.
- Wheezing.
- Chest tightness.

Symptoms worsen over time. COPD has no cure yet. The goals of treatment are to help you feel better, stay more active, and slow the progress of the disease. Treatment includes:

- Stopping smoking.
- Avoiding lung irritants.
- Taking medications that make breathing easier.
- Preventing and treating respiratory infections.

Emphysema

Signs & Symptoms

Emphysema takes years to develop. When symptoms occur, they include:

- Cough with mucus.
- Shortness of breath on exertion. This gets worse over time.
- Wheezing.
- Chest tightness.
- Slight body build with marked weight loss and a rounded chest that doesn't appear to expand when breathing in.

Causes

- Smoking. This causes as much as 90% of cases. Most people with emphysema are cigarette smokers aged 50 or older.
- A genetic problem with a certain protein that protects the lungs from damage.
- Repeated lung infections.
- **Chronic bronchitis.** (See page 98.)
- Heavy exposure to air pollution.
- Years of exposure to chemical fumes, vapors, and dusts. This is usually linked to certain jobs.

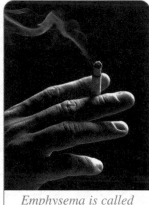

Emphysema is called "the smoker's disease."

Emphysema, Continued

Treatment

- A program, medication, and/or nicotine replacement to stop smoking.

- Physical therapy to loosen mucus in the lungs for chronic bronchitis.

- Medicines, such as bronchodilators, corticosteroids, and antibiotics.

- Flu and pneumonia vaccines.

- Surgery that removes the most severely diseased parts of the lung. A lung transplant may be needed for some persons with very severe disease.

Emphysema can't be reversed. By the time it is found, 50% to 70% of lung tissue may already be destroyed. Prevention is the only way to avoid permanent damage.

Questions to Ask

With emphysema, do you have any of these problems?
- Blue or purple-colored lips or fingertips.
- Severe shortness of breath or you can't say 4 or 5 words between breaths.
- Coughing up true red blood.

YES → Get Medical Care Fast

NO

With emphysema, do your legs and ankles swell more than usual, do you have a fever, or does your cough get worse?

YES → See Doctor

NO

Flowchart continued in next column

Do you have **signs and symptoms of emphysema** listed on page 106?

YES → See Doctor

NO → Use Self-Care

Self-Care / Prevention

- Don't smoke. If you smoke, quit. Avoid secondhand smoke.

- Limit exposure to air pollution and lung irritants. Follow safety measures when working with materials that can irritate your lungs.

- Use a cool-mist vaporizer indoors.

- Drink plenty of fluids.

- Avoid dust, fumes, pollutants, etc.

- Do breathing exercises as advised by your doctor.

- Exercise daily as prescribed by your doctor or exercise therapist.

Get more information from:

American Lung Association
800.LUNG.USA (586.4872)
www.lungusa.org

National Cancer Institute's Smoking Quitline
877.44U.QUIT (448.7848)

National Heart, Lung, and Blood Institute
www.nhlbi.nih.gov

Smokefree.Gov
800.QUIT.NOW (748.8669)
www.smokefree.gov

Hiccups

Hiccups are simple to explain. The diaphragm (the major muscle which sits like a cap over the stomach) goes into spasms. The vocal cords close rapidly. This causes the "hiccup" sound.

Causes

- Eating too fast. Swallowing air with the food.
- Drinking carbonated beverages. Drinking too much alcohol.
- Doing things to make the stomach full enough to irritate the diaphragm, such as eating a lot of fatty foods in a short period of time.

Treatment

Hiccups seldom cause harm. Usually, they don't last very long. Self-Care treats most cases of hiccups. Hiccups that persist could be a sign of a nervous system problem. A doctor needs to diagnose and treat this.

Questions to Ask

Do the hiccups occur with severe abdominal pain and spitting up blood or blood in the stools?

YES → **Get Medical Care Fast**

NO

Have hiccups lasted longer than 8 hours in an adult or 3 hours in a child? Or, have they started only after taking prescribed medicine?

YES → **Call Doctor**

NO

 Use Self-Care

Self-Care / Prevention

Common Remedies for Hiccups

- Swallow 1 teaspoon of dry table sugar. If this doesn't stop the hiccups right away, repeat it 3 times, at 2-minute intervals. {*Note:* For young children (that do not have diabetes), use a teaspoon of corn syrup.}

- Hold your tongue with your thumb and index finger and gently pull it forward.

- Drink a glass of water rapidly. {*Note:* Young children should drink a glass of milk slowly.}

Pneumonia

Pneumonia is lung inflammation. It is one of the leading causes of death in the U.S., especially in the elderly.

Signs & Symptoms

- Chest pain when breathing in.
- Fever and chills.
- Cough, often with bloody, dark yellow, green, or rust-colored sputum.
- Shortness of breath. Rapid breathing.
- Appetite loss.
- Fatigue. Headache. Nausea. Vomiting.
- Bluish lips and fingertips, if severe.

Causes

Viral or bacterial infections are the most common causes. Other causes are fungal infections and chemical irritants like inhaled poisonous gases.

Risk Factors

- Having had pneumonia before.
- Being in the hospital for other problems.
- A suppressed cough reflex after a stroke.
- Smoking.
- Very poor diet, alcoholism, or drug use.
- A recent respiratory infection.
- Emphysema. Chronic bronchitis.
- Radiation treatments, chemotherapy, and any medication or illness that wears down the immune system.

Treatment

Treatment depends on its type (viral, bacterial, or chemical) and location. Treatment includes:

- Medications.
- Oxygen therapy. Hospitalization. Removing fluid from the lungs, if needed.

Questions to Ask

Do you have severe shortness of breath and/or blue or purple-colored lips and fingertips?

YES → Get Medical Care Fast

NO

Do you have **signs and symptoms of pneumonia** listed in the left column?

YES → See Doctor

NO

 Use Self-Care

Self-Care / Prevention

- Get vaccines for influenza and pneumonia. (See **Immunization Schedule** on page 23.)
- Don't smoke. If you smoke, quit. Avoid secondhand smoke.
- Get plenty of rest.
- Use a cool-mist vaporizer in the room(s) in which you spend most of your time.
- Drink plenty of fluids.
- Take medicines as prescribed by your doctor. Take the medicine for pain and/or fever that your doctor advises. Over-the-counter pain relievers should be avoided for some types of bacterial pneumonia.

SARS – Severe Acute Respiratory Syndrome

SARS is a viral respiratory illness. It began in Asia in February 2003 and spread to other countries.

Signs & Symptoms

- Fever higher than 100.4°F.

- Headache. The body aches all over. Diarrhea may occur.

- Dry cough after 2 to 7 days.

- A hard time breathing and/or shortness of breath. Most persons develop pneumonia.

Treatment

Medical treatment is needed for SARS. Persons suspected of having SARS should be quarantined in a hospital.

Cause

SARS is thought to be caused by a certain virus. It is spread by close contact with someone who has the virus. Most likely, this is through coughs and sneezes or from touching objects that have infectious droplets on them.

Questions to Ask

Do you have a fever, higher than 100.4°F, a dry cough, a hard time breathing, and/or shortness of breath <u>and</u> have you been in close contact with someone who has SARS, might have SARS, or who travelled to a SARS site within the last 10 days?

Self-Care / Prevention

- Before you travel, check the CDCs Travelers' Health Web site at www.cdc.gov/travel for updates on SARS.

- If you will be in close contact with a person infected with SARS, follow infection control measures. Wash your hands often or use alcohol-based hand rubs. If you can, wear a surgical mask. Don't share eating utensils, towels, etc. For a more complete list of guidelines, access www.cdc.gov/ncidod/sars/ic-closecontacts.htm.

Get more information from:

Centers for Disease Control and Prevention (CDC)
800.CDC.INFO (232.4636) • www.cdc.gov/ncidod/sars

World Health Organization (WHO)
www.who.int/topics/sars/en/

Wheezing

Wheezing means you are having a problem with breathing. Air is flowing through swollen or tight breathing tubes.

Signs & Symptoms

- A high-pitched squeaky or whistling sound. This is heard more on breathing out than in.
- Chest tightness.

Causes

- Asthma is the number one cause.
- Allergic reactions.
- Respiratory infections.
- Something caught in the windpipe.
- Smoking, air pollution, etc.

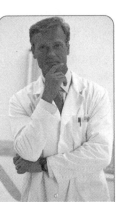

Follow your doctor's advice to treat conditions that cause wheezing.

Treatment

Treatment depends on the cause. Medication to relieve narrowing of the airways is usually given for acute attacks of wheezing.

Questions to Ask

> With wheezing, do you have severe shortness of breath; blue-colored lips, skin, or fingernails; or are you unable to talk?

YES → Get Medical Care Fast

NO

Flowchart continued in next column

> With wheezing, do any of these problems occur?
> - Decreasing level of consciousness or mental status changes.
> - Fever higher than 101°F in a baby less than 3 months old; 104°F or higher in a child between 3 months and 3 years old.
> - The wheezing started in the last few hours and bubbly pink or white phlegm is being coughed up.

YES → Get Medical Care Fast

NO

> Did wheezing begin after an insect sting, taking medication, or exposure to something that caused a severe allergic reaction in the past?

YES → Get Medical Care Fast

NO

> Does wheezing occur in a child between 3 months and 3 years of age who has a fever of 102.2°F and up to 104°F?

YES → See Doctor

NO

Use Self-Care

Self-Care / Prevention

- Take prescribed medicines as directed.
- Drink plenty of fluids.
- Use a cool-mist vaporizer.
- Don't smoke. Avoid secondhand smoke.
- Chew foods well before swallowing. When you eat, try not to laugh and swallow at the same time.
- Keep small objects that can easily be inhaled away from children under age 5.

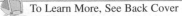

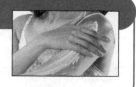

Chapter 12

Skin Conditions

ABC's of Skin Care

About Your Skin

The skin is the body's largest organ.

- It protects tissues inside the body from injury.

- It serves as a barrier against chemicals, germs, hot and cold weather, pollution, the sun, etc.

- It helps regulate body temperature. It seals in moisture.

Basic Skin Care

- Protect your skin from the sun's harmful ultraviolet (UV) rays.
  - Limit exposure to the sun, especially between 10:00 a.m. and 4:00 p.m. standard time; 11:00 a.m. to 5:00 p.m. daylight savings time.

  - When outdoors, wear a water-resistant sunscreen that has a sun protection factor (SPF) number of at least 15. Use one that protects you from both UVA and UVB rays. Apply sunscreen about 30 minutes before going outside. Use sunscreen as directed on the label.

  - Wear protective clothing, such as long sleeves and a wide brimmed hat.

- Don't use tanning beds and heat lamps.

- Don't smoke. If you smoke, quit. Smoking can cause premature wrinkles.

- Eat healthy foods. Drink plenty of water and other fluids.

- Clean your skin daily. Clean it when it gets dirty, too.

- Wash your hands often to avoid picking up germs.

- Wash your skin with warm (not hot) water. Hot water dries the skin.

- Use mild or gentle soaps and cleaning products to prevent dry, irritated skin.

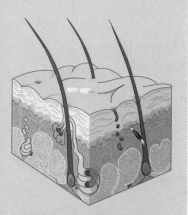

The skin has two basic layers. The outer, protective layer is the epidermis. The thicker, inner layer is the dermis.

Get more information from:

American Academy of Dermatology
888.462.3376
www.aad.org

Skinsight℠
www.skinsight.com

ABC's of Skin Care, Continued

- Moisturize your skin daily and/or when it is dry. Dry, cracked skin lets harmful germs and other irritants in. Use moisturizers that don't have alcohol.

- Protect your skin from the wind and cold weather. Wear gloves, a hat, a scarf, etc.

- Protect your skin from injury. Wear gloves when you garden, work with chemicals, etc. When shaving, soften the beard with a warm washcloth. Use plenty of shaving cream. With a sharp blade, shave in the direction of hair growth. Using a back and forth motion causes skin irritation.

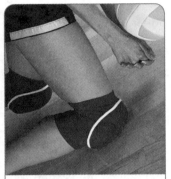

Wear knee pads, etc. during sports to help protect your skin from injury.

- Avoid items that cause allergic reactions and/or irritate the skin.

Cosmetic Safety

With so many products to choose from, how do you know which ones are safe to use? How do you know if they give the results they promote?

- If you have skin concerns or problems, consult your primary care doctor or a dermatologist.

- Before using a cosmetic, read the label. The label must give directions for safe use and/or warning statements. Heed the warnings. For example, products with an alpha hydroxy acid (AHA) may list the following on the label: "Sunburn alert: This product contains an alpha hydroxy acid (AHA) that may increase your skin's sensitivity to the sun and the possibility of sunburn. Use a sunscreen and limit sun exposure while using this product and for a week afterwards."

- Follow directions on the label.

- Test a small amount of a new product on your skin to find out how your skin reacts to it.

- When sampling a cosmetic at a store's cosmetic counter, test it with a new, unused cotton swab.

- Keep make-up containers tightly closed when not in use.

- Throw away any cosmetic that has developed an odor or changed color.

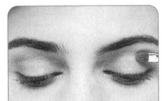

Don't share make-up with others.

- If you have an eye infection, such as pink eye, don't use eye cosmetics. Throw away the ones you were using when you first noticed the infection.

- Use products for your skin type (dry, normal, oily, or sensitive, etc.). If you have dry skin, don't use astringents and products with alcohol. They take moisture away from the skin.

Acne

Acne is a common skin condition. It occurs most often in teenagers and young adults, but can persist into adulthood.

Signs & Symptoms

- Whiteheads and/or blackheads.
- Red and painful pimples.
- Deeper lumps (cysts or nodules).

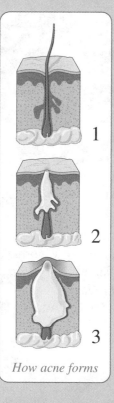

1

2

3

How acne forms

Causes

Acne results when oil ducts below the skin get clogged. Factors that help cause acne include:

- Hormone changes during adolescence, before a female's menstrual period, or during pregnancy.
- Rich moisturizing lotions. Oily makeup.
- Emotional stress.
- Nutritional supplements that have iodine.
- Medications, such as lithium and corticosteroids.
- Illegal (anabolic) steroids. These are used for muscle-building.

Foods and beverages, such as chocolate, nuts, greasy foods, and cola do not cause acne. If you find that eating certain foods make your acne worse, avoid them.

Treatment

Mild acne can be treated with **Self-Care / Prevention** (see page 115). When this is not enough, a doctor may prescribe one or more of these medications:

- A topical cream, gel, or liquid with retinoic acid (Retin-A). {*Note:* Retin-A makes your skin more sensitive to the sun.}
- A topical cream, lotion, or wipe with an antibiotic, such as clindamycin.
- A topical gel with dapsone. A brand name is Aczone™ Gel 5%.
- An antibiotic pill, such as minocycline or tetracycline. {*Note:* These medicines can make birth control pills less effective and make your skin more sensitive to the sun.}
- For some females, a certain birth control pill.
- Isotretinoin. Brand names are Accutane, Amnesteem, Sotret, Claravis. This medicine is usually prescribed for severe acne. {*Note:* This medicine can have serious side effects. These include bone and fracture problems, severe birth defects, depression, psychosis, aggressive and/or violent behaviors, and suicide.}

Acne, Continued

Treatments Other Than Medications
- Chemical peels.
- Laser treatments.
- Surgery for acne scarring.

Questions to Ask

Are you taking isotretinoin and are you planning suicide or making suicidal gestures? Or, do you have repeated thoughts of suicide or death? **YES** Get Medical Care Fast

NO

Is your acne very bad and do you have signs of an infection, such as a fever and swelling at the acne site? **YES** See Doctor

NO

Do you have any of these problems?
- The acne results in scarring.
- The pimples are big and painful or widespread.
- The acne causes a lot of emotional embarrassment.
YES  See Doctor

NO

Have you tried self-care and it doesn't help or does it make your skin worse? **YES** Call Doctor

NO

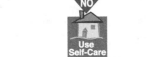
Use Self-Care

Self-Care / Prevention

- Keep your skin clean. Gently wash your skin, where the acne appears, twice a day. Use a mild soap, such as Neutrogena. Use a clean washcloth every time. Work the soap into your skin gently for 1 to 2 minutes and rinse well. Don't scrub.

- Don't squeeze, scratch, or poke at pimples. They can get infected and leave scars.

- Wash after you exercise or sweat.

- Use an over-the-counter lotion or cream that has benzoyl peroxide. (Some people are allergic to benzoyl peroxide. Try a little on your arm first to make sure it doesn't hurt your skin.) Follow the directions as listed.

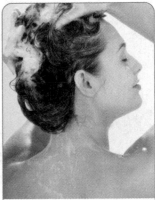

Wash your hair at least every other day.

- Use only oil-free and water-based makeups. Don't use greasy or oil-based creams, lotions, or makeups.

- For males, wrap a warm towel around your face before you shave. Shave along the natural grain of the beard.

- Don't spend too much time in the sun especially if you take antibiotics for acne. Don't use sun lamps.

Get more information from:

American Academy of Dermatology
888.462.DERM (462.3376)
www.aad.org

National Institute of Arthritis and Musculoskeletal and Skin Diseases (NIAMS)
www.niams.nih.gov

Athlete's Foot

Athlete's foot is a fungal infection. It usually affects the skin between the toes.

Signs & Symptoms

- Moist, soft, red or gray-white scales on the feet, especially between the toes.

- Cracked, peeling, dead skin areas.

- Itching.

- Sometimes small blisters on the feet.

Treatment

Self-care treats most cases of athlete's foot.

Get more information from:

HealthyLearn®
www.HealthyLearn.com
Click on MedlinePlus®

American Academy of Dermatology
888.462.DERM
(462.3376)
www.aad.org

Causes

People usually pick up the fungus from walking barefoot over wet floors, around swimming pools and locker rooms, and in public showers.

Questions to Ask

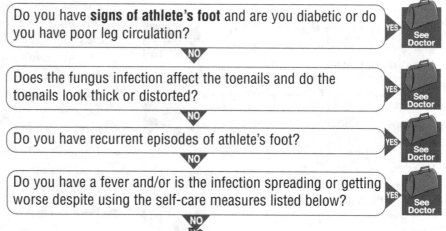

Do you have **signs of athlete's foot** and are you diabetic or do you have poor leg circulation? YES → See Doctor

NO

Does the fungus infection affect the toenails and do the toenails look thick or distorted? YES → See Doctor

NO

Do you have recurrent episodes of athlete's foot? YES → See Doctor

NO

Do you have a fever and/or is the infection spreading or getting worse despite using the self-care measures listed below? YES → See Doctor

NO → Use Self-Care

Self-Care / Prevention

- Wash your feet twice a day, especially between your toes. Dry the area thoroughly. Don't use deodorant soaps.

- Use an over-the-counter antifungal powder, cream, or spray between your toes and inside your socks and shoes.

- Wear clean socks made of natural fibers (cotton or wool). Change your socks during the day to help your feet stay dry. Wear shoes, such as sandals or canvas loafers, that allow ventilation.

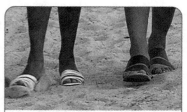

Wear shoes, such as sandals or canvas loafers, that allow ventilation.

- Alternate shoes daily to let each pair dry out.

Blisters

Signs & Symptoms

- Sore bump on the skin that may be filled with fluid. Swelling.

- Pain and tenderness to the touch.

Causes

- Friction on the skin. This is the main cause.

- Skin rashes, frostbite, and second-degree burns.

- Herpes simplex viruses. (See **Cold Sores** on page 346 and **Genital Herpes** on page 249.)

- Allergic reaction to medicine.

- **Epidermolysis bullosa (EB)**. This is a group of blistering skin conditions. With these, the skin is so fragile, even minor rubbing can cause blisters. Blisters can occur inside the body, too.

Treatment

Self-care treats most blisters. Medical care may be needed for blisters that get infected and for ones caused by a skin disorder.

Questions to Ask

Does minor rubbing of the skin result in blisters or do they occur often for no apparent reason? **YES** → See Doctor

NO ↓

Flowchart continued in next column

With a blister, are any of these signs of an infection present?
- Increased redness, warmth or pain.
- White, green, or yellow pus.
- Red streak that extends from the blister.

YES → See Doctor

NO ↓

With blisters, do you have diabetes or peripheral vascular disease? **YES** → Call Doctor

NO ↓

 Use Self-Care

Self-Care / Prevention

To Prevent Blisters
- Wear shoes and socks that fit well. Wear moleskin pads on areas where socks or shoes rub the skin.

- Apply an antiperspirant to the bottom of your feet before an athletic activity.

- Wear gloves for activities that put friction on the hands, such as raking leaves.

To Treat Blisters
- Protect a blister from more friction. Cover it with a loose bandage or a moleskin pad. The skin over the blister protects it from infection.

- If the blister is very painful, drain it. Clean the area with alcohol. Sterilize a needle. Gently, pierce an edge of the blister. Let it drain. If no dirt or pus is under the skin flap, pat it down to protect the skin below it. Wash the area well with soap and water. Apply an antibiotic ointment and cover it with a bandage or gauze and tape. Change this daily. Change it more often if it gets dirty or wet.

Boils are common, but usually minor, skin problems. Most often, they occur in areas where the skin becomes chaffed and where there are hair follicles. This includes the neck, buttocks, armpits, and genitals. A boil can range in size from that of a pea to a ping pong ball.

Boils

Signs & Symptoms

- A round or cone-shaped lump or pimple that is red, tender, painful, or throbs.

- Pus may be visible under the skin's surface after several days.

- The boil usually bursts open on its own after 10 to 14 days.

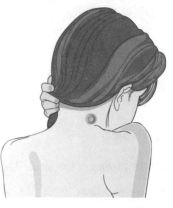

Causes

Boils are caused when a hair follicle or oil gland becomes infected with *staph* bacteria. Boils can be very contagious. Risk factors that make them more likely to occur include:

- Poor hygiene.

- Overuse of corticosteroid medicine.

- Diabetes.

- Short, curly hair that has a tendency to grow back down into the skin.

Treatment

Self-care treats boils. If this is not enough, your doctor may need to lance and drain the boil and prescribe an antibiotic.

Questions to Ask

With a boil, do you have any of these problems?
- **Fever.** (See pages 226 and 227.)
- Red streaks on the skin near the boil.
- Pain that limits normal activity.
- Diabetes.

YES → See Doctor

NO

Flowchart continued on next page

Boils, Continued

Do any of these problems occur?
• Many boils don't drain or heal.
• A boil is on the spine, lip, nose, ear, or eye.
• A boil is on the genitals, pelvis, hand, foot, or face.

YES → Call Doctor

↓ **NO**

Did boils occur after taking antibiotics? **YES** → Call Doctor

↓ **NO**

After using self-care for 3 or more days, do any of these problems occur?
• A boil grows larger.
• New boils occur.
• You get no relief from self-care.

YES → Call Doctor

↓ **NO**

Use Self-Care

Self-Care / Prevention

- Don't scratch, squeeze, or lance boils.
- Put a hot water bottle over a damp washcloth and place it on the boil.
- Soak in a warm tub. Use an antibacterial soap. If boil is ready to burst open, take warm showers instead.

- Take an over-the-counter medicine for pain and swelling as directed.
- Wash your hands after contact with a boil. Keep clothing and other items that were in contact with the boil away from others.
- Once the boil begins to drain, keep it dry and clean. Loosely cover the boil with a sterile gauze dressing. Use first-aid tape to keep it in place. Replace the dressing if it gets moist.

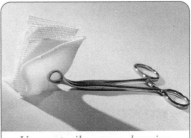
Use a sterile gauze dressing on a boil.

- Wash bed linens, towels, and clothing in hot water. Do not share towels, sports equipment, etc.
- Don't wear tight-fitting clothes over a boil.

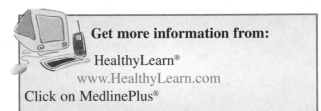

Get more information from:

HealthyLearn®
www.HealthyLearn.com
Click on MedlinePlus®

Cellulitis

Cellulitis is an acute infection of the skin and the tissues beneath the skin. Most often, cellulitis develops on the face, arm, or legs.

Signs & Symptoms

- Redness and swelling of a skin area that worsen as the infection spreads. The skin may look glossy and tight.

- Pain, tenderness, and/or warmth of the skin area.

- Red lines or streaks spread from the wound.

- Lymph nodes near the affected skin area may be swollen.

Treatment

Antibiotics are given by mouth or through an IV. This depends on how serious the infection is. Medicine may be needed to relieve pain.

Causes

A bacterial infection causes cellulitis. Bacteria usually enter the skin layers through a break in the skin, such as a cut or other wound.

Questions To Ask

Do pain, redness, and swelling start and spread quickly? **YES** → Get Medical Care Fast

NO

Are any of these signs present with an existing skin wound?
- Increased redness or blisters form on top of the wound.
- Red lines or streaks spread from the wound.

YES → See Doctor

NO

Are any of these **signs of an infection** present?
- Redness or tenderness of a skin area.
- Hot and/or swollen skin.
- Skin wound with fever, fatigue, muscle aches, or feeling ill.

YES → See Doctor

NO

 Use Self-Care

Self-Care / Prevention

To Prevent Cellulitis
- Keep your skin clean and protect it from injury.

- Clean cuts, abrasions, and other skin injuries thoroughly with soap and water.

- Keep wounds and sores clean, dry, and protected to promote healing.

- If prescribed medication for an infection, take it as directed.

To Treat Cellulitis
- Follow your doctor's treatment plan.

- Rest the area of the body that has cellulitis.

- Elevate the affected body part. This helps to reduce swelling.

- Take an over-the-counter pain reliever as directed.

Cold Hands & Feet

Signs & Symptoms

- Fingers or toes turn pale white or blue, then red, in response to cold temperatures.
- Pain when the fingers or toes turn white.
- Tingling or numbness in the hands or feet.

Causes

Cold hands and feet can be a symptom of the conditions that follow.

- Poor circulation. This is most often due to diseased arteries.
- **Raynaud's disease**. This is a disorder that affects the flow of blood to the fingers and sometimes to the toes.
- Any underlying disease that affects the blood flow in the tiny blood vessels of the skin. Women who smoke may be more prone to this.
- **Frostbite.** (See page 381.)
- Stress.
- A side effect of taking certain medicines
- **Cervical rib syndrome**. This is a compression of the nerves and blood vessels in the neck that affects the shoulders, arms, and hands.

Often the cause is unknown and not serious.

Treatment

Emergency care is needed for frostbite. If a medical condition causes cold hands and/or feet, treatment for the condition is needed.

Questions to Ask

After exposure to cold temperatures, do you have **signs and symptoms of frostbite** listed on page 381?

YES → Get Medical Care Fast

NO ↓

With cold hands and/or feet, do you have weakness in the arms, hands, or feet?

YES → See Doctor

NO ↓

When exposed to the cold or when you are under stress, do your hands or feet turn pale, then blue, then red, and get painful and numb?

YES → See Doctor

NO ↓

 Use Self-Care

Self-Care / Prevention

- Don't smoke. If you smoke, quit.
- Avoid caffeine.
- Don't handle cold objects with bare hands. Use ice tongs to pick up ice cubes, etc.
- Set your indoor thermostat at 65°F or higher.
- Wear mittens and wool socks to keep hands and feet warm.
- Don't wear tight-fitting footwear.
- Wiggle your toes. It may help keep them warm by increasing blood flow.
- Stretch your fingers straight out. Swing your arms in large circles like a baseball pitcher warming up for a game. This may increase blood flow to the fingers. Skip this tip if you have bursitis or back problems.
- Meditate. Learn and practice biofeedback.

Corns & Calluses

Signs & Symptoms

Corns and calluses are extra cells made in a skin area that gets repeated rubbing or squeezing.

- **Corns** are areas of dead skin on the tops or sides of the joints or on the skin between the toes.
- **Calluses** are patches of dead skin usually found on the balls or heels of the feet, on the hands, and on the knees. Calluses are thick and feel hard to the touch.

Causes

Footwear that fits poorly causes corns and calluses. So can activities that cause friction on the hands, knees, and feet.

Treatment

Self-care treats most cases. If not, a family doctor or foot doctor (podiatrist) can scrape the hardened tissue and peel away the corn with stronger solutions. Sometimes warts lie beneath corns and need to be treated, too.

Questions to Ask

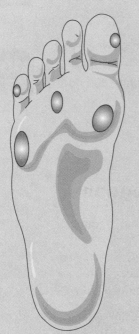

Common sites on the bottom of the foot for corns and calluses.

With a corn or callus, do you have any signs of infection, such as fever, swelling, redness, and/or pus?

YES →  See Doctor

NO

With a corn or callus, do you have circulation problems or diabetes?

YES → See Doctor

NO

Do you have one or both of these problems even after using self-care measures?
- Continued or worse pain.
- No improvement after 2 to 3 weeks.

YES → Call Doctor

NO

 Use Self-Care

See Self-Care / Prevention on next page

Corns & Calluses, Continued

Self-Care / Prevention

{*Note:* Persons with diabetes should see a doctor for treatment for foot problems.}

For Corns

- Don't pick at corns. Don't use toenail scissors, clippers, or any sharp tool to cut off corns.

- Don't wear shoes that fit poorly or that squeeze your toes together.

- Soak your feet in warm water to soften the corn.

- Cover the corn with a protective, nonmedicated pad or bandage which you can buy at drug stores.

- If the outer layers of a corn have peeled away, apply a nonprescription liquid of 5 to 10% salicylic acid. Gently rub the corn off with cotton gauze.

Pointed, tight-fitting boots and shoes can cause corns. Wear footwear that doesn't squeeze the toes together.

- Ask a shoe repair person to sew a metatarsal bar onto your shoe to use when a corn is healing.

For Calluses

- Don't try to cut a callus off.

- Soak your feet in warm water to soften the callus. Pat it dry.

- Rub the callus gently with a pumice stone.

- Cover calluses with protective pads. You can get these at drug stores.

- Don't wear poorly fitting shoes or other sources of friction that may lead to calluses.

- Wear gloves for a hobby or work that puts pressure on your hands.

- Wear knee pads for activities that put pressure on your knees.

Wear gloves when you garden or do other activities that put repeated pressure on your hands.

Get more information from:

HealthyLearn® • www.HealthyLearn.com
Click on MedlinePlus®

American Podiatric Medical Association
800.FOOTCARE (366.8227)
www.apma.org

Dry Skin

Signs & Symptoms

- Itchy skin. The skin can be red from scratching it.
- Chapped skin.
- Skin cracks, peels, and/or flakes.

Causes

- Aging. The body naturally produces less oil and moisture.
- Cold winter weather. Dry air or heat.
- Washing the skin often. Using harsh skin products.
- Chronic and excessive sun exposure.
- Allergies. An underactive thyroid gland. Diabetes. Kidney disease. Other skin conditions, such as psoriasis.

Treatment

Dry skin is not a serious health risk. It can be managed with self-care. When dry skin is a symptom of a health problem, treating the problem treats the dry skin.

Questions to Ask

With dry skin, do you have any of these problems?
- Tight, shiny, or hardened skin.
- Deep cracks on the hands or feet.
- Itchy skin areas that are raised, have red borders, and are covered with large white or silver-white scales.
- **Signs of hypothyroidism** listed on page 260.
- Diabetes and the dry skin is troublesome.

YES → See Doctor

NO ↓

With dry skin, do signs of an infection occur, such as fever, blisters, redness, swelling, pain, tenderness and/or pus?

YES → See Doctor

NO ↓

With dry skin, do you itch all over (without a rash), does itching prevent sleep, or do you get no relief from self-care?

YES → Call Doctor

NO ↓

 Use Self-Care

See Self-Care / Prevention on next page

Get more information from:

HealthyLearn®
www.HealthyLearn.com
Click on MedlinePlus®

American Academy of Dermatology
888.462.DERM
(462.3376)
www.aad.org

Dry Skin, Continued

Self-Care / Prevention

- Drink 8 or more glasses of water a day.

- Apply an oil-based lotion daily.

- Wear rubber gloves when you wash dishes.

- Take showers instead of baths. Use warm (not hot) water. Try sponge baths.

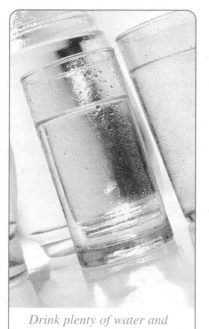

Drink plenty of water and other fluids.

- Apply a moisturizing cream while your skin is damp. Use products with lanolin.

- If you do bathe, do so for only 15 to 20 minutes in lukewarm water. Pat yourself dry. Do not rub.

- Put soap on a washcloth, not right on the skin.

- Use a mild liquid soap, like Cetaphil lotion or use a fatted soap. Avoid deodorant, medicated, or alkaline soaps.

- Don't use moisturizers with fragrances, preservatives, or alcohol.

- Use a night cream for the face.

- Stay out of the strong sun. Do not use tanning salons. When in the sun, use a sunblock with a sun protection factor (SPF) of at least 15.

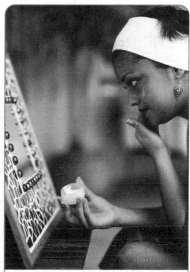

Apply a night cream to the face.

- Don't scratch or rub dry skin.

Hair Loss

Causes

- Normal aging. Family history of hair loss. Hormonal changes, such as with menopause.

- A side effect of some medicines, chemotherapy, and radiation therapy. Crash dieting.

- A prolonged or serious illness. Major surgery. Thyroid disease.

- **Areata.** This causes areas of patchy hair loss. It improves quickly when treated, but can go away within 18 months without treatment.

Questions to Ask

Do you have redness, tenderness, swelling, and/or pain at the site of hair loss? **YES** → **See Doctor**

NO

Do you have **signs of hypothyroidism** listed on page 260? **YES** → **See Doctor**

NO

Has the hair loss occurred suddenly and in patches on the head? Do you have red or gray-green scales on the scalp? **YES** → **See Doctor**

NO

Do you uncontrollably pull out patches of hair? Or, do you want to find out about hair loss treatments? **YES** → **Call Doctor**

NO

Use Self-Care

Self-Care / Prevention

- Try the over-the-counter medication, Rogaine.

- Avoid (or don't use often) hair care practices of bleaching, braiding, cornrowing, dyeing, perming, etc. Avoid hot curling irons and/or hot rollers. Use gentle hair care products.

- Air dry or towel dry your hair. If you use a hairdryer, set it on low.

- Keep your hair cut short. It will look fuller.

- Don't be taken in by claims for products that promise to cure baldness.

Most men have some degree of baldness by age 60. After age 60, 50% of women do.

Signs & Symptoms

- Thinning of hair on the temples and crown.

- Receding hair line.

- Bald spot on back of head.

- Areas of patchy hair loss.

Treatment

- Medications. These include over-the-counter Rogaine and prescribed ones.

- Hair transplant with surgery.

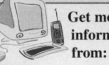

Get more information from:

HealthyLearn®
www.HealthyLearn.com
Click on MedlinePlus®

American Academy of Dermatology
888.462.3376
www.aad.org

Ingrown Toenails

An **ingrown toenail** digs into the skin next to the side of the nail. The most common site is the big toe. Other toes and even fingernails can be affected.

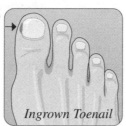

Ingrown Toenail

Signs & Symptoms

- Redness.
- Tenderness.
- Discomfort or pain.

Causes

- Jamming your toes.
- Wearing shoes or socks that fit too tight.
- Clipping toenails too short. The corners can penetrate the skin as the nail grows out.
- Having wider-than-average toenails.

Treatment

Self-care usually treats ingrown toenails. If this fails to work, a doctor or podiatrist may have to remove a portion of the nail.

Questions to Ask

Does the skin next to the side of your toenail show any signs of infection, such as pain, redness, tenderness, and/or pus? **YES** → **See Doctor**

NO ↓

Flowchart continued in next column

With an ingrown toenail, do you have diabetes or circulation problems? **YES** →  **See Doctor**

NO ↓

Do you get ingrown toenails often? **YES** → **Call Doctor**

NO ↓

Use Self-Care

Self-Care / Prevention

- Cut nails straight across. Don't cut the nails shorter at the sides than in the middle. {*Note:* If you have diabetes or circulation problems, follow your doctor's advice about clipping your toenails.}

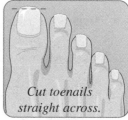

Cut toenails straight across.

- File the nails if they're sharp after clipping them.
- Wear shoes and socks that fit well.

To Treat an Ingrown Toenail
- Soak your foot in warm, soapy water for 5 to 10 minutes, 1 to 3 times a day.
- Gently lift the nail away from the reddened skin at the outer corners with the tip of a nail file.
- Soak a small piece of cotton in an antiseptic, such as Betadine. Place it just under the outer corners of the toenails, if you can.
- Repeat the previous 3 steps, daily, until the nail begins to grow correctly and pressure is relieved. Wear roomy shoes during this time.

Insect Stings

Signs & Symptoms

- Quick, sharp pain.
- Swelling.
- Itching.
- Redness at the sting site.
- **Hives.** (See page 136.)

Insect stings can even result in a severe allergic reaction. (See "Signs of a Severe Allergic Reaction" below.)

Signs of Severe Allergic Reaction

- Fainting or decreasing level of consciousness.
- Shortness of breath or difficulty breathing or swallowing.
- Severe swelling all over or of the face, lips, tongue, and/or throat.
- Pale or bluish lips, skin, and/or fingernails.
- Wheezing.
- Dizziness, weakness, and/or numbness.
- Cool, moist skin or sudden onset of pale skin and sweating.

Causes

Insect stings come from bumblebees, honeybees, hornets, wasps, yellow jackets, and fire ants.

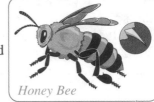

Honey Bee

Treatment

Self-care treats mild reactions to insect stings. A severe allergic reaction needs immediate care. Symptoms of a severe allergic reaction usually happen soon after or within an hour of the sting.

If you have had a severe allergic reaction to an insect sting, you should carry an emergency insect sting kit, prescribed by your doctor. You should also wear a medical alert tag that lets others know that you are allergic to insect stings. Persons who have had severe reactions to bee or wasp stings should ask their doctor about allergy shots.

Questions to Ask

After an insect sting, do any of these problems occur?
- **Signs of a severe allergic reaction** listed at left.
- The sting was in the mouth, inside the throat, or on the tongue.
- Dizziness, muscle spasms, diarrhea, or vomiting occur with many insect stings. (This is 10 or more in a teenager or adult; 5 or more in a child.)
- Hoarseness.
- Red, severe hives occur all over.

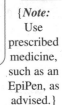

YES ▶ Get Medical Care Fast

{*Note:* Use prescribed medicine, such as an EpiPen, as advised.}

NO

Flowchart continued on next page

Insect Stings, Continued

After an insect sting, do you have any of these problems?
- The area around the sting is increasingly red, warm, and/or tender to touch, or reddish streaks extend from the site.
- Severe or increased pain or swelling at the site.
- Drainage or pus at the site.
- **Fever.** (See pages 226 and 227.)

YES See Doctor

NO

Do self-care measures not treat symptoms or make symptoms worse?

YES Call Doctor

NO

 Use Self-Care

Self-Care / Prevention

To Avoid Insect Stings
- Keep food and drink containers tightly covered. (Bees love sweet things, like soft drinks.)

- Don't wear perfume, colognes, or hair spray when you are outdoors.

- Don't wear bright colors, like white or yellow. Choose neutral colors, like tan or khaki. Wear snug clothing that covers your arms and legs.

- Don't go barefoot. If camping, look for insects in your shoes before you put them on.

- Wear an insect repellent, especially if you are sensitive to insect stings.

- Be careful when you work outdoors, pull weeds, mow tall grass, and work around shutters. Bees often build hives behind shutters.

- If an insect that stings gets in your car, stop the car. Put the windows down. Once the insect leaves, resume driving.

- Check for and repair openings in your window screens.

To Treat an Insect Sting Without a Severe Allergic Reaction
- For a bee sting, gently scrape out the stinger as soon as possible. Use a blunt knife, credit card, or a fingernail. Yellow jackets, wasps, and hornets don't lose their stingers.

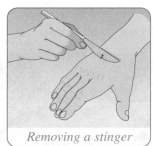
Removing a stinger

- Don't pull the stinger out with your fingers or tweezers. Don't squeeze the stinger. It contains venom. You could re-sting yourself.

- Clean the sting area with soapy water.

- Remove jewelry from bitten fingers, wrists, etc. It may be difficult to remove jewelry once swelling occurs.

- Put a cold compress (ice in a cloth, etc.) on the sting. Don't put ice directly on the skin. Hold the cold compress on the site for 10 to 15 minutes.

- Keep the sting area lower than heart level.

- Take an over-the-counter medicine for pain as directed on the label.

- For itching and swelling, apply a topical 1% hydrocortisone cream and/or take an over-the-counter antihistamine, such as Benadryl, if okay with your doctor. Follow directions on the labels. Also, see information on "Antihistamine" use on page 28.

Poison Ivy, Oak & Sumac

Poison ivy, oak, and sumac are the most common plants that cause a skin rash. A sap that comes from these plants causes the rash. The sap is not really a poison, but can cause an allergic reaction in some people.

Signs & Symptoms

The skin rash comes a day or two after contact with the plant. Symptoms that follow can range from mild to severe.

- Itching.
- Redness.
- Burning feeling.
- Swelling.
- Blisters.

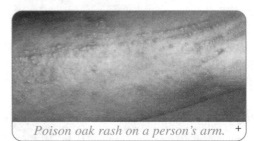

Poison oak rash on a person's arm. +

+ Photo courtesy of the Public Health Image Library (PHIL) of the Centers for Disease Control and Prevention.

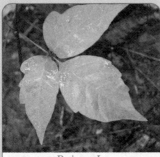

Poison Ivy

Causes

You can get poison ivy, oak, or sumac when you touch one of these plants or touch pets, clothes, shoes, etc. that have the sap on them. Contact with the smoke of these burning plants can also cause a rash.

Treatment

Self-care treats most cases of poison ivy, oak, and sumac. For severe cases, your doctor may prescribe medicine(s).

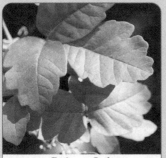

Poison Oak

Questions to Ask

After contact with poison ivy, oak, or sumac, do you have any of these problems?
- The skin is a very bright red color.
- Severe itching, swelling, or blisters.
- A rash on large areas of the body or the face.
- A rash that has spread to the mouth, eyes, or genitals.
- Pus.

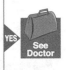
YES — See Doctor

NO — Use Self-Care

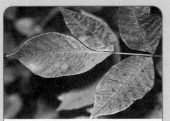

Poison Sumac

USDA, NRCS. 2009. The PLANTS Database (http://plants.usda.gov).

See Self-Care / Prevention on next page

Poison Ivy, Oak & Sumac, Continued

Self-Care / Prevention

To Prevent Getting a Rash

- Know what these plants look like and avoid them. (See illustrations on page 130.)

  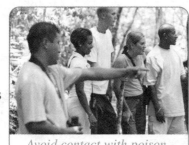

  Avoid contact with poison ivy, oak, and sumac.

  - Poison ivy and poison oak both have 3 leaflets per stem. This is why you may have heard the saying, "Leaflets three, let them be."

  - Each branch of poison sumac has 7 to 13 leaflets on a reddish stem. A single leaf is on the end of the stem. The others are paired along each side of the stem. Poison sumac grows in wetlands.

- Use an over-the-counter lotion (IvyBlock), which blocks skin contact with the sap. Use it as directed.

- Wear pants and long-sleeved shirts.

- To help prevent an allergic reaction, do the things listed below. Do them within 6 hours of contact with one of the plants.

  - Remove all clothes and shoes that have touched the plant.

  - Wash your skin with soap and water.

  - Apply rubbing alcohol or alcohol wipes to the parts of the skin that are affected.

  - Use an over-the-counter product (e.g., Tecnu) that removes poison ivy sap.

  - Rinse the affected area with water.

To Treat Poison Ivy, Oak, or Sumac

- Take a cold shower, put the rash area in cold water, or pour cold water over it. Use soap when you shower.

- To relieve itching, take an over-the-counter antihistamine, such as Benadryl. Follow the label's directions.

- For weeping blisters, mix 2 teaspoons of baking soda in 4 cups of water. Dip squares of gauze in this mixture. Cover the blisters with wet gauze for 10 minutes, 4 times a day. Do not apply this to the eyes.

- Wash all clothes and shoes with hot water and a strong soap. Bathe pets that have come in contact with the plant. The sap can stay on pets for many days. Clean items used to wash clothing and pets. Wear rubber gloves when you do all these things.

- Keep your hands away from your eyes, mouth, and face.

- Do not scratch or rub the rash.

- Apply any of these to the skin rash:
  - Calamine (not Caladryl) lotion.

  - Over-the-counter hydrocortisone cream. Follow the directions on the label.

  - A paste of 3 teaspoons of baking soda and 1 teaspoon of water.

- Take baths with lukewarm water. Add an over-the-counter product called Aveeno colloidal oatmeal.

Shingles

Shingles (herpes zoster) is a skin condition. It is triggered by the chicken pox virus, which is thought to lie dormant in the spinal cord until later in life. Most often, shingles occurs in people over 50 years old.

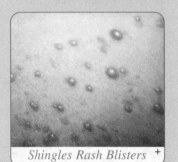

Shingles Rash Blisters +

+ Photo courtesy of the Public Health Image Library (PHIL) of the Centers for Disease Control and Prevention.

Signs & Symptoms

- Pain, itching, or a tingling feeling before a rash appears.
- A rash of painful red blisters. These later crust over. Most often, the rash appears in a band on one side of the body or in a cluster on one side of the face.
- Fever and general weakness can occur.
- The crusts fall off, usually within 3 weeks.
- Pain can persist in the area of the rash. This usually goes away within 1 to 6 months. Chronic pain called **postherpetic neuralgia (PHN)** can last longer, even for years. The older you are, the greater the chance that this is the case. The recovery time may also take longer.
- Blindness can occur if the eye is affected.
- Most cases of shingles are mild.

Causes

The virus that causes chicken pox – varicella zoster virus (VZV) causes shingles. To get shingles, you must have had chicken pox. You are more likely to get shingles after an illness or taking medicine that lowers the immune system. Stress or trauma can also increase the risk for shingles.

Treatment

If you think you might have shingles, see your doctor right away! He or she can prescribe:

- An oral antiviral medicine. This can make symptoms less severe and help you get better sooner. To help, this medicine needs to be started within 24 to 72 hours after the rash first appears.
- Medicine for pain. This includes over-the-counter pain relievers and capsaicin topical cream. Prescribed medicine may be needed for pain. A skin patch called Lidoderm may be helpful for PHN.
- Other medicines to treat symptoms.

Shingles, Continued

Questions to Ask

With shingles, are any of these statements true?
- You are over age 60.
- You take medications that weaken the immune system.
- You have a chronic illness, such as diabetes or HIV/AIDS.

YES → See Doctor

NO ↓

Are any of these problems present?
- Shingles has affected an eye.
- Blisters itch all the time or are very painful.
- Fever and/or general weakness occurs.
- You think you might have shingles.

YES → See Doctor

NO ↓

 Use Self-Care

Self-Care / Prevention

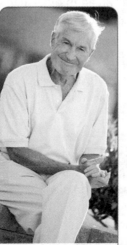

Wear loose-fitting clothes over the rash area.

- A Zoster vaccine may help prevent getting shingles. It can also reduce the pain due to shingles. The vaccine is advised for persons age 60 and older.

- Unless your doctor has prescribed pain medicine, take an over-the-counter one as directed.

- Don't wear clothing that irritates the skin area where sores are present.

- Keep sores open to the air. Until the blisters are completely crusted over, do not go near children or adults who have not yet had the chicken pox. Do not go near persons who have a condition which weakens their immune system. Examples are cancer, HIV/AIDS, and chronic illnesses. They could get chicken pox from exposure to shingles.

- Wash blisters. Don't scrub them.

- To relieve itching, apply calamine lotion to the affected area. You can also use a paste made of 3 teaspoons of baking soda mixed with 1 teaspoon of water.

- Avoid drafty areas.

- Put a cool compress, such as a cold cloth dipped in ice water, on the blisters. Do this for 20 minutes at a time.

- Drink lots of liquids.

Get more information from:

HealthyLearn® • www.HealthyLearn.com
Click on MedlinePlus®

National Institute of Allergy and Infectious Diseases (NIAID)
www.niaid.nih.gov

National Shingles Foundation
212.472.3181
www.vzvfoundation.org

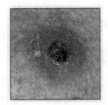

Skin Cancer

Skin cancer is the most common kind of cancer in the U.S. When found early, skin cancer can be treated with success.

Causes

- Recurrent exposure to ultraviolet (UV) radiation from the sun is the main cause.

- Artificial sources of UV radiation, such as sun lamps and tanning beds.

Risk Factors

- Having skin cancer in the past.

- A family history of skin cancer.

- Having fair skin that freckles easily, especially with red or blond hair and blue or light-colored eyes.

Skin Cancer Warning Signs

Contact your doctor if you notice any of these following signs:

For **basal cell** and **squamous cell** skin cancers (types that seldom spread to other parts of the body):

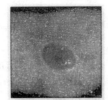 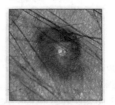 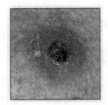

Small, smooth, shiny, pale, or waxy lump   Firm red lump   A lump that bleeds or develops a crust

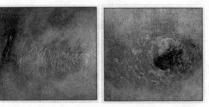

A flat, red spot that is rough, dry, or scaly

For **melanoma** (can spread to other parts of the body and be fatal if not treated early). Look for any of these signs in an existing mole:

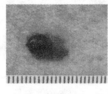

A. **Asymmetry** - The shape of one half does not match the other.

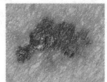

C. **Color** - The color is uneven.

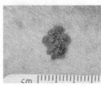

B. **Border** - The edges are ragged, notched or blurred.

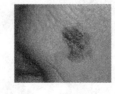

D. **Diameter** - The size changes and is often bigger than a pencil eraser.

E. **Evolving lesion** - This is one that changes size, shape, shades of color or symptoms or has surface bleeding.

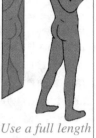

Skin Cancer, Continued

Treatment

Depending on the size, type, and stage of the cancer, treatment includes:

- Surgery. There are many types.
- Laser therapy.
- Chemotherapy. One form is a cream or lotion with anticancer drugs that is applied to the skin. Other forms are given through an IV.
- Radiation therapy.
- Interferon drugs.
- Skin grafting.

Questions to Ask

Do you have any **skin cancer warning sign** listed on page 134?

Self-Care / Prevention

Prevention should start in childhood to prevent skin cancer later in life.

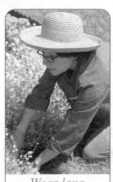

Wear long sleeves, sun hats, etc. to block out the sun's harmful rays.

- Avoid exposure to midday sun (10:00 a.m. to 4:00 p.m. standard time; 11:00 a.m. to 5:00 p.m. daylight savings time).
- Use a sunblock with a sun protection factor (SPF) of 15 or higher as directed.
- Avoid sun lamps and tanning salons.

Skin Self-Exam

- Do a skin self-exam monthly. The best time to do this is after a shower or bath. To check your skin, use a well-lit room, a full-length mirror, and a hand-held mirror.
- Locate your birthmarks, moles, and blemishes. Know what they look like. Check for a sore that does not heal.
- Check all areas.

  Use a full length mirror to do a skin self-exam.

  1. Look at the front and back of your body in the mirror. Then, raise your arms and look at the left and right sides.

  2. Bend your elbows and look carefully at the palms of your hands. Make sure to look at both sides of your forearms and upper arms.

  3. Look at the back and front of the legs. Look between the buttocks and around the genital area.

  4. Look at your face, neck, and scalp. Use a comb or blow dryer to move hair so that you can see the scalp better.

  5. Sit and closely examine the feet. Look at the soles and the spaces between the toes.

{*Note:* Get a skin exam from your doctor or health care provider as often as advised.}

Get more information from:

HealthyLearn® • www.HealthyLearn.com
Click on MedlinePlus®

National Cancer Institute
800.4.CANCER (422.6237) • www.cancer.gov

Skin Rashes

Skin Rash Chart			
Signs & Symptoms	**What It Could Be/Cause**	**What To Do**	**Self-Care**
Red or pink, raised areas on the skin (weals) that can change shape, fade, then rapidly reappear. May come and go anywhere on the body. Itching.	**Hives**, usually due to an allergic reaction.	Call 9-1-1 if hives come with a hard time breathing or swallowing, wheezing, severe swelling all over or of the face, lips, tongue and/or throat (severe allergic reaction). {*Note:* If you have an emergency kit for an allergy, give the shot from the kit and follow other instructions before medical care.} For hives without a severe allergic reaction, see doctor for severe hives or for attacks of hives that recur.	Avoid substance that caused allergic reaction. Take an over-the-counter (OTC) antihistamine as advised by your doctor. Take a lukewarm (not hot) shower or bath. Add baking soda or an oatmeal bath product to bath water. Apply a cold compress or calamine lotion to itchy areas. Wear loose-fitting clothes. Don't take aspirin, ibuprofen, ketoprofen, or naproxen sodium. Relax as much as you can.
Rash of deep red or purple spots that don't fade when the skin is pressed. Other symptoms include high fever; stiff neck; severe headache that persists; vomiting; lethargy; seizure; sensitivity to light; and bulging of the fontanelle (soft spot of the skull) in an infant.	Meningococcemia from a **meningitis** infection.*	Get medical care fast!	After medical care, follow your doctor's advice.
* These conditions are contagious.			

Skin Rashes, continued on next page

Skin Rashes, Continued

Skin Rash Chart			
Signs & Symptoms	**What It Could Be/Cause**	**What To Do**	**Self-Care**
Rash on the trunk of the body with fever, headache, bodyaches, and swollen lymph glands.	**West Nile virus**, 3 to 15 days after a bite from a mosquito infected with the virus.	See doctor right away.	Follow your doctor's advice.
Pink to red rash on the arms, legs, and palms of the hands. Often starts near the wrists and ankles, then spreads inward. Rash darkens in color, spreads, and can bleed. Sudden high fever with chills, severe headache, and delirium also occur.	**Rocky mountain spotted fever**, 1 to 14 days after a bite from an American dog tick or Rocky Mountain woodtick.	Contact doctor right away.	Follow your doctor's advice.
Rash of painful red blisters (most often on only one side and in only one area of the body). Pain, itching, burning, or tingling feeling before the rash appeared.	**Shingles** from the herpes zoster virus.* (Persons who have not had chicken pox or a vaccine for it can get chicken pox from exposure to shingles.) See **Shingles** on pages 132 and 133.	See doctor or health care provider within 24 to 72 hours for an oral antiviral medicine. This can shorten the course of shingles and make symptoms less severe. {*Note:* All adults 60 years of age and older are advised to get a vaccine that can help prevent shingles and reduce the pain due to shingles.}	Take pain relievers as advised by your doctor. For itching, apply calamine lotion or a paste made of 3 teaspoons of baking soda mixed with 1 teaspoon of water to the affected area. Apply a cool, wet compress to blisters for 20 minutes at a time. Wash (don't scrub) blisters until they crust over. Drink plenty of liquids.
* These conditions are contagious.		Skin Rashes, continued on next page	

+ These skin rash photos are courtesy of the Public Health Image Library (PHIL) of the Centers for Disease Control and Prevention.

Skin Rashes, Continued

Skin Rash Chart			
Signs & Symptoms	**What It Could Be/Cause**	**What To Do**	**Self-Care**
Rough, bright red rash (feels like sandpaper) on the face, neck, elbows, armpits, and groin. It spreads rapidly to entire body. A high fever and weakness occur before the rash. Other symptoms include sore throat, peeling of the skin, vomiting, and swollen tongue.	**Scarlet fever**. This is caused by a bacterial infection.*	See doctor or health care provider for diagnosis. Can be treated with an antibiotic.	Take acetaminophen for fever. Rest and drink plenty of fluids.
A fever and red rash 3 days to 2 weeks after a deer tick bite. The rash has raised edges with pale centers. It fades after a few days. Joint pain may develop later.	**Lyme disease**. This is caused by a deer tick bite.	See doctor or health care provider for diagnosis. Can be treated with an antibiotic.	Follow your doctor's advice.
Widespread red rash on the palms of the hands, soles of the feet, and sometimes around the mouth and nose. The small, red, scaly bumps do not itch. Other types of rashes, swollen lymph nodes, fever, and flu-like symptoms may also occur.	**Syphilis**. This is a sexually transmitted disease caused by a specific bacterial infection.*	See doctor or health care provider for diagnosis. Can be treated with an antibiotic.	Follow your doctor's advice.

* These conditions are contagious.

Skin Rashes, continued on next page

+ These skin rash photos are courtesy of the Public Health Image Library (PHIL) of the Centers for Disease Control and Prevention.

Skin Rashes, Continued

Skin Rash Chart			
Signs & Symptoms	**What It Could Be/Cause**	**What To Do**	**Self-Care**
Tiny red pimples that itch intensely, usually between the fingers, on the wrists and genitals; in the armpits; and along the belt line. Scabs and sores may form.	**Scabies**. This is caused by skin parasites called itch mites.* +	See doctor or health care provider for diagnosis. Can be treated with a prescribed topical medicine.	Follow your doctor's instructions. Wash clothing and bedding in hot water and detergent.
Redness, itchy, scaly patches on the skin or scalp that are round with distinct edges that grow outward as the infection spreads. Moistness in the folds of the skin (under the breasts or in the groin area). Bald spots may appear on the scalp.	**Ringworm**. This is caused by a fungal infection.* + *Ringworm on the scalp.*	See doctor or health care provider for diagnosis and treatment, especially if you have not had this before or if ringworm occurs on the scalp or in several patches on the skin.	Follow your doctor's advice.
Dry, red, itchy patches of skin. Blisters which may drain and then crust over.	**Contact dermatitis**. Causes are direct contact with poison ivy, oak, or sumac or contact with an irritant (cleaning product, cosmetic, jewelry, etc.). + *Poison Ivy Rash on Arm*	See doctor or health care provider if self-care measures don't bring relief or if there are signs of infection (e.g., red streaks, fever, pus, increased redness, swelling, or pain).	Try to identify the irritant and avoid direct contact with it. Don't scratch the rash. For itching, apply calamine lotion or OTC hydrocortisone cream to the affected area. Bathe in warm (not hot) water. Add an oatmeal product to the water. Pat (don't rub) the skin dry. Take an OTC antihistamine as advised.
* These conditions are contagious.		Skin Rashes, continued on next page	

+ These skin rash photos are courtesy of the Public Health Image Library (PHIL) of the Centers for Disease Control and Prevention.

Skin Rashes, Continued

Skin Rash Chart			
Signs & Symptoms	**What It Could Be/Cause**	**What To Do**	**Self-Care**
Patches of skin that are dry, red, scaly, blistered, swollen, and sometimes thick, discolored, or oozing and crusting. Commonly occurs in the bend of the elbow or behind the knee.	**Eczema (atopic dermatitis).** This tends to run in families. It is common in persons with asthma or allergies. Contact with irritants may worsen eczema.	See doctor or health care provider if self-care measures don't bring relief or if there are signs of infection (e.g., red streaks, fever, pus, increased redness, swelling, or pain).	Use an OTC hydrocortisone cream on the affected area. Don't scratch. Don't bathe too often. When you do, use warm (not hot) water and a mild soap (or no soap). Use a light, nongreasy, unscented lotion (without alcohol) after you wash. Avoid items that worsen the eczema.
Red rash on the face. Red nose that looks swollen and puffy cheeks. May have pus-filled spots without blackheads or whiteheads.	**Rosacea (adult acne).** The exact cause is not known. It may result from overuse of corticosteroid creams or alcohol use.	See doctor or health care provider if rosacea affects large areas of skin and/or if self-care measures don't bring relief.	Avoid hot and/or spicy foods, alcohol, and caffeine. Don't rub or massage the face. Avoid strong sunlight.
Itchy, red patches covered with silvery-white flaky skin. Common sites are the scalp, elbows, forearms, knees, and legs.	**Psoriasis.** This is a chronic skin disease that tends to run in families. The exact cause is not known. +	See doctor or health care provider if psoriasis affects large areas of skin and/or if self-care measures don't bring relief.	To prevent dryness, use a moisturizer. Use an OTC hydrocortisone or coal tar cream or ointment. If psoriasis affects your scalp, use an antidandruff shampoo. Take a bath with mineral salts or an oatmeal bath product.

* These conditions are contagious.

Skin Rashes, continued on next page

+ These skin rash photos are courtesy of the Public Health Image Library (PHIL) of the Centers for Disease Control and Prevention.

Skin Rashes, Continued

Skin Rash Chart			
Signs & Symptoms	**What It Could Be/Cause**	**What To Do**	**Self-Care**
Flat, red spots that become raised and look like small pimples. These develop into small blisters that break and crust over. Fatigue and mild fever occur 24 hours before rash appears. Itching may be intense.	**Chickenpox**. This is caused by the varicella-zoster virus.*	See doctor or health care provider if it occurs in an adult; if self-care measures don't bring relief in children; or if there are signs of infection (e.g., pus, increased redness, swelling, or pain). A vaccine is given to prevent this disease.	Keep from scratching affected areas. Apply cool, wet washcloths with baking soda or calamine lotion to affected areas. Take acetaminophen for fever. Take an OTC antihistamine as advised by your doctor if itching is intense. Chickenpox can be prevented with a chickenpox vaccine.
Scaly, oily rash with small, reddish-yellow patches. Areas affected are usually oily ones (the edge of the scalp, forehead, nose, and eyebrows) and the back and chest.	**Seborrhea**. This is a type of dermatitis. The glands in the skin make too much oil.	See doctor or health care provider if self-care measures don't bring relief or if there are signs of infection (e.g., red streaks, fever, pus, increased redness, swelling, or pain).	Use an OTC antidandruff shampoo with salicylic acid on the scalp area. Use OTC hydrocortisone cream on the affected skin areas. Handle the skin gently. Don't scratch. Don't use irritants like detergents.
Small patches of rough skin and tiny pimples (in babies), on the buttocks, thighs, and/or genitals. Soreness without itching.	**Diaper rash**. This is due to dampness and the interaction of urine and the skin.	See doctor or health care provider if there are blisters or small red patches outside the diaper area (e.g., the chest). Otherwise, use self-care.	Change diapers as soon as they are wet. Wash the area with warm water. Don't use throwaway wipes. Keep the skin dry. Apply a little zinc oxide ointment to the skin. Don't use plastic pants until the rash is gone.
* These conditions are contagious.		Skin Rashes, continued on next page	

Skin Rashes, Continued

Skin Rash Chart			
Signs & Symptoms	**What It Could Be/Cause**	**What To Do**	**Self-Care**
In infants, pus-filled blisters and red skin. In older children, golden crusts on red sores. Areas affected are the arms, legs, face, and around the nose first, then most of body. Sometimes fever. Occasional itching.	**Impetigo**. This is caused by a bacterial infection.* +	See doctor or health care provider, especially if self-care measures don't bring relief, if blisters are larger than 1 inch across, or if a red streak runs from the infection. An antibiotic may need to be prescribed.	Clean the area with an antibacterial soap several times a day. Apply an OTC antibiotic ointment 3 times a day <u>after</u> the scab falls off. Wash your hands after contact with the rash area. Don't share towels, etc.
Flat, rosy red rash on the chest and abdomen. A high fever occurs 2 to 4 days before the rash. The child feels only mildly ill when the fever is present.	**Roseola**. This is caused by the Herpes type-6 virus. +	See doctor or health care provider if high fever causes febrile seizure.	Take acetaminophen for fever. Apply cool, wet washcloths or take baths with tepid (not cold) water.
Blotchy red rash that starts on the face and spreads to the rest of the body. Rash lasts about 7 days. These signs come before the rash: Fever; runny nose; sneezing; cough; eyes that look red and are sensitive to light; and blue-white spots in the mouth.	**Measles.** This is caused by a virus.* MMR vaccines prevent measles. +	Call doctor right away to be sure the problem is measles. If it is, follow the doctor's advice. Let the child's school and the local health department know.	Rest until fever and rash go away. Drink lots of liquids. For fever, take acetaminophen. Treat cough (see page 105). Avoid lights, TV, reading, etc. while eyes are sensitive to light. Usually okay to return to school about 7 to 10 days after rash and fever are gone.

* These conditions are contagious.

Skin Rashes, continued on next page

+ These skin rash photos are courtesy of the Public Health Image Library (PHIL) of the Centers for Disease Control and Prevention.

Skin Rashes, Continued

Skin Rash Chart			
Signs & Symptoms	**What It Could Be/Cause**	**What To Do**	**Self-Care**
Red rash of varying shades that fades to a flat, lacy pattern. Rash comes and goes. It usually starts on the facial cheeks and then on the arms and legs. This is a mild disease, usually with no other symptoms.	**Fifth Disease**. This is caused by the Human parvovirus B19.* +	Use self-care, but no special treatment is required.	Avoid hot or even warm baths or showers. Keep cool.
Rash with small red pimples, pink blotchy skin, and itching. Common sites are between skin folds (armpits, under the breasts, the groin).	**Heat rash (prickly heat)** or chafing. This occurs from too much sweating.	Use self-care.	Bathe in cool water without soap every couple of hours. Let your skin air dry. Put cornstarch in body creases or apply calamine lotion to very itchy spots. Don't use ointments and creams that can block sweat gland pores. Stay in a cool, dry area.
Scaly, crusty rash (in newborns) that starts behind the ears and spreads to the scalp.	**Cradle cap**. This is due to hormones that pass through the placenta before birth.	Use self-care.	Apply mineral oil to the scalp to soften the hard crusts, then use an antidandruff shampoo. Do this 2 to 3 times a week, massaging the scalp with a soft brush or washcloth for 5 minutes. Be sure to wash all of the oil out.

* These conditions are contagious.

+ These skin rash photos are courtesy of the Public Health Image Library (PHIL) of the Centers for Disease Control and Prevention.

Get more information from:

MedlinePlus® • www.medlineplus.gov

American Academy of Dermatology
888.462.DERM (462.3376) • www.aad.org

To Learn More, See Back Cover

Splinters

Signs & Symptoms

- An opening near the skin where the splinter entered.

- Pain may not be felt and the splinter may or may not be visible.

- Bleeding, swelling, and/or pain at the wound area, especially for splinters stuck deep under the skin.

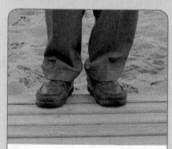

Wear shoes when walking outdoors, on wooden floors, etc.

Causes

Splinters are pieces of wood, glass, metal, or other matter that lodge under the skin.

Treatment

Remove splinters so they don't cause an infection. Self-care takes care of most splinters. A doctor may need to remove a splinter if it is not visible, if it is deep in the skin, or if it is in a person with diabetes.

Questions to Ask

With a splinter, are any of these problems present?
- Red lines or streaks that spread from the wound.
- Swelling, redness, or warmth at the wound site.
- Pus.
- Fever.

YES → See Doctor

NO ↓

With a splinter, are any of the following present?
- The splinter is deeply embedded in the skin, you cannot get it out, and you have diabetes.
- The splinter is still embedded in the skin, you cannot get it out, and it is painful.

YES → See Doctor

NO ↓

Is your tetanus immunization (DTaP or Td) not up-to-date? (See **Immunization Schedule** on page 23.)

YES → See Doctor

NO ↓

With a splinter, is a fever present? (See pages 226 and 227.)

YES → See Doctor

NO ↓

Use Self-Care

See Self-Care / Prevention on next page

Splinters, Continued

Self-Care / Prevention

To Prevent Getting Splinters

- Wear shoes out-of-doors at all times and whenever you walk on unfinished floors.

- Sand, varnish, and/or paint handrails to keep from getting splinters in the hands.

- Clean up all broken glass and metal shavings around the house. Be careful when you handle broken glass. Wear hard-soled shoes when glass has been broken.

- Wear work gloves when you handle plants with thorns, sharp tips, or spines.

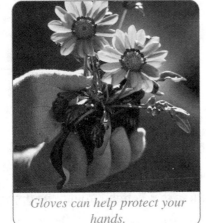

Gloves can help protect your hands.

To Remove a Splinter

- Wash your hands, but don't let the area around a wooden splinter get wet. A wooden splinter that gets wet will swell. This will make it harder to remove.

- Sterilize tweezers. Place the tips in a flame. Wipe off the blackness on the tips with sterile gauze if you use a lit match for the flame.

- Use the tweezers to gently pull the part of the splinter that sticks out through the skin. It should slide right out. If necessary, use a magnifying glass to help you see close up.

- If the splinter is buried under the skin, sterilize a needle and gently slit the skin over one end of the splinter. Then, use the needle to lift that end and pull the splinter out with the tweezers.

  - Check to see that all of the splinter has been removed. If not, repeat the above step.

  - If you still can't get the splinter out, soak the skin around the splinter in a solution made with 1 tablespoon of baking soda mixed in 1 cup of warm water. Do this 2 times a day. After a few days, the splinter may work its way out.

  - Once the splinter is removed, clean the wound by washing it with soap and water. Blot it dry with a clean cloth or sterile gauze pad. Apply a sterile bandage.

  - To remove a large number of close-to-the-surface splinters, such as cactus spines, apply a layer of hair removing wax or white glue, such as Elmer's, to the skin. Let it dry for 5 minutes. Gently peel it off by lifting the edges of the dried wax, gel, or glue with tweezers. The splinter(s) should come up with it.

  - Contact your doctor if you still have the splinter(s) after using self-care measures. Also, see that your tetanus immunizations are up-to-date. See **Immunization Schedule** on page 23.

Varicose Veins

Varicose veins may occur in almost any part of the body. They are most often seen in the back of the calf or on the inside of the leg between the groin and the ankle. Hemorrhoids (veins around the anus) can also become varicose.

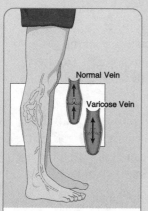

With varicose veins, valves don't work like they should. Blood is able to pool downward. This causes some veins to overfill with blood and swell.

Signs & Symptoms

- Swollen and twisted veins look blue and are close to the surface of the skin.
- Veins bulge and feel heavy.
- The legs and feet can swell.
- The skin can itch.

Causes

- Obesity.
- Pregnancy.
- Hormone changes at menopause.
- Activities or hobbies that require standing or lifting heavy objects for long periods of time.
- A family history of varicose veins.
- Often wearing clothing that is tight around the upper thighs.
- Body positions that restrict lower leg blood flow for long periods of time. One example is sitting on an airplane, especially in the economy class section on a long flight.
- Past vein diseases, such as **thrombophlebitis**. This is inflammation of a vein before a blood clot forms.

Treatment

Medical treatment is not required for most varicose veins unless problems result, such as deep-vein blood clot or severe bleeding which can be caused by injury to the vein. Problems can occur without an injury, as well.

An X-ray of the vein (venogram) or a special ultrasound can tell if there are any problems.

Varicose Veins, Continued

Medical Treatment Includes

- Surgery, to remove all or part of the vein.

- Sclerotherapy. This uses a chemical injection into the vein causing it to close up.

- Laser therapy. This causes the vein to fade away.

Questions to Ask

Does it look like the varicose vein has broken open and is bleeding a lot under the skin? {*Note:* Apply direct pressure on the skin area over the varicose vein.} **YES** → See Doctor

NO ↓

Has the varicose vein become swollen, red, very tender, or warm to the touch? **YES** → See Doctor

NO ↓

With varicose veins, do sores or a rash occur on the leg or ankle? **YES** → See Doctor

NO ↓

Do varicose veins cause chronic, achy pain in the legs? **YES** → Call Doctor

NO ↓

Do you want to find out about cosmetic treatments for varicose veins? **YES** → Call Doctor

NO ↓

Use Self-Care

See Self-Care / Prevention in next column

Self-Care / Prevention

- Don't cross your legs when sitting.

- Exercise regularly. Walking is a good choice. It improves leg and vein strength.

- Keep your weight down.

- Avoid standing for prolonged periods of time. If your job or hobby requires you to stand, shift your weight from one leg to the other every few minutes. Just wiggling your toes can help, too.

- Wear elastic support stockings or support hose as advised by your doctor.

- Don't wear clothing or undergarments that are tight or constrict your waist, groin, or legs.

- Eat high-fiber foods, like bran cereals, whole grain breads, and fresh fruits and vegetables to promote regularity. Constipation may be a factor in varicose veins.

- To prevent swelling, cut your salt intake.

- Exercise your legs. From a sitting position, rotate your feet at the ankles, turning them first clockwise, then counterclockwise, using a circular motion. Next, extend your legs forward and point your toes to the ceiling, then to the floor. Then, lift your feet off the floor and gently bend your legs back and forth at the knees.

- Elevate your legs when resting.

- Get up and move about every 35 to 45 minutes when traveling by air or even when sitting in an all-day conference. Opt for an aisle seat in such situations.

- Stop and take short walks at least every 45 minutes when taking long car rides.

Warts

Warts are small skin growths. Most are harmless and painless. They can appear on any part of the body.

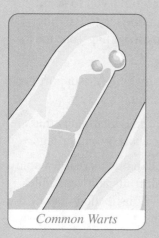

Common Warts

Signs & Symptoms

- *Common warts.* These are firm and often have a rough surface. They are round or have an irregular shape. They are found on places subject to injury, such as the hands, fingers, and knees. Common warts are flesh-colored to brown. They may spread, but are not cancer.

- *Flat warts.* These are smooth and flesh-colored. They are found mainly on the hands and face and may itch.

- *Plantar warts.* These occur on the soles of the feet. They look like corns or calluses and may have little black dots in the center. They can be painful.

- *Digitate warts.* These threadlike warts grow on the scalp.

- *Filiform warts.* These are long, narrow, small growths. They appear mainly on the neck, eyelids, or armpits.

- *Genital warts.* See **Sexually Transmitted Infections (STIs) – Human Papillomavirus (HPV)** on page 250.

Causes

Warts are caused by human papillomaviruses. One of these viruses may enter the body through a cut or nick in the skin. Scratching or picking at warts may spread them to other sites. Some persons are more prone to getting warts than others. People who cannot fight off disease are also more at risk for warts. You cannot get warts from frogs or toads.

Treatment

Treatment for warts depends on their location, type, and severity and how long they have been on the skin. About 50% of warts go away in 6 to 12 months without treatment.

Self-care measures can be used for warts not on the face or genitals. Medical treatment includes liquid nitrogen, chemical injections, topical medicines, laser surgery, and minor surgery. For genital warts, see **Treatment** in **Sexually Transmitted Infections (STIs) – Human Papillomavirus (HPV)** on page 250.

Warts, Continued

Questions to Ask

Are any of these problems present?
- The wart is near the genital or anal area.
- The wart is painful.
- The wart has changed its shape or color.
- Signs of infection, such as redness, swelling, pain, drainage, warmth, or red streaks occur at the wart site.
- The location of the wart limits normal movement.
- The wart is a new wart on a person over 45 years old.

YES  See Doctor

NO

Do any of these problems occur?
- The wart is bothersome and has not responded to self-care measures.
- The wart has been irritated or ripped off.
- The wart is on the face and you want it removed.
- Multiple warts are present.

YES Call Doctor

NO

 Use Self-Care

See Self-Care / Prevention in next column

Self-Care / Prevention

■ Don't touch, scratch, or pick at warts.

■ Never cut or burn a wart off.

■ Try an over-the-counter wart remover with salicylic acid. This can be a liquid or it can be in a medicated wart pad or patch. {*Note:* Do not use these wart removers on the face or genitals.} Follow package directions. A pumice stone helps remove the dead skin during this treatment.

■ Ask your doctor about Retin A for flat warts.

■ During treatment for plantar warts, put pads or cushions in your shoes. This can help relieve the pain when you walk.

To Prevent Warts

■ Don't touch warts on yourself or others.

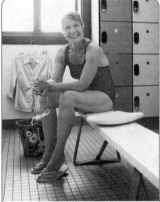

Wear plastic sandals or shower shoes in locker rooms or public pool areas.

■ When you shave a skin area that has a wart, use an electric shaver instead of a razor blade. Or, use an over-the-counter hair remover cream or lotion.

■ Change shoes often to air them out.

■ See **Self-Care / Prevention** for **Genital Herpes** on page 253.

Chapter 13

Digestive & Urinary Problems

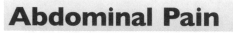

Abdominal Pain

Causes

Abdominal pain can be a symptom of a problem that affects any of the organs shown in the boxes on the right side of this page. Causes of abdominal pain include:

- Artery diseases, such as a blocked artery or an aneurysm.

- Celiac disease.

- Constipation.

- Crohn's disease.

- Food poisoning.

- Gallstones.

- Heartburn. Indigestion.

- Infections, such as ones in the digestive tract and urinary tract.

- Irritable bowel syndrome (IBS).

- Kidney stones.

- Menstrual cramps or ovarian cysts in females.

- Reflux.

- Stomach ulcers.

The abdomen is the body region between the lower ribs and the pelvis. Many vital organs make up this body region.

Signs & Symptoms

- Mild to severe pain. It can feel dull or sharp.

- Acute (sudden) pain.

- Chronic pain. This is constant pain or pain that recurs over time.

The type of pain, its location, and other symptoms that come with it point to the cause.

Treatment

Treatment depends on the cause. The key is knowing when it's just a minor problem like a mild stomach ache or when it's something worse. Pain that persists can be a sign of a medical condition or illness. Very severe abdominal pain usually needs immediate medical care.

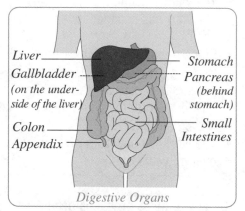

Digestive Organs

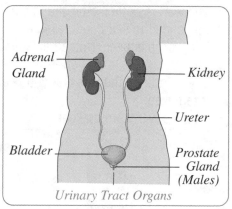

Urinary Tract Organs

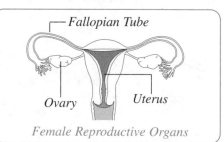

Female Reproductive Organs

Abdominal Pain, Continued

Questions to Ask

With abdominal pain, is any **heart attack warning sign** listed on page 387 present?

 YES — Get Medical Care Fast

NO

With abdominal pain, are any of these problems present?
- You vomit without stopping or you vomit blood or material that looks like coffee grounds.
- You vomit, have a fever and shaking chills, and feel pain in one or both sides of your mid back or shoulders.
- You have dry mouth, excessive thirst, little or no urination, and dry skin that doesn't spring back after you pinch it.
- Your stools have blood or are tarlike and black in color.
- You had a recent injury to the abdomen.
- Pain is so bad that you can't move or it gets a lot worse when you move.
- You have heavy vaginal bleeding and you are pregnant.

 YES — Get Medical Care Fast

NO

With abdominal pain, do you have any of these problems?
- The pain spreads to the back, chest, or shoulders.
- You feel a mass in the abdomen that throbs or pulsates.
- Your abdomen is very tender when touched.
- You don't know why your abdomen is swollen but it keeps getting worse.

YES — Get Medical Care Fast

NO

Flowchart continued in next column

Is the abdominal pain very severe or sudden, extreme, and constant?

YES — Get Medical Care Fast

NO

Are all of these **symptoms of appendicitis** present?
- You have not had your appendix removed.
- Pain and tenderness usually start in the upper part of the stomach or around the belly button and moves to the lower right part of the abdomen. The pain can be sharp, severe, and felt more when the lower right abdomen is touched.
- Nausea, vomiting, or no appetite.
- Mild fever.

 YES — Get Medical Care Fast

NO

With abdominal pain, are **symptoms of a kidney infection** listed on page 178 present?

YES — Get Medical Care Fast

NO

With abdominal pain, are these **symptoms of a kidney stone** present?
- The pain started in your side or back before it moved to your abdomen or groin.
- The pain can be constant or come and go. The pain may be severe.
- Your urine is bloody, cloudy, or dark-colored.
- Nausea and vomiting.
- Chills and fever, if you also have an infection. (See **Fever** on pages 226 and 227.)

 YES — See Doctor

NO

Flowchart continued on next page

Abdominal Pain, Continued

Crohn's Disease is a chronic problem that can cause abdominal pain and diarrhea. Other symptoms are fever, fatigue, and, at times, rectal bleeding or drainage. Symptoms occur when the disease flares up. This is followed by periods when symptoms go away or lessen.

With Crohn's disease, any part of the GI tract, from the mouth to the anus, can be inflamed. Usually, the colon and the last part of the small intestine, the ileum, are affected.

Treatment for Crohn's disease includes medicines, nutrition supplements, and surgery.

With abdominal pain, do you have any of these problems?
- The whites of your eyes or your skin looks yellow.
- Recurrent pain in the upper abdomen is temporarily relieved by antacids.
- Severe diarrhea or constipation lasts for more than a week.
- Skin on the abdomen is sensitive or you have a skin rash on one side of the abdomen.
- You have a bulge and/or discomfort (when pressed) anywhere in the abdomen.

YES **See Doctor**

NO

With the abdominal pain, are any **symptoms of a bladder infection** listed on page 178 present?

YES **See Doctor**

NO

Is swelling or discomfort in the groin made worse when you cough or lift heavy objects?

YES **Call Doctor**

NO

With abdominal pain, do you have any of these problems?
- Continued belching, nausea, gas, or gurgling noises.
- Pain worsens when you bend over or lie down.

YES **Call Doctor**

NO

Are you female? Do you have abdominal pain and could you be pregnant?

YES **Call Doctor**

NO

 Use Self-Care

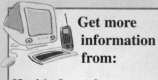
Self-Care / Prevention

- Find a comfortable position. Relax.
- Take an over-the-counter pain medicine as directed on the label.
- Apply a heating pad set on low (adults only).
- Don't wear clothes that fit tight.
- Don't exercise too hard.

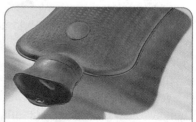
Use a hot water bottle on the area that aches.

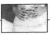

Constipation

Constipation is having trouble passing stool or having hard stools. "Regularity" does not mean that you have a bowel movement every day. Normal bowel habits range from 3 movements a day to 3 each week. What is more important is what is normal for you.

Signs & Symptoms

- A hard time passing stool. Not being able to pass stool. Having very hard stool.
- Straining to have a bowel movement.
- Abdominal swelling. The feeling of continued fullness after passing stool.

Causes

- Drinking too few fluids. Not eating enough dietary fiber.
- Not being active enough.
- Not going to the bathroom when you have the urge to pass stool.
- Misuse of laxatives.
- A side effect of some heart, pain, and antidepressant medicines, as well as, antacids, antihistamines, and water pills.
- Chronic illnesses that slow the digestive tract. Examples are diabetes and an underactive thyroid.
- Cancer or other diseases of the bowel.

Treatment

Self-care usually treats constipation. You may also need to talk to your doctor about health problems and medicines that could cause the problem.

Questions to Ask

With constipation, do you have any of these problems?
- Abdominal pain, especially on the lower left side, that occurs often.
- Very narrow stools.
- Recent change in bowel movement pattern.
- Nausea or vomiting.

YES See Doctor

 NO

Did constipation occur after taking prescribed or over-the-counter medicines, vitamins, herbal products, etc.? Or, does it worsen or not improve after 1 week of self-care?

YES Call Doctor

NO

 Use Self-Care

Self-Care / Prevention

- Eat foods high in dietary fiber. Examples are bran, whole-grain breads and cereals, and fresh fruits and vegetables.
- Drink at least 1$\frac{1}{2}$ to 2 quarts fluids every day. Have hot water, tea, etc. to stimulate the bowel.
- Get enough exercise.
- Don't resist the urge to pass stool.
- If you take antacids or iron supplements and get constipated easily, discuss the use of these with your doctor.
- Take stool softeners (e.g., Colace), fiber supplements (e.g., Metamucil), "stimulant" laxatives (e.g., Ex-Lax), or enemas, as directed on the label and by your doctor.

Diarrhea

Diarrhea occurs when body wastes are discharged from the bowel more often and in a more liquid state than usual.

Signs & Symptoms

- Frequent watery, loose stools.
- Cramping or pain in the abdomen.

Causes

Common causes are infections that affect the digestive system, food allergies, overuse of laxatives or alcohol, and taking some antibiotics. Diarrhea is also a symptom of lactose intolerance, diverticulitis, food poisoning, ulcerative colitis, Crohn's disease, and irritable bowel syndrome (IBS).

Treatment

Self-care treats most cases of diarrhea. If it is caused by a medical condition, treatment for the condition usually treats the diarrhea.

Questions to Ask

With diarrhea, does an adult have any of these problems?
- Bloody, maroon, or tarlike stools.
- Very severe abdominal or rectal pain.
- **Signs of severe dehydration** listed on page 372.

YES → Get Medical Care Fast

NO ↓

With diarrhea, does an infant or a child have any of these problems?
- Sunken eyes.
- Dry skin that doesn't spring back when pinched.
- Dry diaper for more than 3 hours in an infant.
- Passing no urine for more than 6 hours in a child.
- Weak cry. Acting very weak and very sleepy.
- Acting very upset or cranky.

YES → Get Medical Care Fast

NO ↓

Has the diarrhea lasted 48 hours or more and/or is a fever present? (See **Fever** on pages 226 and 227.)

YES → See Doctor

NO ↓

Does an infant or sick, elder person have diarrhea more than 8 times per day?

YES → Call Doctor

NO ↓

Flowchart continued on next page

Get more information from:

HealthyLearn®
www.HealthyLearn.com
Click on MedlinePlus®

National Institute of Diabetes and Digestive and Kidney Diseases (NIDDK)
www.niddk.nih.gov

Diarrhea, Continued

Are medicines being taken? (Medicines you take may not be working because of the diarrhea. Or, prescribed or over-the-counter ones, including herbal products, may be causing the diarrhea.)

YES Call Doctor

NO

Did diarrhea occur when you were in another country or shortly after coming back?

YES Call Doctor

NO

Use Self-Care

Self-Care / Prevention

- If you are also vomiting, treat this first. (See **Vomiting & Nausea** on pages 180 and 181.)

- Follow a light diet if there are no signs of dehydration. (See **Dehydration** on page 372.)

- Until the diarrhea subsides, avoid caffeine, milk products, and foods that are greasy, high in fiber, or very sweet.

- Don't exercise too hard until the diarrhea is gone.

- Adults can try an over-the-counter medicine, such as Imodium A-D or Pepto-Bismol. Follow the directions listed on the label. {*Note:* Stools can become black after taking Pepto-Bismol. Also, do not give aspirin or any medication that has salicylates, such as Pepto-Bismol, to anyone under 19 years of age, due to the link to Reye's Syndrome.}

- Wash your hands after you go to the toilet and before you prepare food. Use paper towels to dry your hands. Throw the towels away.

If There Are Signs of Dehydration

- Stop solid foods. Drink clear liquids. Fluids of choice are:
  - Broths; sport drinks like Gatorade; and Kool-Aid (this usually has less sugar than juices and soda pop).
  - For children under 2, give over-the-counter mixtures, such as Infalyte and Pedialyte as advised.
  - If you breast-feed, give only as much milk as your baby wants. Feed every 2 hours.

- Avoid giving these liquids:
  - High "simple" sugar drinks like apple juice, grape juice, regular colas, other sodas, and gelatin. These can pull water into the gut and make the diarrhea persist. If necessary, dilute clear juices and sodas with water.
  - Milk, especially if it is boiled.

- Avoid caffeine and alcohol.

- Adults should have around 2 cups of fluid per hour (if vomiting isn't present). For children under age 2, consult their doctor about the amount and type of fluids. For children over age 2, give up to 6 cups of fluid per day.

- Don't give just clear liquids for more than 48 hours.

- Start eating more solid meals within 12 hours. Start with foods that are easy to digest, such as rice, potatoes, crackers, and toast.

- Eat yogurt with live cultures of lactobacillus acidophilus (unless you are lactose intolerant). Choose foods that don't upset your stomach.

- Avoid fatty and fried foods.

- You don't need to follow a B.R.A.T. diet. The B.R.A.T. diet is having just bananas (ripe), rice, applesauce, and toast (dry). It is okay to eat these foods, though.

Diverticulosis & Diverticulitis

Sometimes small pouches bulge outward through weak spots in the colon. This is called **diverticulosis**. The pockets (called diverticula) can fill with intestinal waste. With **diverticulitis**, these pockets and areas around them get inflamed or infected.

Signs & Symptoms

For Diverticulosis
Often this has no symptoms. Some persons may have:

- Mild cramps.
- Bloating
- Constipation.
- Blood in the stool.

For Diverticulitis

- Severe cramping and bloating in the abdomen, usually on the lower left side. The pain is made worse with a bowel movement.
- Tenderness over the abdomen.
- Nausea.
- Fever.

Causes

A low fiber diet is thought to be the main cause. Constipation and overuse of laxatives may also play a role.

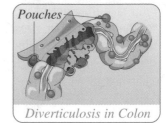
Pouches
Diverticulosis in Colon

Treatment

Diverticulitis needs medical treatment. *Diverticulosis* can't be cured, but self-care measures can reduce symptoms and prevent serious problems.

Questions to Ask

Do you have any of these problems?
- Very severe abdominal pain.
- **Signs of an intestinal obstruction**: Inability to pass stool or even gas; mild fever and weakness; abdominal cramps that come and go; the abdomen gets more and more swollen with increasing pain; hiccups that don't stop; and vomiting.
- Blood in the stool, tarlike, or maroon-colored stool.

YES **Get Medical Care Fast**

NO

Do you have any of these problems?
- Changes in bowel habits last longer than 2 weeks.
- Tenderness, pain, mild cramping, or a bloated feeling. These are usually felt in the lower left side of the abdomen.
- Gas. Nausea. Constipation.
- Pain in the abdomen and a fever. (See Fever on pages 226 and 227.)

YES **See Doctor**

NO

Use Self-Care

Self-Care / Prevention

- Get regular exercise. Drink 1½ to 2 quarts of water daily. Eat a diet high in fiber, but avoid foods that bother you (e.g., corn, nuts, etc.).

- Avoid the regular use of "stimulant" laxatives, such as Ex-Lax. Ask your doctor about taking bulk-forming laxatives like Metamucil.

- Try not to strain when you have bowel movements.

Flatulence (Gas)

Flatulence is passing gas through the anus. For the average adult, this happens about 6 to 20 times a day.

Signs & Symptoms

- Pressure or discomfort in the lower abdomen or anal area.
- Passing gas. A foul odor occurs sometimes.

Causes

Gas is caused by swallowing air and digesting foods. Eating high fiber foods like beans, peas, and whole-grains create more gas than other foods. Dairy foods can create large amounts of gas in some people.

Gas may signal other problems, too. These include lactose intolerance, taking certain antibiotics, and abnormal muscle movement in the colon.

Gas can also be a symptom of **celiac disease**. With this, the lining of the small intestine is damaged from eating **gluten**. This is a protein in wheat, barley, and rye. Other symptoms of celiac disease are pain and bloating in the abdomen; diarrhea; weight loss; anemia; and a certain skin rash. Treatment is a gluten-free diet. Find out about celiac disease from www.celiac.nih.gov.

Treatment

Self-care treats most cases of gas. If the gas is due to another problem, treating the problem reduces or gets rid of the gas.

Questions to Ask

With gas, do you have a steady pain in the upper abdomen with nausea and vomiting? Or, do the whites of your eyes or your skin look yellow?

YES →  **See Doctor**

NO ↓

Do you get a lot of gas only after taking a prescribed antibiotic?

YES → **Call Doctor**

NO ↓

 Use Self-Care

Self-Care / Prevention

- Try not to swallow air. Don't have carbonated drinks and chewing gum. These can cause more air to get into your stomach.
- When you add fiber to your diet, do so gradually.
- When you pass gas, note which foods you have eaten. Eat less of the foods that often cause gas. Common ones are apples, bran, whole-wheat foods, cabbage-family vegetables, eggs, dairy products, prunes, and beans.
- To prevent getting gas from many "gassy" foods, try an over-the-counter product, such as Beano. This helps prevent gas from beans, bran, nuts, onions, soy, and many vegetables.
- Try an over-the-counter medicine with simethicone, such as Gas-X.
- Release the gas when you need to. Go to another room if it will help you be less embarrassed.

Food Poisoning

Food Poisoning Chart		
Cause	**Signs & Symptoms**	**Prevention**
Botulism. Toxin from bacteria usually from eating improperly canned foods. Also found in honey and oils infused with garlic. Grows only in little or no oxygen.	Blurred vision. Double vision. A hard time speaking and swallowing. Breathing problems. Muscle weakness. Paralysis. Signs occur within 4 to 36 hours.	Follow proper canning methods. Boil home-canned food for 10 or more minutes. Don't eat foods from cans with leaks or bulges. Refrigerate oils infused with garlic or herbs. Don't give honey to children less than 1 year old.
E. coli. Bacteria from contaminated water, raw milk, raw or rare ground beef, unpasteurized apple juice or cider, or contact with contaminated animal feces.	Diarrhea or bloody discharge. Abdominal cramps. Nausea. Signs occur within 2 to 5 days and last about 8 days.	Don't drink unpasteurized milk and apple cider. Wash your hands after using the bathroom and cleaning up animal feces.
Listeria. Bacteria from unpasteurized milk, uncooked meats, foods contaminated during processing (cold cuts, hot dogs, soft cheeses).	Fever. Chills. Headache. Backache. Abdominal pain. Diarrhea. Often, signs occur within 48 to 72 hours, but can take up to 3 weeks to occur.	Don't drink unpasteurized milk. Cook beef to an internal temperature of 160°F.
Salmonella. Bacteria from raw or undercooked eggs, poultry, and meat and from food that comes in contact with contaminated surfaces.	Stomach pain. Diarrhea. Nausea. Chills. Fever. Headache. Signs occur within 8 to 12 hours and last up to 1 or 2 days.	Don't have unpasteurized milk, raw and undercooked eggs. Cook eggs to 160°F (the white and yolk are firm). Use clean utensils and surfaces.
Staphylococcal enterotoxin. Toxin from bacteria usually from meats, dairy foods, eggs, etc. that are not kept cold (e.g., unrefrigerated, at picnics, etc.) Also spread by human contact.	Severe nausea. Abdominal cramps. Diarrhea. Vomiting. Signs occur within 1 to 6 hours and last up to 3 days. Signs last longer if severe dehydration occurs.	Keep foods that can spoil cold (40°F or below) or hot (140°F or higher). Don't eat foods kept for more than 2 hours between 40°F and 140°F. Don't eat foods that look or smell spoiled. Wash your hands often. Use clean utensils and surfaces.
Chemicals. From foods with pesticides and eating poisonous mushrooms or poisonous plant leaves or berries.	Sweating. Dizziness. Mental confusion. Very teary eyes. Watery mouth. Stomach pain. Vomiting. Diarrhea. Signs start to occur within 30 minutes.	Wash raw fruits and vegetables before eating them. Don't store food or liquids in containers with lead-based paints. Don't store alcohol in lead crystal containers.

Food Poisoning Chart, continued on next page

Food Poisoning, Continued

Food Poisoning Chart		
Cause	**Signs & Symptoms**	**Prevention**
Hepatitis A virus. From contaminated water, raw and undercooked shellfish, oysters, clams, mussels, scallops, etc.	Appetite loss. Nausea. Vomiting. Fever. Jaundice and dark urine after 3 to 10 days. Liver damage and death from severe infection.	Hepatitis A vaccine. Don't eat raw or undercooked shellfish, oysters, etc.
Norwalk-like viruses. From food and touching objects contaminated with the virus. Direct contact with an infected person.	Nausea. Vomiting. Diarrhea. Stomach cramps. Signs occur within 12 to 48 hours and last up to 2 days.	Wash your hands often, especially after using the bathroom, changing diapers, and before handling food. Disinfect contaminated surfaces.
Mercury. From eating contaminated fish (e.g., shark, swordfish, tuna, king mackerel, tilefish).	Numbness and tingling in the lips, fingers, and toes. A hard time walking and speaking. Muscle weakness. Memory loss. Mental changes. Tremors.	Check local health department for safety of fish. Limit fish high in mercury. Pregnant women need to follow the advice of their doctor.

Treatment

Self-care treats most cases. Botulism, chemical food poisoning, and severe bacterial food poisoning need immediate care.

Questions to Ask

Do you have any of these problems?
- **Botulism symptoms** on page 158.
- **Signs of dehydration** listed on page 372.
- You vomit bright red blood or matter that looks like coffee grounds.
- You have bright red blood in diarrhea.
- You have a severe headache that persists, a stiff neck, or a convulsion.
- You are confused.

YES ▸ Get Medical Care Fast

NO

Flowchart continued in next column

Do you have any of these problems?
- Severe vomiting. Blood-streaked stools.
- Fever over 101°F.
- Pain has lasted for several hours or the pain gets worse.

YES ▸ See Doctor

NO

Do you vomit after having only ice chips for 12 hours? Or, do you still have diarrhea after using self-care for 2 days?

YES ▸ Call Doctor

NO

Use Self-Care

Self-Care / Prevention

- For chemical food poisoning, call the Poison Control Center (800.222.1222).

- See **Self-Care / Prevention** for **Vomiting and Nausea** on page 181; **Diarrhea** on page 155.

- Heed warnings for food products that could be harmful. News reports list these items. So does the FDA at *www.fda.gov*.

Gallstones

Signs & Symptoms

The gallbladder stores bile. This substance helps digest fats. **Gallstones** form when bile hardens

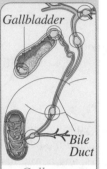

Gallbladder

Bile Duct

Gallstones

into pieces of stone-like material. These deposit in the gallbladder or bile ducts (which carry bile to the small intestine). The stones can range in size from less than a pinhead to 3 inches across.

- Feeling bloated and gassy, especially after eating fried or fatty foods.
- Steady pain in the upper right abdomen lasting 20 minutes to 5 hours.
- Pain between the shoulder blades or in the right shoulder.
- Indigestion. Nausea. Vomiting. Severe abdominal pain with fever. Sometimes a yellow color to the skin and/or the whites of the eyes.

{*Note:* Gallstone symptoms can be hard to tell apart from heart-related or other serious problems. A doctor should evaluate any new symptoms.}

Causes

- A family history of gallbladder disease. Middle age.
- Obesity. Very rapid weight loss.
- Being female. Having had many pregnancies. Taking estrogen.
- Having diabetes. Having diseases of the small intestine.

Treatment

- A low-fat diet.
- Medicines to dissolve the stones.
- **Lithotripsy**. This is the use of sound waves to shatter the stones.
- Surgery to remove the gallbladder. This is the most common treatment. You can still digest foods without a gallbladder.

Questions to Ask

Do you have any of these problems?
- The skin and the whites of your eyes are yellow in color.
- Pain in your upper right abdomen with vomiting and/or a fever. Or, the pain goes away and comes back.

YES See Doctor

NO Use Self-Care

Self-Care / Prevention

- Avoid high-fat foods. Don't eat large meals.
- Get to and stay at a healthy body weight. If you are overweight, lose weight slowly (1 to 1½ pounds per week). Do not follow a rapid weight loss diet unless under strict medical guidance.
- Eat a high fiber, low-fat diet.

Heartburn & Indigestion

Heartburn has nothing to do with the heart. It involves the esophagus and the stomach. The esophagus passes behind the breastbone alongside the heart. The irritation that takes place there feels like a burning feeling in the heart. **Indigestion** is a general term for discomfort in the abdomen that comes after eating.

Signs & Symptoms

- A burning feeling behind the breastbone occurs after eating.

- Chest pain is felt when you bend over or lie down.

- Your mouth has a bitter, hot, or sour taste.

Causes

Gastric acids from the stomach splash back up into the lower portion of the esophagus. This causes pain. The medical term for this is **gastroesophageal reflex disease (GERD)**. The digestive acids don't harm the stomach. It has a coating to protect it. The esophagus doesn't. Acids there cause pain.

Common Heartburn Triggers

- Aspirin, ibuprofen, naproxen sodium, arthritis medicine, or corticosteroids.

- Heavy meals. Eating too fast. Chocolate. Garlic. Onions. Peppermint. Tomatoes and citrus fruits.

- Smoking or lying down after eating.

- Drinking alcohol or coffee (regular or decaffeinated).

- Being very overweight.

- Wearing tight clothing.

- Swallowing too much air.

- Stress.

- Hiatal hernia. (See page 167.)

- Pregnancy.

Treatment

Self-care treats most cases of this common problem. Heartburn symptoms can be confused, though, with ones of a heart attack or other medical problems.

Questions to Ask

Does the heartburn come with any **heart attack warning sign** listed on page 387? **YES** → Get Medical Care Fast

NO ↓

Do you vomit blood or material that looks like coffee grounds? Or, are your stools tarlike, maroon, or bloody in color? **YES** → Get Medical Care Fast

NO ↓

With heartburn symptoms, do you also have pain that goes through to your back or a gripping pain in your upper abdomen? Or, do you feel lightheaded or did you faint? **YES** → Get Medical Care Fast

NO ↓

Flowchart continued on next page

Heartburn & Indigestion, Continued

With heartburn symptoms, is it hard for you to swallow? Has the heartburn occurred often over 3 days and/or has self-care brought no relief?

Self-Care / Prevention

■ Sit straight while you eat. Stand up or walk around after you eat. Bending over or lying down after you eat makes it too easy for stomach acids to move up to the esophagus.

■ Don't smoke.

■ Lose weight if you are overweight.

■ If heartburn bothers you at night, raise the head of the bed. Put the head of your bed up on 6-inch blocks. You can also buy a special wedge that is made to be placed between the mattress and box spring. Don't just prop your head up with pillows. This makes the problem worse by putting pressure on your stomach.

■ Don't wear garments that fit tight around the abdomen.

■ Eat small meals. Limit alcohol.

■ Limit foods and drinks with air. Examples are whipped cream and carbonated drinks.

■ Don't eat or drink for 2 to 3 hours before bedtime.

■ If you take aspirin, ibuprofen, naproxen sodium, or arthritis medicines, take them with food.

■ If other treatments fail, take antacids, such as Tums. If these don't bring relief, take an over-the-counter acid controller, such as Pepcid AC, Tagamet HB, etc. These prevent and relieve heartburn. {*Note:* Read labels before taking antacids or acid controllers. Check with your doctor, too. Adverse side effects are more likely and more severe in older persons who take some acid controllers, such as Tagamet HB.}

■ Don't take baking soda. It may help at first, but when its effects wear off, the acid comes back even worse.

Get more information from:

HealthyLearn®
www.HealthyLearn.com
Click on MedlinePlus®

National Institute of Diabetes and Digestive and Kidney Diseases (NIDDK)
www.niddk.nih.gov

Hemorrhoids

Hemorrhoids are veins in or outside of the anus that may become dilated or swollen.

Signs & Symptoms

- Bright red blood on or in the stool, on toilet paper, or in the toilet.
- Anal or rectal tenderness. Anal itching.
- Uncomfortable, painful bowel movements, especially with straining.
- A lump can be felt at the anus.
- Mucus passes from the anus.

Causes

Hemorrhoids are usually caused by repeated pressure in the rectal or anal veins. Often this is due to repeated straining to pass stool.

The risk for getting hemorrhoids increases with:
- Prolonged sitting on the toilet and straining to have a bowel movement.
- Constipation.
- A low dietary fiber intake.
- Obesity.

Treatment

Hemorrhoids are common. They are not likely to be a serious health problem. Most people have some bleeding from them once in a while.

Don't assume that rectal bleeding is "just hemorrhoids." See your doctor to find out the cause.

If symptoms of hemorrhoids are not relieved with self-care or with time, medical care may be needed. This includes:
- Laser heat or infrared light.
- Rubber band ligation. A rubber band is placed around the base of the hemorrhoid inside the rectum. The band cuts off blood flow to the hemorrhoid.
- Surgery.
- Cryosurgery. This freezes the affected tissue.

Questions to Ask

Do you have severe rectal bleeding that is nonstop or are you weak or dizzy because of it?

YES → Get Medical Care Fast

NO ↓

Do you have any of these problems?
- Rectal bleeding occurs with or without bowel movements and you don't know why.
- A hard lump is felt where a hemorrhoid used to be.
- Rectal pain is severe or lasts longer than a few days.
- The bleeding from a hemorrhoid lasts longer than 2 weeks despite using self-care.

YES → See Doctor

NO ↓

 Use Self-Care

Self-Care / Prevention continued on next page

Hemorrhoids, Continued

Self-Care / Prevention

- Drink at least 6 to 8 cups of fluid per day.

- Eat foods with good sources of dietary fiber, such as bran, whole-grain breads and cereals, vegetables, and fruits.

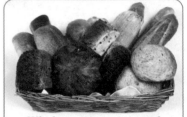

Whole grains are a good source of dietary fiber.

- Add bran to your foods. Add about 3 to 4 tablespoons per day.

- Eat prunes. Drink prune juice.

- Lose weight if you are overweight.

- Get regular exercise.

- Pass stool as soon as you feel the urge. If you wait and the urge goes away, your stool could become dry and hard. This makes it harder to pass.

- Don't strain to pass stool.

- Don't hold your breath when trying to pass stool.

- Keep the anal area clean. Use moist towelettes or wet (not dry) toilet paper after you pass stool.

- Don't sit too much. This can restrict blood flow around the anal area. Don't sit too long on the toilet. Don't read while on the toilet.

- For itching or pain, put a cold compress on the anus for 10 minutes at a time. Do this up to 4 times a day.

- Take warm baths or use a sitz bath with hot water. A sitz bath is a basin that fits over the toilet. Get one at a medical supply or drug store.

- Check with your doctor about using over-the-counter products, such as:

  - Stool softeners.
  - Zinc oxide or anesthetic (numbing) products, such as Preparation H.
  - Medicated wipes, such as Tucks.
  - Suppositories.

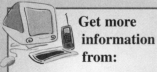

Get more information from:

HealthyLearn®
www.HealthyLearn.com
Click on MedlinePlus®

Hernias

A **hernia** occurs when body tissue "bulges" through a weak area or hole in a muscle. Often, this happens in the wall of the abdomen.

Common Hernias Include

- *Hiatal hernia.* (See page 167.)

- *Inguinal hernia.* A part of the intestine bulges through a muscle near the groin or scrotum.

- *Incisional hernia.* This is a bulge through a muscle at the site of a past surgical scar.

- *Femoral hernia.* This is a bulge in the top front of a thigh. It is most common in obese women.

- *Ventral hernia.* This is a bulge in the middle of the abdomen, usually near the navel.

Signs & Symptoms

- A bulge in the skin. The bulge may be more easy to see when you cough, lift, or strain, or when you lie flat on your back. The bulge may feel soft.

- Mild pain or discomfort at the hernia site. The pain may only be felt when you strain, lift, or cough. The pain can be extreme when the hernia bulges out and can't be pushed back in.

- For an inguinal hernia, weakness, pressure, burning, or pain in the groin area. A lump in the groin near the thigh may be seen when standing.

- Swelling of the scrotum.

Causes

A weakness in the wall of the abdomen is often the cause. Some persons are born with this problem. Hernias can run in families. Other causes include:

- Lifting heavy objects. Heavy coughing.

- Obesity.

- Straining to pass stool.

- Abdominal surgery.

- Being male or elderly.

Treatment

Treatment depends on the type and symptoms. Some hernias can be put back into the body. Others may need treatment with surgery.

Questions to Ask

Do you have any of these problems?
- Sudden, severe pain in the groin, scrotum, or the area of an existing hernia.
- You are unable to have a bowel movement or to pass gas.

YES — Get Medical Care Fast

NO

Do you have any of these problems?
- A bulge or swelling in the abdomen or groin.
- Mild groin pain lasts longer than a week.

YES — See Doctor

NO

Use Self-Care

Self-Care / Prevention continued on next page

Hernias, Continued

Self-Care / Prevention

▬ Don't smoke. If you smoke, quit. Avoid secondhand smoke.

▬ Maintain a healthy diet. Lose weight if you are overweight.

▬ Avoid constipation. (See **Self-Care / Prevention** in **Constipation** on page 153.) Don't strain to pass stool.

▬ Exercise to keep abdominal muscles strong. Follow your doctor's advice.

▬ When you do sit ups, keep your knees bent and your feet flat on the floor.

▬ Follow proper lifting techniques. (See the **Do's and Don'ts of Lifting** in **Back Pain** on page 187.)

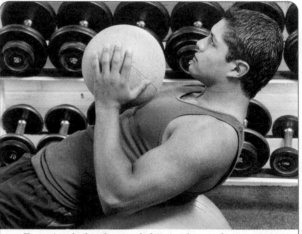

Exercise helps keep abdominal muscles strong.

▬ Wear a weight lifting belt to support the back when lifting.

▬ Wear a truss. This is a device that holds a hernia in place.

▬ For mild pain, take an over-the-counter medicine for pain. If even mild pain lasts longer than a week, see your doctor.

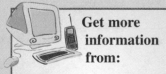

Get more information from:

HealthyLearn®
www.HealthyLearn.com
Click on MedlinePlus®

Hiatal Hernia

With a **hiatal hernia**, the normal action that closes off the top of the stomach does not work well. Food or stomach acids back up into the esophagus. This is known as **Gastroesophageal reflux disease (GERD)**.

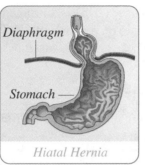

Diaphragm

Stomach

Hiatal Hernia

Signs & Symptoms

Many people have no symptoms with a hiatal hernia. Others have one or more of these problems:

- **Acid reflux.** Stomach acid backs up into the esophagus.

- Chest pain. {*Note:* Don't assume that chest pain is due to a hiatal hernia. See **Chest Pain** on page 216.}

- Pain in the esophagus. Heartburn.

- Hiccups. Belching after meals.

- A hard time swallowing.

Causes

The actual cause is not known. Risk factors are obesity, being a woman, or being middle aged. Smoking, lifting, strong coughing, and straining with bowel movements also increase the risk. So does having spicy foods, alcohol, and caffeine.

Treatment

Hiatal hernias are usually not serious problems. Often they can be treated with self-care. If not, surgery is an option.

Questions to Ask

Does a hiatal hernia cause pain at night often? Does it still bother you after using antacids and/or self-care?

YES → See Doctor

NO ↓

Use Self-Care

Self-Care / Prevention

- Don't smoke. If you smoke, quit.

- Get regular exercise. This helps keep abdominal muscles in shape.

- Lose weight if you are overweight.

- Eat 5 to 6 small meals a day instead of 3 larger meals.

- Avoid alcohol, caffeine, and spicy foods.

- Don't lie down after eating. Wait 2 to 3 hours.

- Raise the head of the bed 6 inches. Put 6 inch blocks under the legs of the head of the bed or put a 6 inch wedge between the mattress and box springs at the head portion. Don't prop your head up with pillows. Doing this puts pressure on your stomach area and can help force acid up into the esophagus.

- Don't strain to pass stool.

- Take over-the-counter antacids or acid controllers, such as Pepcid AC or Tagamet HB. {*Note:* Read the labels before taking. Check with your doctor, too. Adverse side effects are more likely and more severe in older persons who take some acid controllers, such as Tagamet HB.}

- If you take aspirin, ibuprofen, or naproxen sodium, take it with food.

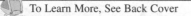

Irritable Bowel Syndrome (IBS)

Irritable bowel syndrome (IBS) is a problem that mostly affects the bowel (the large intestine). A person with IBS has bowel habit problems and abdominal pain. These are not caused by any other bowel disease.

Signs & Symptoms

- Gas, bloating, or pain in the abdomen. Crampy urge, but not being able to move the bowels.
- Constipation, diarrhea, (or both).
- Mucus in the stool.

Causes

The cause is not known. A person with IBS has a sensitive colon that responds strongly to stress, anxiety, smoking, certain foods, alcohol, and caffeine.

Treatment

Self-care helps in many cases. When this is not enough, medicines and psychotherapy may be prescribed to reduce spasms of the colon and to help relieve distress.

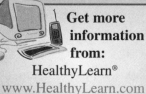

Get more information from:
HealthyLearn®
www.HealthyLearn.com
Click on MedlinePlus®

Questions to Ask

Do you have very severe abdominal pain or tarlike, maroon, or bloody-colored stools? **YES** **Get Medical Care Fast**

NO

Do you have any of these problems?
- A lot of mucus in your stools.
- A fever with cramps, pain in the abdomen, or diarrhea.
- Unwanted weight loss.
- IBS symptoms change a lot or get worse.

YES **See Doctor**

NO

Use Self-Care

Self-Care / Prevention

- Don't smoke. If you smoke, quit. Avoid secondhand smoke.
- Keep a log of when symptoms occur. Avoid things that trigger symptoms. Common ones are having: Large meals; fried foods; kidney and other beans; cabbage; broccoli; dairy products with milk sugar (lactose); chocolate; spicy foods; and the artificial sweetener sorbitol.
- Manage stress. (See **Manage Stress** on page 53.)
- Eat foods with dietary fiber (whole-grain breads and cereals and fruits and vegetables). Kidney beans and other beans are a good source if they do not cause IBS symptoms for you. Talk to your doctor about over-the-counter fiber pills or powders that you mix with water. {*Note:* Add all types of fiber slowly. Too much, too soon, can worsen symptoms.}
- Drink lots of water. Don't have alcohol and caffeine.
- Get enough rest. Get regular exercise.
- Take an over-the-counter pain reliever as directed. Put a hot water bottle or heating pad (set on low) on your abdomen. Try to relax.

Kidney Stones

Kidney stones are hard masses of mineral deposits formed in the kidney(s). They can be as small as a tiny pebble or an inch or more across. They are more common in men.

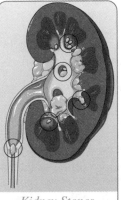

Kidney Stones

Signs & Symptoms

Some kidney stones cause no symptoms. Small ones can be passed, without pain, when you urinate. When symptoms occur, they include:

- Crampy pain that comes and goes. The pain starts in the lower back, travels down the side of the abdomen, and into the groin area. The pain can be severe.

- Bloody, cloudy, or dark-colored urine.

- You may need to pass urine often. You may pass only small amounts of urine. You may only be able to pass urine in certain positions.

- Nausea and vomiting. Fever and chills (if an infection is also present).

Causes

- Too much calcium in the urine or in the blood.

- High levels of uric acid in the blood. (See **Gout** on page 182.)

- A diet high in oxalic acid. This is in spinach, leafy vegetables, rhubarb, and coffee.

- Repeated urinary tract infections.

- Mild dehydration that persists.

- Family history of kidney stones.

- Living in certain parts of the U.S. Areas of the southeast have the highest rates.

In some cases, the cause is not known.

Treatment

Treatment includes drinking plenty of fluids and taking medicines to reduce stone-forming substances in the blood and urine. **Lithotripsy** may be done. With this, shock waves break the stone into fragments. A urologist may retrieve a stone by inserting a catheter and scope into the urinary tract.

Questions to Ask

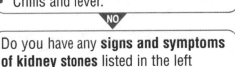

Do you have these problems?
- Severe pain in your back or side that does not go away.
- Chills and fever.

YES → Get Medical Care Fast

NO

Do you have any **signs and symptoms of kidney stones** listed in the left column of this page?

YES → See Doctor

NO

Use Self-Care

Self-Care / Prevention

- Drink lots of fluids. Drink at least 8 to 10 glasses of water a day.

- Eat a well-balanced diet. Vary food choices.

Save any stone you pass so your doctor can have it tested. If you've had a kidney stone, you're prone to getting more. Follow your doctor's advice for diet and prescribed medicines.

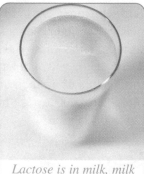

Lactose Intolerance

Lactose is the natural sugar in milk. A person with **lactose intolerance** lacks enough of the enzyme, lactase, to digest this sugar.

Signs & Symptoms

- Nausea.
- Cramps.
- Bloating.
- Gas.
- Diarrhea.

These symptoms start about 30 minutes to 2 hours after you eat or drink foods with lactose.

Treatment

Symptoms can be controlled with self-care measures.

Causes

- The body can't make the enzyme lactase. This can occur from birth or over time.
- Digestive diseases.
- Injury to the small intestine.

Asian Americans, African Americans, and American Indians are more prone to lactose intolerance.

Lactose is in milk, milk products, and dairy whey.

Questions to Ask

Are nausea, cramps, bloating, gas, and/or diarrhea not controlled with self-care?

 YES See Doctor

 NO Use Self-Care

Self-Care / Prevention

- Eat fewer dairy foods. Some people with lactose intolerance can tolerate dairy foods if they have small amounts at a time.
- Have lactose-free dairy products. Have ones that reduce lactose with bacterial cultures. Examples are buttermilk, yogurt, and acidophilus milks.
- Take over-the-counter drops or pills that have the enzyme lactase when you have dairy foods.
- If the above measures don't help, don't have products with milk, milk solids, and dairy whey. Have soy milk instead. Products marked "parve" are milk free.
- Read food labels. Many food products contain small amounts of lactose. These include bread and other baked goods, instant mashed potatoes, breakfast and diet drinks and bars, and mixes for biscuits, cookies, and pancakes.

Get more information from:

HealthyLearn®
www.HealthyLearn.com
Click on MedlinePlus®

Peptic Ulcers

A **peptic ulcer** is a sore in the stomach or first part of the small bowel.

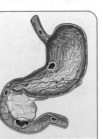

Peptic Ulcers

Signs & Symptoms

- A gnawing or burning pain is felt in the abdomen between the breastbone and navel. The pain often occurs between meals and in the early hours of the morning. It may last from a few minutes to a few hours and may be relieved with eating or antacids.

- Appetite and weight loss.

- Nausea or vomiting dark, red blood or material that looks like coffee grounds.

- Bloody, black, or tarry stools.

- Paleness and weakness if anemia is present.

Causes

- An infection with *Helicobacter pylori* (*H. pylori*) bacteria. This is the main cause.

- The repeated use of aspirin and other nonsteroidal anti-inflammatory drugs (NSAIDs), such as ibuprofen and naproxen sodium.

A small percentage of peptic ulcers are caused by **Zollinger-Ellison Syndrome**. With this rare disorder, the body makes excess acid.

Family history, smoking, caffeine, and making excess digestive acids play a role in peptic ulcers. So does stress, especially some types of physical stress (e.g., severe burns and major surgery).

Treatment

Treatment includes medicines to treat the problem and surgery, if needed.

Questions to Ask

Do you have any of these problems?
- Sudden, severe pain in the abdomen. It may be felt in the upper left stomach area below the ribs or below the ribs on the right side.
- You vomit bright red blood or material that looks like coffee grounds.
- Your stools are bloody, black, or tarry and you are very tired, pale, and weak.

YES Get Medical Care Fast

NO

Do you still have symptoms after getting treatment? Or, do you still have problems after using self-care?

YES See Doctor

NO

 Use Self-Care

Self-Care / Prevention

- Take medications as prescribed.

- Eat healthy foods. Include foods high in fiber.

- Don't have coffee (regular and decaffeinated); tea and soft drinks with caffeine; and fruit juices high in acid like tomato juice. Don't have alcohol or foods that bother you.

- Don't use aspirin and other NSAIDs. Follow your doctor's advice for prescribed NSAIDs.

- Try over-the-counter antacids or acid controllers (with your doctor's okay). Use them on a short-term basis. Don't try to self-medicate an ulcer.

- Don't smoke. If you smoke, quit.

Rectal Problems

The rectum is the lowest part of the large bowel (colon). The opening of the rectum is the anus. Stool are passed from the anus.

Signs & Symptoms

- Rectal pain.
- Rectal bleeding.
- Anal itching.
- Redness, swelling, or a rash in the rectal area.

Causes

For Anal / Rectal Pain and/or Bleeding

- Constipation. Straining to pass stool. Hemorrhoids.
- Anal fissures. These are splits or tears in the skin around the anus.
- Polyps or small growths.
- Injury due to anal intercourse or the insertion of a foreign object.
- Blockage in the intestines.
- Colon or rectal cancer.

For Anal / Rectal Itching

- Dry skin. Products that irritate or cause a skin allergy in the anal area. Examples are over-the-counter anesthetic ointments that end in "caine," such as benzocaine.
- **Hemorrhoids.** (See page 163.)
- **Psoriasis**. This is a chronic skin disease. With this, itchy, scaly red patches form on a part of the body.
- **Pinworms**. These are intestinal parasites. They usually affect children. The anal itching is at night and can be painful.
- A fungal infection.

Often there is no clear cause. Persons with diabetes and liver disease are more prone to rectal itching.

Treatment

Treatment for rectal problems depends on the cause. Any sign of rectal bleeding should be evaluated by a doctor. This includes blood on toilet paper. Colon cancer should be checked for, despite the person's age or family history of this disease.

Rectal Problems, Continued

Questions to Ask

Do you have any of these problems?
- Bright red blood in the stools (not just on toilet paper) with dizziness, nausea and vomiting, shortness of breath, and/or severe abdominal pain, cramps, and swelling.
- Rectal bleeding is heavy or dark maroon or black in color.
- Rape or sexual abuse has occurred.
- A foreign object is not able to be removed from the rectum.

YES → Get Medical Care Fast

NO

Does rectal bleeding occur with any of these conditions?
- Sudden onset of severe and constant pain and a purple-colored hemorrhoid that bleeds easily.
- Bright red blood after an injury, intercourse, or having something put up the rectum.
- Between bowel movements.
- After taking a new medicine or returning from another country.

YES → See Doctor

NO

Does rectal pain occur with any of these problems?
- The pain is severe or lasts longer than a few days.
- Anal spasms occur after passing stool.
- Diarrhea or mucus discharge.
- Swelling or itching in the anal area.

YES →  See Doctor

NO

Flowchart continued in next column

Are any of these problems present, especially in a child?
- Small (¼ to ½ inch) white worms in the stools or around the anal area.
- Pain and itching at night.
- Acting cranky. Restless sleep.

YES → Call Doctor

NO

Do rectal pain and/or itching still bother you after using self-care?

YES → Call Doctor

NO

 Use Self-Care

Self-Care / Prevention

For Anal / Rectal Bleeding
- Don't lift heavy things.
- Stop taking anti-inflammatory medicines and/or aspirin (unless prescribed and monitored by your doctor).
- Don't strain to pass stool.

For Anal / Rectal Itching
- Practice good hygiene. Clean the rectal area daily.
- Use an over-the-counter ointment, such as one with zinc oxide or one for hemorrhoids, such as Preparation H. Follow package directions.
- Wear clothes and undergarments that fit loosely.
- Take a warm bath or sitz bath. A sitz bath is a shallow, warm water bath. You can get a sitz bath device from a medical supply company and some drug stores. Then dry the rectal area well. Use talcum powder, as needed.

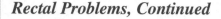

Rectal Problems, Continued

Limiting these items may help with anal / rectal itching:
- Caffeine.
- Colas.
- Citrus fruits.
- Chocolate.
- Alcohol.
- Spicy foods.

■ Take warm tub baths.

■ Lose weight if you are overweight.

■ If you are diabetic, keep blood sugar under control.

■ For pinworms:
- Check for pinworms in this way: In a dark room, a few hours after bedtime, shine a flashlight on the anus. Pinworms, if present, will go back into the anus when the flashlight is shined on them.

- Wash the hands often.

- Keep fingernails closely trimmed.

- Try to get your child to not suck his thumb and not bite his nails.

- Wash underwear and bed linen in hot soapy water.

- If medication for pinworms is prescribed, use it as directed.

For Rectal Pain

■ Take warm baths.

■ Use a warm water sitz bath for 15 minutes, 2 to 3 times a day.

■ Put towels soaked in warm water on the anal area. Or, apply a cold compress to the painful area, if this helps with the pain.

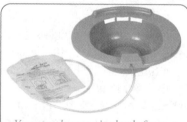

You can buy a sitz bath from a medical supply or drug store.

■ Follow measures to prevent **constipation**. (See page 153.)

■ Don't strain to pass stool.

■ Keep the rectal area clean.

■ Use soft, plain, unscented, two-ply toilet paper. Take your own toilet paper to work or other places that may use harsh paper. Use wet, not dry, toilet paper, if that helps.

■ Use an over-the-counter wipe, such as Tucks, after using toilet paper.

■ Don't sit for long periods of time. When you do sit, raise your legs, as often as you can.

■ If needed, take an over-the-counter medicine for pain as directed.

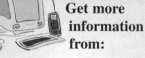

Get more information from:

HealthyLearn®
www.HealthyLearn.com
Click on MedlinePlus®

Urinary Incontinence

Urinary incontinence means you lose bladder control or can't store urine like you should.

This problem is not a normal part of aging. It often affects older persons because muscles used in bladder control don't work as well with aging.

Signs, Symptoms & Causes

For Acute Incontinence

This form comes on suddenly. Often, it is a symptom of a new illness or problem. Examples are a bladder infection, diabetes (new or out-of-control), and inflammation of the prostate, urethra, or vagina. It can also be a side effect of some medicines, such as water pills.

This form is often easily reversed when the problem that caused it is treated.

For Persistent Incontinence

This form comes on gradually over time. It lingers or remains, even after other problems have been treated. There are many types of this form. The ones below cause 80% of cases.

- *Stress Incontinence.* Urine leaks out when there is a sudden rise in pressure in the abdomen. This can happen when you cough, sneeze, laugh, lift, jump, run, or strain to pass stool. This type is more common in women than in men.

- *Urge Incontinence.* With this type, the urge to pass urine is so strong and comes on so fast, that the urine is released before you can get to the toilet. This type can be caused by an enlarged prostate gland, a spinal cord injury, or an illness, such as Parkinson's disease.

- *Mixed Incontinence.* This type is a mix of stress and urge types of incontinence.

- *Overflow Incontinence.* This is the constant dribbling of urine because the bladder overfills. This may be due to an enlarged prostate, diabetes, or multiple sclerosis.

- *Functional Incontinence.* With this type, you have trouble getting to the bathroom fast enough, even though you have bladder control. This can happen in a person who is physically challenged.

- *Total Incontinence.* This is a rare type with complete loss of bladder control. Urine leakage can be constant.

Treatment

The first step is to find out if another problem causes the incontinence and to treat that problem. Other treatments include:

- Pelvic floor exercises, called **Kegel exercises**. (See page 177.)

- Medication.

- Collagen injections. These treat a certain type of stress incontinence.

- Surgery, as needed, to correct the problem.

Urinary Incontinence, Continued

Overactive Bladder

With this condition, you have at least 2 of these problems:

- An urgency to pass urine.
- Urge incontinence. (See page 175.)
- You pass urine 8 or more times a day and 2 or more times during night.

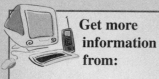

Get more information from:

HealthyLearn®
www.HealthyLearn.com
Click on MedlinePlus®

National Association for Continence (NAFC)
800.BLADDER
    (252.3337)
www.nafc.org

American Urological Association (AUA) Foundation
866.RING.AUA
(866.746.4282)
www.auafoundation.org

Questions to Ask

Does loss of bladder control occur with any of these problems?
- A spine or back injury.
- Slurred speech or not being able to speak.
- Loss of sight. Double or blurred vision.
- Sudden, severe headaches.
- Paralysis, weakness, or loss of feeling in an arm or leg, and/or the face on the same side of the body.
- Change in personality, behavior, and/or emotions.
- Confusion and dizziness.
- Sudden new seizures with collapse and shaking of the limbs.

YES → Get Medical Care Fast

NO ↓

Does loss of bladder control come with **symptoms of a kidney infection** listed on page 178?

YES →  Get Medical Care Fast

NO ↓

With loss of bladder control, are any of these problems present?
- Recent surgery or injury to the abdomen.
- It burns when you pass urine or you pass urine often.
- Urine is cloudy or has blood in it.
- Pain in the abdomen or mid back.
- Fever and/or chills.
- Diabetes or **signs and symptoms of diabetes** listed on page 220.

YES → See Doctor

NO ↓

For men, are **signs and symptoms of prostate problems** listed on page 294 present?

YES → Call Doctor

NO ↓

Do you leak urine when you cough, sneeze, laugh, jump, run, or lift heavy objects?

YES → Call Doctor

NO ↓

Did you lose bladder control after you took a new medicine or took a higher dose of one you were already taking?

YES → Call Doctor

NO ↓

 Use Self-Care

See Self-Care / Prevention on next page

Urinary Incontinence, Continued

Self-Care / Prevention

- Don't have caffeine. Limit or avoid fluids 2 to 3 hours before bedtime.

- Limit carbonated drinks, alcohol, citrus juices, greasy and spicy foods, and items with artificial sweeteners.

- Empty your bladder before you leave the house, take a nap, or go to bed.

- Go to the bathroom often, even if you don't feel the urge. When you pass urine, empty the bladder as much as you can. Relax for 1 to 2 minutes. Then try to pass urine again.

- Keep a diary of when you leak urine. If you find that you have accidents every 3 hours, empty your bladder every 2 hours. Use an alarm clock or wristwatch with an alarm to remind you.

- Wear clothes you can pull down easily when you use the bathroom. Wear elastic-waist bottoms. Wear items with velcro closures or snaps instead of buttons and zippers.

- Wear absorbent pads or briefs, if needed.

- Keep the pathway to your bathroom free of clutter and well lit. Leave the bathroom door open until you use it. Use a night light in the bathroom when it is dark.

- Use an elevated toilet seat and grab bars if these will make it easier for you to get on and off the toilet.

- Keep a bedpan, plastic urinal (for men), or portable commode chair near your bed.

- Ask your doctor if your type of incontinence could be managed by using self-catheters. These help to empty your bladder all the way. A doctor needs to prescribe self-catheters.

Kegel Exercises

Kegel exercises are pelvic floor exercises. These help treat or cure stress incontinence. Persons who have leaked urine for years can benefit greatly from these exercises. How do you do them?

- First, start to urinate, then hold back and try to stop. If you can slow the stream of urine, you are using the right muscles. You should feel muscles squeeze around the urethra and the anus. The urethra is the tube through which urine is passed. The anus is the opening through which stool is passed.

- Next, relax your body, and close your eyes. Imagine that you are going to pass urine, but hold back from doing so. You should feel the muscles squeeze like you did in the step before this one.

- Squeeze the muscles for 3 seconds. Then relax them for 3 seconds. When you squeeze and relax, count slowly. Start out doing this 3 times a day. Gradually work up to 3 sets of 10 contractions. Hold each one for 10 seconds at a time. You can do them when you lie down, and/or stand.

- When you do these exercises, do not tense the muscles in your belly or buttocks. Do not hold your breath, clench your fists or teeth, or make a face.

- Squeeze your pelvic floor muscles right before and during whatever it is (coughing, sneezing, jumping, etc.) that causes you to lose urine. Relax the muscles once the activity is over.

- Women can also use pelvic weights prescribed by their doctor. A women inserts a weighted cone into the vagina and squeezes the correct muscles to keep the weight from falling out.

It may take several months to benefit from pelvic floor exercises. They should be done daily.

Urinary Tract Infections (UTIs)

Urinary tract infections (UTIs) are ones that occur in any organs that make up the urinary tract. The kidneys filter waste products from the blood and make urine. Ureters connect the kidney to the bladder. This holds urine until it is passed.

Signs & Symptoms

- A strong need to pass urine.

- You pass urine more often than usual.

- A sharp pain or burning feeling when you pass urine.

- Bloody or cloudy urine.

- It feels like your bladder is still full after you pass urine.

- Pain in the abdomen, back, or sides.

- Chills. Fever.

- Nausea or vomiting.

- A change in mental status, especially if you are over age 70.

Sometimes there are no symptoms with a UTI.

Causes

UTIs result when bacteria infect any part of the urinary tract. The bladder is the most common site.

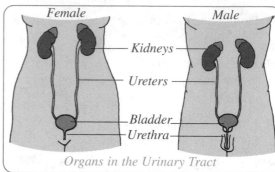

Organs in the Urinary Tract

Persons at Greater Risk for UTIs

- Sexually active females.

- Females who use a diaphragm for birth control.

- Males and females who have had UTIs in the past.

- Anyone with a condition that doesn't allow urine to pass freely. An enlarged prostate gland (in males) and kidney stones are examples.

Treatment

An antibiotic is prescribed to treat the specific infection. Pain relievers are taken as needed. If you get UTIs often, your doctor may order medical tests to find out the problem.

Questions to Ask

Do you have these **symptoms of a kidney infection**?
- Fever and shaking chills.
- Pain in one or both sides of your mid back.
- Nausea and vomiting.

YES → 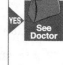 Get Medical Care Fast

NO ↓

Do you have any of these **symptoms of a bladder infection**?
- It burns or stings when you pass urine.
- You pass urine a lot more often than usual, often in small amounts.
- Your urine is bloody, cloudy, or foul-smelling.
- You have pain in the abdomen or over your bladder.

YES → See Doctor

NO ↓

Flowchart continued on next page

Urinary Tract Infections (UTIs), Continued

Have you had more than 3 bladder infections within 6 months or more than 4 bladder infections in the same year? **YES** See Doctor

NO

After taking prescribed medicine for a UTI, do symptoms not clear up over 3 days? Or, did the prescribed medicine give you side effects, such as a skin rash or a vaginal yeast infection? **YES** Call Doctor

NO

 Use Self-Care

Self-Care / Prevention

To Treat a Urinary Tract Infection (UTI)

■ Drink at least 8 glasses of water a day.

■ Drink juice made from unsweetened cranberry juice concentrate. Take cranberry tablets. (Get these at health food stores.)

■ Don't have alcohol, spicy foods, and caffeine.

■ Get plenty of rest.

■ Take an over-the-counter (OTC) medicine for pain or one that relieves pain and spasms that come with a bladder infection (e.g., Uristat). {*Note:* Uristat helps with symptoms, but doesn't get rid of the infection. See your doctor for diagnosis and treatment.}

■ Go to the bathroom as soon as you feel the urge. Empty your bladder all the way.

■ Don't have sex until the infection is cleared up.

To Help Prevent UTIs

■ Drink plenty of water and other fluids every day. Cranberry juice may help prevent bladder infections.

■ Empty your bladder as soon as you feel the urge.

■ Drink a glass of water before you have sex. Go to the bathroom as soon as you can after sex.

■ If you're prone to UTIs, don't take bubble baths.

■ If you're female, wipe from front to back after using the toilet. This helps keep bacteria away from the opening of the urethra. If you use a diaphragm, clean it after each use. Have your health care provider check your diaphragm periodically to make sure it fits properly.

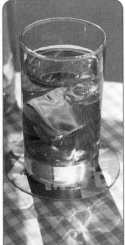

Drink cranberry juice and other liquids that do not have caffeine.

 Get more information from:

HealthyLearn®
www.HealthyLearn.com
Click on MedlinePlus®

National Institute of Diabetes and Digestive and Kidney Diseases (NIDDK)
www.niddk.nih.gov

Vomiting & Nausea

Signs & Symptoms

- **Vomiting** is throwing up the stomach's contents. Dry heaves may precede or follow vomiting.

- **Nausea** is when you feel like you're going to throw up.

Causes

- Viruses in the intestines. Eating spoiled food or eating or drinking too much.

- A side effect of some medications, such as certain antibiotics.

- Motion sickness. Morning sickness in pregnant females.

- **Labyrinthitis.** This is inflammation of an area in the ear. Often, a respiratory infection causes this.

- **Migraine headaches.** (See page 228.)

- **Acute glaucoma.** (See page 72.)

- Stomach ulcers. (See **Peptic Ulcers** on page 171.)

- Bowel obstruction.

- A concussion from a head injury.

- **Hepatitis.** (See page 236.)

- **Meningitis.** This is inflammation of membranes that cover the brain and spinal cord.

Questions to Ask

With vomiting, do you have any of these problems?
- Any **heart attack warning sign** listed on page 387.
- One or more **symptoms of meningitis** listed on page 101.
- You vomit true, red blood or material that looks like coffee grounds.

YES → Get Medical Care Fast

NO

With vomiting, do you have any of these problems?
- Sudden, severe pain in and around one eye, blurred vision, headache, and you see rainbow-colored halos around lights.
- Fainting or decreased level of consciousness.
- A head or abdominal injury happened a short time ago.

YES → Get Medical Care Fast

NO

Do you have **signs of dehydration** listed on page 372? **YES** → Get Medical Care Fast

NO

Flowchart continued on next page

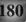

Vomiting & Nausea, Continued

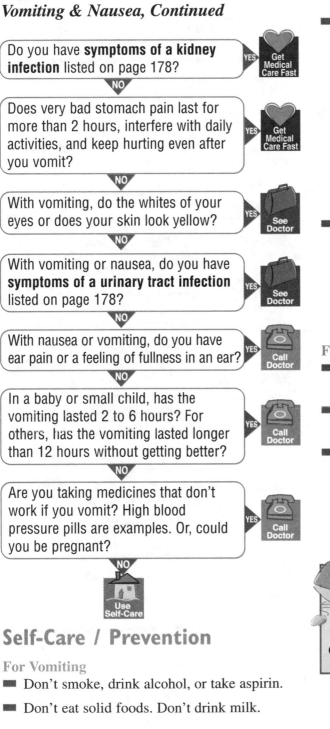

Do you have **symptoms of a kidney infection** listed on page 178?

YES → Get Medical Care Fast

NO ↓

Does very bad stomach pain last for more than 2 hours, interfere with daily activities, and keep hurting even after you vomit?

YES → Get Medical Care Fast

NO ↓

With vomiting, do the whites of your eyes or does your skin look yellow?

YES → See Doctor

NO ↓

With vomiting or nausea, do you have **symptoms of a urinary tract infection** listed on page 178?

YES → See Doctor

NO ↓

With nausea or vomiting, do you have ear pain or a feeling of fullness in an ear?

YES → Call Doctor

NO ↓

In a baby or small child, has the vomiting lasted 2 to 6 hours? For others, has the vomiting lasted longer than 12 hours without getting better?

YES → Call Doctor

NO ↓

Are you taking medicines that don't work if you vomit? High blood pressure pills are examples. Or, could you be pregnant?

YES → Call Doctor

NO ↓

Use Self-Care

Self-Care / Prevention

For Vomiting

- Don't smoke, drink alcohol, or take aspirin.

- Don't eat solid foods. Don't drink milk.

- Drink clear liquids at room temperature (not too hot or cold). Good examples are water; sport drinks, such as Gatorade; diluted fruit juices; ginger ale, etc. Take small sips. Drink only 1 to 2 ounces at a time. Stir carbonated beverages to get all the bubbles out before you sip them. Suck on ice chips if nothing else will stay down. {*Note:* For children, contact your child's doctor about using over-the-counter (OTC) mixtures, such as Pedialyte.}

- Gradually return to a regular diet, but wait about 8 hours from the last time you vomited. Start with foods like dry toast, crackers, rice, and other foods that are easy to digest. Or, eat foods as tolerated. Avoid greasy or fatty foods.

For Nausea Without Vomiting

- Drink clear liquids. Eat small amounts of dry foods, such as soda crackers, if they help.

- Avoid things that irritate the stomach, such as alcohol and aspirin.

- For motion sickness, use an over-the-counter medicine, such as Dramamine. You could also try Sea-Bands, a wrist band product that uses acupressure on a certain point on the wrist to control motion sickness. Sporting goods stores and drugstores sell Sea-Bands.

Get more information from:

HealthyLearn® • www.HealthyLearn.com
Click on MedlinePlus®

Chapter 14

Muscle & Bone Problems

Arthritis

Arthritis refers to over 100 disorders of the joints. The chart below gives information on common types of arthritis.

Types of Arthritis	Signs & Symptoms	Causes & Risk Factors
Osteoarthritis. This is the most common type.	• Joint pain and stiffness in the hands, knees, ankles, etc. • Finger joints with knobby growths. • Swollen joints (sometimes).	• Wear and tear on joints. • Injuries and overuse of joint(s). • Being overweight. • Family history of the disease.
Rheumatoid Arthritis (RA). This is the most disabling type. Besides the joints, RA can affect the lungs, eyes, spleen, skin, and heart.	• Morning stiffness that lasts longer than an hour. • Swelling in 3 or more joints. • Swelling of the same joints on both sides of the body, such as both knees or both wrists. • Joint tenderness, warmth, or redness.	The exact cause is not known. It may be due to a fault in the immune system that causes the body to attack its own cells. Risk factors include: • Chronic swelling of the membranes that line the joints. • Family history of the disease.
Gout. This is most common in men over age 30. In women, it usually occurs after menopause.	• Sudden, intense pain in a joint, often in the big toe. • Swollen joint. • The joint area is red or purple in color, feels warm, and is tender to the touch. An attack can last hours to days.	Gout occurs when crystals from high blood levels of a body waste product (uric acid) form in the joints. The body's immune system treats these crystals like a foreign substance.
Ankylosing Spondylitis. This type most often affects young men between the ages of 15 and 45.	• Stiff backbone. • Low back pain. • Stiff, bent posture. • Breathing problems. • Swelling of the iris of the eye.	• Family history of the disease. • In some cases, it has been linked with inflammatory bowel disease. • Joints in the spine start growing together.

Arthritis, Continued

Treatment

Treatment depends on the type and how severe it is. In general, treatment includes:

- An exercise program, as needed. Exercises done in water are very helpful and soothing.

- Medicines to help relieve pain and reduce swelling. For gout, medicine to lower blood uric acid.

- Healthy diet. Weight loss, if overweight.

- Physical therapy.

- Surgery. When needed, damaged joints can be repaired or replaced with artificial ones.

Questions to Ask

Do you have black, tarry stools, and/or stomach pain after taking medicines for arthritis? **YES** → See Doctor

NO ↓

Is the skin over a joint red and shiny or do you have these problems?
- Increased pain, redness, and/or swelling of one or more joints.
- Fever and you feel sick.
YES → See Doctor

NO ↓

In a child with joint pain or swelling, do any of these problems occur?
- Pain and swelling about 2 inches below the knee cap.
- The child limps from pain in a knee or hip or the child cannot run or use an arm or hand.
YES → See Doctor

NO ↓

Are **signs and symptoms of any type of arthritis** listed on page 182 present? **YES** → See Doctor

NO ↓

Flowchart continued in next column

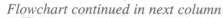
To Learn More, See Back Cover

Do joint pain and stiffness prevent normal activities? Or, do symptoms not improve with prescribed treatment? **YES** → Call Doctor

NO ↓

Use Self-Care

Self-Care / Prevention

- Follow your doctor's advice on exercise.

- Take OTC and prescribed medicines as your doctor advises. Ask about supplements, such as glucosamine and flaxseed oil. Discuss products that promise to "cure" arthritis with your doctor. Do this before you try any of them.

- Follow a healthy diet. Lose weight if you are overweight. Do not fast, though. This can raise uric acid levels and increase the risk for gout.

- Don't do activities that put too much stress on your joints. Take regular breaks. Protect the joints from injury. Wear knee pads, etc.

To Prevent Osteoarthritis
- Get to and stay at a healthy weight.

- Get regular exercise. (See **Be Physically Active** on page 42.) Don't overdo it, though. If you feel pain, stop.

- Prevent falls (see page 54) and sports injuries (see page 406).

Get more information from:

HealthyLearn® • www.HealthyLearn.com
Click on MedlinePlus®

Arthritis Foundation
800.283.7800 • www.arthritis.org

Back Pain

Signs & Symptoms

Back pain can be:
- Sharp.
- Dull.
- Acute.
- Chronic.

There may also be swelling in the back area.

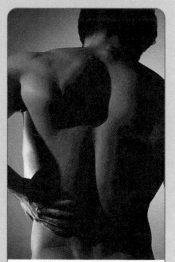

Back pain can be felt on one or both sides of the back.

Causes

The most common cause is muscle strain of the lower back. Other causes include back injuries, osteoarthritis, osteoporosis, and bladder infections.

Treatment

Most backaches are caused by strained muscles and ligaments and can be treated with self-care. (See **Self-Care / Prevention** on pages 185 to 187.) Other causes need a medical evaluation and treatment specific to the problem.

The goals of treatment are to treat the cause, relieve the pain, promote healing, and avoid re-injury.

Questions to Ask

Did the back pain start inside the chest and move to the upper back? (This could be a sign of a heart attack.) **YES** Get Medical Care Fast

NO

Is the back pain extreme and felt across the whole upper back? Did it come on suddenly (within about 15 minutes) without a reason, such as an injury or back strain? (These may be **symptoms of a dissecting aortic aneurysm**.) **YES** Get Medical Care Fast

NO

Was the back pain sudden with a cracking sound? Or, does the pain occur with passing out and/or severe abdominal pain? **YES** Get Medical Care Fast

NO

Did the pain come after a recent fall, injury, or violent movement to the back and are you having a hard time moving your arm or leg? Do you also have numbness or tingling in your legs, feet, toes, arms, or hands, and/or loss of bladder or bowel control? **YES** Get Medical Care Fast

NO

Flowchart continued on next page

Back Pain, Continued

Did the pain come on all of a sudden after being in a wheelchair or a long stay in bed or are you over 60 years old? **YES** See Doctor

NO

Is the pain severe (but not a result from a fall or injury to the back) and has it lasted for more than 5 to 7 days? Or, is there also a sense of weakness, numbness, or tingling in the feet or toes? **YES** See Doctor

NO

Do you have **symptoms of kidney stones** listed on page 169 or **symptoms of a bladder infection** listed on page 178? **YES**  See Doctor

NO

Does the pain travel down the leg(s), especially below the knee(s)? **YES** See Doctor

NO

Does it hurt more when you move, cough, sneeze, lift, or strain? **YES** See Doctor

NO

Is the pain felt on one side of the small of your back, just above your waist, and do you feel sick and have a fever of 101°F or higher? **YES** See Doctor

NO

With back pain, do you have any of these problems?
- Fever, joint stiffness, and pain.
- Fever, redness, heat, or swelling in affected joints.
- Fever, cracking or grating sounds with joint movement.

YES See Doctor

NO

Use Self-Care

See Self-Care / Prevention in next column

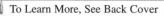
To Learn More, See Back Cover

Self-Care / Prevention

Relieve the Pain
Take an over-the-counter medicine for pain. Acetaminophen will help with pain, but not with swelling.

Don't "overdo it" after taking a painkiller. You can hurt your back more and then it will take longer to heal.

Activity
Continue your regular activities as much as you can, but stop activities that increase pain. Rest the back if you must, but don't rest in bed more than 1 to 2 days even if your back hurts a lot. Your back muscles can get weak if you don't use them or if you stay in bed longer than 2 days. Bed rest should only be used for persons with severe limitations (due mostly to leg pain).

Other Tips
- Get comfortable when you lie down, stand, and sit. For example, when you lie on your back, keep your upper back flat, but your hips and knees bent. Keep your feet flat on the bed. Tip your hips down and up until you find the best spot.

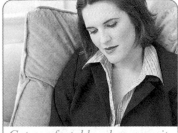
Get comfortable when you sit.

- Put a pillow under your knees or lie on your side with your knees bent. This will take pressure off your lower back.

- When you get up from bed, move slowly, roll on your side, and swing your legs to the floor. Push off the bed with your arms.

Back Pain, Continued

More Tips

- Try some mild stretching exercises (in the morning and afternoon) to make your stomach and back muscles stronger. Ask your doctor for his or her advice on exercising.

- Don't sit in one place longer than you need to. It strains your lower back.

- Sleep on a firm mattress. Don't sleep on your stomach. Sleep on your back or side with your knees bent.

- If your back pain is chronic or doesn't get better on its own, see your doctor who can evaluate your needs. Your doctor may refer you to a chiropractor, physical therapist, or physiatrist (a physical therapy doctor).

Cold Treatment

Cold helps with bruises and swelling. For the first 48 hours after back symptoms start, apply a cold pack (or bag of ice) to the painful area. Lie on your back with your knees bent and put the cold pack under your lower back. Do this for 5 to 10 minutes at a time, several times a day.

Heat Treatment

Heat makes blood flow which helps healing. Heat also helps relieve muscle spasm. Don't use heat on a back strain until 48 or more hours after back symptoms start. Use cold treatment first

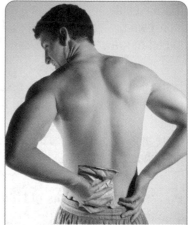

Apply ice or a cold pack for the first 48 hours after symptoms start.

(see "Cold Treatment" above). If used sooner, heat can make the pain and swelling worse. Use a moist heating pad, a hot-water bottle, hot compresses, a hot tub, hot baths, or hot showers. Use heat for 10 minutes at a time. Do this several times a day. Be careful not to burn yourself.

Braces or Corsets

Braces and corsets help to support your back and keep you from moving it too much. They do what strong back muscles do, but they won't make your back stronger.

Massage

Massage won't cure a backache, but it can loosen tight muscles.

Spinal Manipulation

This treatment, usually done by a chiropractor or osteopath, uses the hands to apply force to "adjust" the spine. This may be especially helpful for some people the first month they have low back symptoms. Consult your doctor about spinal manipulations. Your health insurance plan may require a referral from your doctor before it pays anything for spinal manipulation.

Back Pain, Continued

Lifting Do's and Don'ts to Prevent Back Strain

Do's

- Wear good shoes with low heels, not sandals or high heels.

- Stand close to the thing you want to lift.

- Plant your feet squarely, shoulder width apart.

- Bend at the knees, not at the waist. Keep your knees bent as you lift.

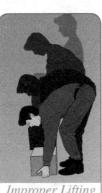

Proper Lifting

- Pull in your stomach and rear end. Keep your back as straight as you can.

- Hold the object close to your body.

- Lift slowly. Let your legs carry the weight.

- Get help or use a dolly to move something that is too big or very heavy.

Don'ts

- Don't lift if your back hurts.

- Don't lift if you have a history of back trouble.

- Don't lift something that's too heavy.

- Don't lift heavy things over your head.

- Don't lift anything if you're not steady on your feet.

Improper Lifting

- Don't bend at the waist to pick something up.

- Don't arch your back when you lift or carry.

- Don't lift too fast or with a jerk.

- Don't twist your back when you are holding something. Turn your whole body, from head to toe.

- Balance the load. Don't lift something heavy with one hand and something light with the other.

- Don't try to lift one thing while you hold something else. For example, don't try to pick up a child while you are holding a bag of groceries. Put the bag down or lift the bag and the child at the same time.

Sciatica

Sciatica is inflammation of the sciatic nerve, which starts in the lower spine and goes down the back of the legs. Pressure on the nerve (from tight muscles, herniated disk, etc.) causes a sharp pain that can be felt in the buttock and may extend to the thigh, knee, or foot. To prevent sciatica:

- Don't strain the muscles in your lower back. (See **Lifting Do's and Don'ts to Prevent Back Strain** in the left column.)

- Do exercises to strengthen your stomach muscles. These exercises help make your back stronger.

Treatment for mild sciatica is rest, heat, and over-the-counter medicine for pain. Physical therapy may be helpful. In some cases, surgery to repair a herniated disk may be needed.

Get more information from:

HealthyLearn® • www.HealthyLearn.com
Click on MedlinePlus®

National Institute of Arthritis and Musculoskeletal and Skin Diseases (NIAMS)
www.nih.gov/niams

Fibromyalgia

Fibromyalgia is a chronic, arthritis-like illness. It affects the muscles, not the joints.

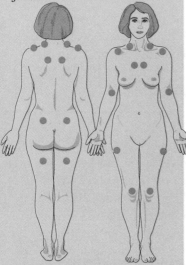

Tender points of fibromyalgia

Treatment

- Exercise therapy.
- Medication to treat symptoms.
- Massage therapy.

Get more information from:

HealthyLearn®
www.HealthyLearn.com
Click on MedlinePlus®

Co-Cure Information Exchange
www.co-cure.org

Signs & Symptoms

- Chronic widespread pain on both sides of the body. This lasts for at least 3 months. It is not due to any other problem. Muscle pain can be severe.
- Pain in 11 or more of 22 "tender points." (These are shown at left.)
- Fatigue. Disturbed sleep. Anxiety. Depression.

These symptoms are also linked to fibromyalgia:
- Memory lapses. Problems concentrating. Feeling confused.
- Chronic headaches. Jaw pain. A tingling feeling in the limbs.
- Irritable bowel. Swelling and pain in the abdomen. Gas. Constipation. Diarrhea.

Causes

The exact cause is not known. Factors thought to play a role include:
- An illness caused by an infection. Emotional or physical trauma.
- Hormones. Women are affected more often than men.
- Brain chemicals and muscles don't function like they should.

Questions to Ask

Does a person with fibromyalgia have severe pain, depression, or anxiety? Is prescribed treatment not helping?

YES → See Doctor

NO ↓

Do symptoms get worse or do you have new symptoms?

YES →  Call Doctor

NO ↓

 Use Self-Care

Self-Care / Prevention

- Follow the treatment plan advised by your doctor.
- Use biofeedback. Use relaxation techniques. Meditate.
- Take warm baths. Use a heating pad. Massage sore muscles.

Foot Problems

Some foot problems are due to years of wear and tear on your feet. Others can be due to shoes that do not fit well or trimming your toenails too close to your skin. Circulation problems and diseases, such as diabetes, can lead to foot problems, too.

Foot Problems Chart		
Signs & Symptoms	**What It Could Be**	**What to Do**
These problems appear in a matter of hours to a few days: • The skin of your foot or toe is gray to black in color. • You cannot feel sensation in your foot.	**Gangrene.**	Get medical care fast!
Pain from a fall or injury to your foot (not just a toe) with any of these problems: • Severe bleeding. • Your foot is misshaped. • You can't move your foot. • Your foot looks blue or pale and is cold and numb. • Your foot is so painful and/or swollen that you can't put any weight on it.	**Broken bone(s)** in the foot (not just a toe).	Get medical care fast! See **Broken Bones / Dislocations** on page 365.
Sudden onset of pain in your feet and legs. The skin on your feet rapidly changes color: white, red, blue, grayish, or black.	**Peripheral vascular disease.**	Get medical care fast! See **Frostbite & Hypothermia** on page 381 and **Cold Hands & Feet** on page 121.
Toes turn white then red in response to cold. Tingling. Numbness.	**Frostbite** (if signs occurs after cold exposure).	Contact doctor for an appointment right away.
The bottom of the foot is red and swollen and feels warm and tender.	**Cellulitis.**	See **Cellulitis** on page 120.
Cut or puncture from a dirty or contaminated object, such as a rusty nail or other object in the soil.	**Cut or puncture wound.**	See **Skin Injuries/Wounds** on page 402.

+ This photo is courtesy of the Public Health Image Library (PHIL) of the Centers for Disease Control and Prevention.

Foot Problems Chart, continued on next page

To Learn More, See Back Cover

Foot Problems, Continued

Foot Problems Chart		
Signs & Symptoms	**What It Could Be**	**What to Do**
A foot wound with: Fever; redness, tenderness, or warmth; swelling; pain; and/or pus.	**Infection.**	See doctor.
Severe pain in foot joint, often the big toe. The pain is not due to an injury. The joint hurts a lot when anything touches it. The area is red, swollen, and tender.	**Gout.**	See doctor.
Joint pain and morning stiffness in joints that lasts more than 1 hour. Fatigue.	**Rheumatoid arthritis.**	See doctor.
Pain in only one toe after an injury to the toe.	**Broken or sprained toe.**	See **Self-Care/Prevention–For Injuries** on page 193.
Open sores (ulcers) on the toes. Pain on the instep and cold, pale skin color which improves with rest.	**Buerger's Disease.**	See doctor.
Tenderness and pain under the heel bone.	**Heel spur.**	See doctor.
Moist, soft, red, or gray-white scales on the feet, especially between the toes. Cracked, peeling, dead skin area. Itching. Sometimes small blisters on the feet.	**Athlete's foot.**	See **Athlete's Foot** on page 116.
White, brown, or yellow toenail. The nail can thicken, then get soft and weak. It may tear away from the nail bed or look deformed.	**Toenail fungus.**	See doctor.
Sharp and burning pain on the ball of the foot.	**Morton's neuroma.** This is thickening of nerve tissue, usually between the third and fourth toes.	See **Self-Care/Prevention–For Morton's Neuroma** on page 193.

Foot Problems Chart, continued on next page

Foot Problems, Continued

Foot Problems Chart		
Signs & Symptoms	**What It Could Be**	**What to Do**
Painful growth on the ball or heel of the foot. Black pinholes or spots in the center.	**Plantar wart.**	See **Warts** on page 148.
Thickened skin on the ball or heel of the foot. Usually no pain.	**Callus.**	See **Corns & Calluses** on page 122.
Discomfort, pain, tenderness, and/or redness under the corner of a toenail and nearby skin.	**Ingrown toenail.**	See **Ingrown Toenails** on page 127.
The big toe points inward or outward. A bony bulge at side of the big toe. Thickened skin. Possible fluid build-up near the big toe. Stiffness or pain.	**Bunion.**	See **Self-Care/Prevention– For Bunions** on page 192.
Thickened skin on tops of and between toes where rubbing is constant. Feels hard to the touch and looks round. Small, clear spot (hen's eye) may appear in the center.	**Corn.**	See **Corns & Calluses** on page 122.
Pain between the heel and the ball of the foot. Often this is due to walking, running, or putting weight on the foot.	**Planter Fasciitis.** This is a problem with ligaments and tissues in the foot arch.	See **Self-Care/Prevention– For Plantar Fasciitis** on page 193.
Red, sometimes fluid-filled sores caused by shoes that rub the foot.	**Blisters.**	See **Self-Care/Prevention– For Blisters** on page 192.
Charley horse or muscle spasm in the foot. Often, this occurs at bedtime.	**Foot cramp.**	See **Self-Care/Prevention– For Foot Cramps** on page 192.
Curled or claw-like position in a toe (usually the 2nd toe). A corn forms on the top of the toe. Pain.	**Hammertoe.**	See **Self-Care/Prevention– For Hammertoes** on page 193.

{*Note:* If you have diabetes or circulation problems, contact your doctor for any foot problems.}

Foot Problems, Continued

See also, **Self-Care / Prevention** for:
- **Athlete's Foot** on page 116.
- **Cold Hands & Feet** on page 121.
- **Corns & Calluses** on page 123.
- **Skin Injuries/Wounds** on page 403.
- **Ingrown Toenails** on page 127.
- **Splinters** on page 145.

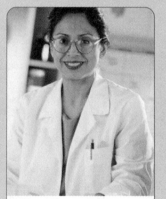

If you have diabetes or circulation problems, contact your doctor for any foot problem.

Self-Care / Prevention

For Blisters
- Don't break a blister. If it breaks on its own, apply an antibacterial spray or ointment and cover with a bandage or sterile dressing.
- Don't cut away or pull off the broken blister's loose skin. This protects the new skin below it.

For Bunions
- Don't wear high heels or shoes with narrow toes.
- Wear sandals.
- Use moleskin or padding to separate overlapped toes.
- Try arch supports to reduce pressure.
- Use ring-shaped pads over a bunion.
- Cut out an old pair of shoes to wear in the house.
- Soak your feet in warm water.
- If needed, take an over-the-counter pain reliever as directed.

For Foot Cramps
- Stretch the foot muscles.
- Pull the foot back into a flexed position.
- Push the foot into the floor.

For Heel Spurs
- Use a cushion or heel cup under the heel.
- Do not jog or run. Avoid prolonged standing.
- Lose weight, if overweight.
- Roll a tennis ball under ball of the foot.
- Put ice on the heel for 10 minutes. Remove it for 10 minutes. Repeat many times.
- If needed, take an over-the-counter pain reliever as directed.

Foot Problems, Continued

For Hammertoes
- Wear wide, roomy shoes.
- Massage the toes or get a foot rub.
- Change shoes during the day. Try athletic shoes.
- Use small pads over the center of the toe to lessen pressure.

For Injuries
Use **R.I.C.E.** (See page 197.)
- For an injured toe, tape it to the toe next to it. Do this for 7 to 10 days.
- Take an over-the-counter medicine to reduce swelling and pain as directed.

For Minor Infections
- Soak the foot in warm, soapy water for 20 minutes, 4 to 6 times a day. Pat the infected area dry. Use extra care if you have peripheral vascular disease. Make sure the water is not hot.
- Apply an over-the-counter antibiotic ointment, such as Neosporin. Cover with a sterile cloth or bandage.

For Morton's Neuroma
- Wear wide shoes with soft insoles.
- Put pads or arch supports in your shoes. These help take pressure off the area.
- Take an over-the-counter medicine for pain as directed.
- See your doctor if the above measures don't bring relief.

For Plantar Fasciitis
- Rest the foot as much as you can.
- Use **R.I.C.E.** (See page 197.)
- Take an over-the-counter medicine for pain and swelling as directed.
- Wear shoes with a solid arch support.

For Plantar Warts
- Try salicylic acid plasters or other over-the-counter products, such as Wart-Off. Follow package directions.
- Use cushions in shoes.
- Wash your hands after touching warts to avoid re-infection.
- Wear sandals in the shower or public areas, such as pools.
- Do not pick at plantar warts.

To Help Prevent Foot Problems
- Wear shoes that fit well. Don't wear shoes with pointed toes or ones that fit too tightly.
- Wash and dry your feet daily.
- Keep your feet moisturized.
- Inspect your feet daily for early signs of problems.
- Rest your feet by elevating them.
- Persons with diabetes and/or circulation problems need to take special care of their feet. Good foot care can prevent some foot infections. It may be necessary for a health care professional to cut the toenails.

{*Note:* If self-care measures do not help or if your foot problem gets worse, contact your doctor.}

Leg Pain & Ankle Pain

Pain in the legs or ankles can range from mild to severe. The type and amount of pain depends on the cause.

Leg Pain & Ankle Pain Chart		
Signs & Symptoms	**What It Could Be**	**What to Do**
Pain, redness (may have shades of red, purple, and blue), or swelling in one ankle or leg. May be followed by severe shortness of breath that came on all of a sudden. May include coughing up blood or pink-frothy sputum. Chest pain.	**Deep-vein thrombosis (DVT)** with or without a blood clot to the lung.	Get medical care fast!
Swelling of both ankles at the same time. Shortness of breath. May have a dry cough or a cough with pink, frothy mucus.	**Heart failure.**	Get medical care fast!
Muscle pain in one or both legs. Fatigue in the thighs, calves, and feet. This improves with rest. Open sores on the lower leg, ankles, or toes. Weak or no pulse in the affected limb. Cold or numb feet. Pale, bluish-colored toes.	**Peripheral vascular disease.**	Get medical care fast!
Any of the signs that follow occur after a leg or ankle injury. A bone sticks out or bones in the injured limb make a grating sound. The injured limb looks deformed, crooked, or the wrong shape. You lose feeling in the injured limb. The skin under the affected injured area is cold and blue. The limb is very painful and/or swollen or you can't bear weight on the limb or move it.	**Broken bone or dislocation.**	See **Broken Bones/Dislocations** on page 365.

Leg Pain & Ankle Pain Chart, continued on next page

Leg Pain & Ankle Pain, Continued

Leg Pain & Ankle Pain Chart		
Signs & Symptoms	**What It Could Be**	**What to Do**
Pain in the leg or ankle after an injury that does not keep you from moving the limb.	**Sprain, strain, or sport injury**. Other overuse injury.	See **Sprains, Strains & Sports Injuries** on page 404.
Pain with fever, redness, tenderness, warmth and pus at a wound site. A red streak up the leg (rarely).	**Infection.** Could also be **Cellulitis.**	See doctor. Get an appointment right away for a red streak up the leg.
Sudden, severe pain in a toe, knee, or ankle joint. The pain can be felt even when clothing is rubbed against the joint. The joint area is swollen, red, or purplish in color. It also feels warm, and is very tender to the touch.	**Gout.**	See doctor.
Leg pain that radiates from the lower back. Pain or stiffness in the knees. Bowing of the legs or other bone deformity. Unexplained bone fractures. May have headache, dizziness, hearing loss, and/or ringing in the ears.	**Paget's disease**. This is a bone disorder that progresses slowly. Most persons with this disease do not develop symptoms.	See doctor.
Sharp pain from the buttocks down the leg. Numbness and tingling in the leg.	**Sciatica.**	See **Sciatica** on page 187.
Pain, stiffness, and swelling, usually in both knees or ankle joints. The joint looks deformed. Weakness and fatigue. Dry mouth and dry, painful eyes.	**Rheumatoid arthritis.**	See **Arthritis** on page 182.
Pain, stiffness, and sometimes swelling of the knee or ankle joints. Often, the joint has gotten tender over months or years and may look enlarged or deformed.	**Osteoarthritis.**	See **Arthritis** on page 182.

Leg Pain & Ankle Pain Chart, continued on next page

Leg Pain & Ankle Pain, Continued

Leg Pain & Ankle Pain Chart		
Signs & Symptoms	**What It Could Be**	**What to Do**
Leg or ankle pain with gradual loss of height; stooped posture; backache; and/or past bone fractures, especially in the wrists and hips.	**Osteoporosis.**	See **Osteoporosis** on page 199.
Pain or itching in the legs with swollen and twisted veins that look blue and are close to the surface of the skin. The veins bulge and feel heavy. Swelling in the legs and ankles.	**Varicose veins.**	See **Varicose Veins** on page 146.
Muscle or joint pain and chronic swelling of the knee joints. These problems develop months or years after a deer-tick bite and a bulls-eye red rash with pale centers.	**Lyme disease.**	See doctor.
Pain and swelling around the knee joint. The pain gets worse with movement. Fever (maybe).	**Bursitis.**	See doctor. See also, **Self-Care / Prevention–For Bursitis, Tendinitis, or an Injury That Does Not Appear Serious** on page 206.
Aches in leg muscles and joints with fever and/or chills. Headache. Dry cough. Sore throat. Fatigue.	**Flu.**	Follow guidelines for **Colds & Flu** on pages 100 to 103.
Sudden, sharp, tightening pain in the leg, often the calf. The muscle feels hard to the touch. The pain subsides after a minute or so and the muscle relaxes.	**Leg cramp.**	See **Self-Care / Prevention–For Leg Cramps** on page 197.

Leg Pain & Ankle Pain, Continued

Self-Care / Prevention

For Pain, in General

- Take an over-the-counter medicine for pain as directed on the label. If the pain is not better after a few doses, call your doctor.

- Use a heating pad (set on low), a hot pack, or a moist, warm towel on the area of pain. If the pain is due to an injury, don't use heat for 48 hours. Use R.I.C.E. (See below.)

R.I.C.E.

- **R**est the injured area for 24 to 48 hours.

- **I**ce the area as soon as possible and keep doing so for 10 minutes every 2 hours for the first 48 hours. Use an ice pack, ice in a heavy plastic bag with a little water, a bag of frozen vegetables, etc.

- **C**ompress the area. Wrap with an elastic bandage. Do not cut off circulation. Remove the bandage every 3 to 4 hours, for 15 to 20 minutes each time.

- **E**levate the area above heart level, if possible. Place it on a pillow, folded blanket, stack of newspapers, etc.

For Paget's Disease

- If needed, take an over-the-counter medicine for pain as directed on the label.

- Take other medicines as prescribed by your doctor.

- Get regular checkups to detect hearing loss.

To Help Prevent Leg Pain & Ankle Pain

- Get to and stay at a healthy weight.

- Get regular exercise. This helps to keep ankle and leg muscles strong.

- Before you exercise, stretch and warm up your muscles. When you are done, cool them down.

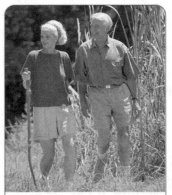

When you can, walk on grass instead of concrete.

- Protect your knees. Use knee pads when you garden or kneel. Always land on bent knees when jumping. Avoid deep knee bend exercises.

- Don't wear high-heeled shoes. Keep your shoes in proper shape.

- Take good care of your feet.

For Leg Cramps

- Walk on the leg.

- Shake the leg and then elevate it.

- Sit with your leg flat on the floor. Flex your foot upward, then toward your knee. Reach for your toes and pull them toward your knee. This stretches the calf muscles.

- Have someone massage the cramped muscle gently, but firmly.

- Apply a heating pad (set on low), a hot pack, or moist, warm towel to the muscle cramp.

- Rub the muscle that is cramping. Rub upward from the ankle toward the heart. (***Note:*** Do not rub a leg if you suspect phlebitis or thrombosis.)

Leg Pain & Ankle Pain, Continued

Good Sources of Calcium

- Nonfat milks.
- Cheeses.
- Yogurts.
- Calcium-fortified cereals and juices.
- Collard greens, broccoli, and spinach.
- Tofu, if calcium is used in processing.

Good Sources of Potassium

- Citrus fruits and juices.
- Bananas.
- Potatoes.
- Bran cereals.
- Fish.

Good Sources of Magnesium

- Whole grain breads and cereals.
- Dried beans.
- Black-eyed peas.
- Nuts, especially peanuts.
- Wild rice.
- Tofu.

To Prevent Leg Cramps

- Get good sources of calcium, potassium, and magnesium. See lists at left. Take calcium, potassium, and magnesium as advised by your doctor.

- Drink plenty of water and other fluids. Limit drinks with caffeine. Avoid drinks with alcohol. Doing these things can help prevent dehydration which could cause leg cramps.

- Warm up your muscles before you exercise. Cool down your muscles when you are done.

- With your doctor's okay, wear elastic stockings while you are awake.

- Before you go to bed, stretch your calf muscles. Here's one way to do this:
  - Stand an arm's length away from a wall. Lean against it with the palms of your hands.
  - Bend your left knee. Keep your right leg straight behind you. Keep both feet flat on the floor and your back straight.
  - Lean forward. Feel your right calf muscle stretch. Hold the stretch as you count to 10 slowly.
  - Repeat, switching leg positions.

- Another way to stretch your calf muscles is to ride a stationary bicycle for a few minutes.

- Take a warm bath before bedtime.

- Sleep with loose-fitting blankets and night clothes. Keep your legs warm.

- If you have severe leg cramps or get them often, tell your doctor. Ask if any medication you take could cause your leg cramps. Ask for ways to treat your leg cramps.

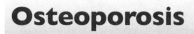

Osteoporosis

Osteoporosis is a loss in bone mass and bone strength. Bones become weak and brittle. This makes them more prone to fractures. Any bone can be affected. The hips, wrists, and spine are the most common sites.

Signs & Symptoms

Osteoporosis is a "silent disease." It can occur without seeing changes taking place inside the body. Often the first sign is a fracture of the hip, wrist, or spine. When signs and symptoms occur, they include:

- Gradual loss of height.
- Rounding of the shoulders.
- Sudden back pain.
- Stooped posture.
- Dowager's hump.

Causes

The actual causes are not known. Risk factors include:

- Being female. Women are 4 times more likely to develop osteoporosis than men.
- Low estrogen level. This occurs with menopause or with surgery that removes a women's ovaries.
- Low testosterone level in men.

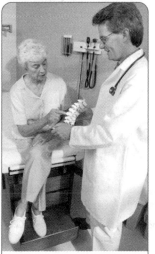

Osteoporosis is more common in women than in men.

- Aging.
- Family history of osteoporosis or broken bones in adulthood.
- Having a thin, small-framed body.
- Lack of physical activity, especially weight-bearing exercises, such as walking and dancing.
- Long-term bed rest.
- Low calcium and vitamin D intake or absorption.
- Smoking cigarettes.
- Drinking too much alcohol. Heavy drinkers often eat poorly, too. They are also more prone to fractures from falls.
- Long-term use of certain medicines, such as oral corticosteroids and antacids with aluminum.
- Having certain health problems, such as anorexia nervosa, kidney disease, an over active thyroid gland, and rheumatoid arthritis. People with Crohn's disease, ulcerative colitis, and celiac disease are at an increased risk, too.
- Exercising too much to the point where menstrual periods cease.

Treatment

There is no cure. The focus of treatment is to:
- Prevent the disease.
- Prevent further bone loss.
- Build new bone.

Osteoporosis, Continued

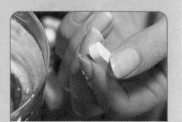

Follow your doctor's advice about taking calcium and vitamin D supplements.

Special X-rays, such as one known as a DXA or DEXA scan, can measure bone mass in the hip, spine, or wrist. These tests are safe and painless. They help doctors decide if and what kind of treatment is needed. This includes:

- Treating medical problems that increase the risk for osteoporosis.

- Medications. There are different kinds. Your doctor will prescribe one(s) best suited for your needs.

- Exercises, as advised by your doctor.

- Proper posture.

- A balanced diet with enough calcium and vitamin D.

- Calcium and vitamin D supplements.

- Fall prevention measures. (Examples are listed on page 54 and on page 201.)

Questions to Ask

After a fall, are you not able to get up or do you have wrist, hip, or back pain? **YES** Get Medical Care Fast

↓ NO

Do you have **signs of osteoporosis** listed on page 199? Do you want to find out about medicines to prevent and/or treat osteoporosis? **YES** See Doctor

↓ NO

Are you a female age 65 or older and have you not had a bone mineral density test? **YES** Call Doctor

↓ NO

Are you a female between ages 60 and 65, do you have risk factors for osteoporosis listed on page 199, and have you not had a bone mineral density test? **YES** Call Doctor

↓ NO

Are you an elderly male and have you used corticosteroid medicine long-term; are you physically inactive and of a low body weight and/or have you had a bone facture possibly due to osteoporosis? **YES** 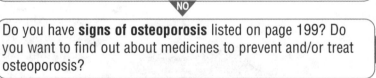 Call Doctor

↓ NO

 Use Self-Care

Get more information from:

HealthyLearn®
www.HealthyLearn.com
Click on MedlinePlus®

National Osteoporosis Foundation
202.223.2226
www.nof.org

Osteoporosis and Related Bone Disease National Resource Center
800.624.BONE
(624.2663)
www.osteo.org

See Self-Care / Prevention on next page

Osteoporosis, Continued

Self-Care / Prevention

To Treat, Slow, and Prevent Osteoporosis

- Take medicines, as prescribed.

- Eat a balanced diet. Get your recommended Adequate Intake (AI) for calcium every day.

Adequate Intakes (AIs) for Calcium*	
Age	Milligrams (Mgs.) Day
1–3 years	500
4–8 years	800
9–18 years	1,300
19–50 years	1,000
51+ years	1,200
Pregnant and breast-feeding women: 18 years and younger 1,300 Over 18 years 1,000	

* Source: The Institute of Medicine (IOM). Follow your doctor's advice for calcium.

- Choose high-calcium foods daily:
  - Skim and low-fat milks, yogurts, and cheeses. {*Note:* If you are lactose intolerant, see information for **Lactose Intolerance** on page 170.}
  - Soy milks and yogurts with added calcium.
  - Soft-boned fish and shellfish, such as salmon, sardines, and shrimp.
  - Broccoli, kale, and collard greens.
  - Beans and bean sprouts, as well as, tofu (soybean curd), if processed with calcium.
  - Calcium-fortified foods, such as some juices and ready-to-eat cereals.

* Check for updates on calcium and vitamin D needs from www.iom.edu.

- Take calcium and vitamin D supplements, as advised by your doctor.

- Get vitamin D from sunshine (15 minutes of midday sunshine may meet daily needs) and from foods (fortified milks and cereals, egg yolks, saltwater fish, liver, and cod liver oil).

Adequate Intakes (AIs) for Vitamin D*	
Age	International Units (IUs)/Day
Birth–50 years	200 IUs
51–70 years	400 IUs
71+ years	600 IUs

* Source: The Institute of Medicine (IOM). The American Academy of Pediatrics advises 400 IUs for children and adolescents. *Note:* The National Osteoporosis Foundation advises 400-800 IUs for adults under age 50; 800-1,000 IUs for adults age 50 and older. Follow your doctor's advice for vitamin D.

- Do regular, weight-bearing exercise, such as walking, at least 3 or 4 times a week. A person with osteoporosis should exercise as advised by his or her doctor. Practice good posture.

- Don't smoke. Limit alcohol.

- Use fall prevention measures:
  - Ask your doctor how to deal with any medications you take that could cause you to fall.
  - Use grab bars and safety mats in your tub and shower. Use handrails on stairways.
  - Pick things up by bending your knees and keeping your back straight. Don't stoop.
  - Wear flat, sturdy, nonskid shoes.
  - If you use throw rugs, use ones with nonskid backs.
  - Use a cane or walker, if necessary.
  - Keep halls, stairways, and entrances well lit. Use night lights in hallways and rooms.

Repetitive Motion Injuries

Repetitive motion injuries (RMIs) are also called **repetitive strain injuries (RSIs)**. They result from doing the same activity over and over for a long period of time. This can be at work, at home, during sports, and/or with hobbies.

Signs & Symptoms

Signs and symptoms depend on the injury.

For Carpal Tunnel Syndrome (CTS)

- Thumb, index, middle, and ring fingers feel numb.
- Tingling feeling in the hand(s).
- Pain is felt in the thumb and fingers. The pain may be worse at night. It can wake you up.
- Pain starts in the hand and spreads to the arm. The pain can even travel to the shoulder.
- The fingers swell. It feels like your fingers are swollen. Your hands feel weak in the morning.
- You have trouble holding on to things. You drop things.
- You have a hard time writing with a pencil or pen, opening a jar, buttoning a blouse, etc.

For back strain, see **Back Pain** on pages 184 to 187.

For **Eyestrain from Computer Use**, see page 70.

For tendinitis, see **Shoulder Pain & Neck Pain** on pages 205 to 207.

Causes

In general, RMIs are caused by repeated movements that involve:
- Drilling or hammering.
- Lifting.
- Pushing or pulling.
- Squeezing.
- Twisting.
- Wrist, finger, and hand movements.

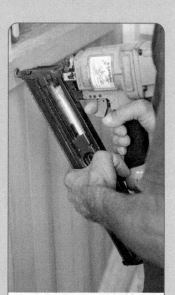

Repeated use of tools that vibrate the hand and wrist can lead to RMIs.

Repetitive Motion Injuries, *Continued*

For Carpal Tunnel Syndrome (CTS)

Repeated motions, typing vibrations, etc. cause swelling of the tendons inside the carpal tunnel. This is the narrow tunnel in the wrist. The swelling puts pressure on the nearby nerves.

Treatment

For Carpal Tunnel Syndrome (CTS)

This is easier to treat and less likely to cause future problems if it is found early. Women are more likely to get CTS than men, because their carpal tunnel is usually smaller. Once diagnosed, CTS can be treated with:

■ Preventing further damage.

■ Wearing a wrist brace, splint, etc. as advised. It may need to be worn while you sleep and during the day.

■ Over-the-counter medicines to reduce pain and swelling. Examples are aspirin, ibuprofen, and naproxen sodium.

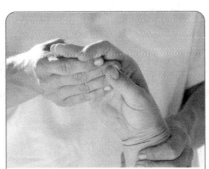

A physical therapist can show you what exercises to do at work and at home to treat CTS.

■ Physical therapy.

■ Occupational therapy.

■ Cortisone shots in the wrist area.

■ Surgery, if needed.

Questions to Ask

Do any of these problems occur?
- Severe or persistent pain, swelling, or spasm.
- Tenderness or stiffness and limited motion in the affected area, such as the shoulder, arm, or wrist.

YES → See Doctor

NO ↓

Does pain in your hand, shoulder, etc. wake you from sleep?

YES → Call Doctor

NO ↓

Have you had one or both of these problems?
- Pain, numbness, and tingling in your hand for more than 2 weeks.
- You haven't been able to make a fist for a couple of weeks.

YES → Call Doctor

NO ↓

Do you drop things often and does your thumb feel weak?

YES → Call Doctor

NO ↓

 Use Self-Care

Self-Care / Prevention

For Preventing Wrist and Hand Injuries

Whenever your hands and wrists do the same activity time and again, you increase your risk for CTS and tendinitis. Change how you do a task and you may avoid some of these injuries.

■ Follow **Proper Position and Support for Computer Users** on page 59.

■ Do not hold an object in the same position for a long time. Even simple tasks, such as hammering nails, can cause injury when done over a period of time.

Repetitive Motion Injuries, Continued

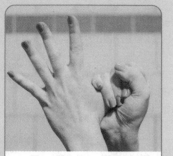

Exercise your hands and wrists often during the day.

- Give your hands a break. Rest them for a few minutes each hour.

- Lift objects with your whole hand or with both hands. Gripping or lifting with the thumb and index finger puts stress on your wrist.

- If your line of work causes pain in your hands and wrists, alternate the stressful tasks with other work.

- Exercise your hands and wrists as often as you can. Here are two examples:
  - Place your hands in front of you. Spread your fingers as far apart as possible. Hold for 5 seconds. Relax. Repeat 5 times with each hand.
  - Turn your wrists in a circle, palms up and then palms down. Relax your fingers and keep your elbows still. Repeat 5 times.

For Carpal Tunnel Syndrome

- Follow **Self-Care / Prevention** tips already listed in this topic.

- Lose weight. CTS is linked to obesity.

- Take an over-the-counter medicine to reduce the pain and swelling as directed.

- Use a wrist splint. Many drug and medical supply stores carry splints that keep the wrist angled slightly back with the thumb parallel to the forearm. This position helps to keep the carpal tunnel open.

Other Tips

- Keep your head upright and your ears, shoulders, and hips in a straight line.

- Keep your work within reach without having to stretch or strain your arms, shoulders, or back. Don't stretch to reach items on an assembly line. Wait for the items to reach you.

- Change positions or tasks often. This avoids repeated stress on a single body part.

- Use the proper tools for the job. Use tools made to reduce vibration and/or pressure, if needed.

Get more information from:

HealthyLearn®
www.HealthyLearn.com
Click on MedlinePlus®

National Institute of Arthritis and Musculoskeletal and Skin Diseases (NIAMS)
www.nih.gov/niams

Shoulder Pain & Neck Pain

Signs & Symptoms

- The pain can be mild to severe. It can be felt in one spot, in a large area, or travel to another area. Movement can cause the pain or make it worse.

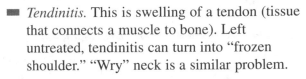

- Stiffness and/or swelling may occur.

Causes

Tension can cause neck muscles to go into spasms.

- Overuse and wear and tear on neck and shoulder muscles and joints.

- Strains. Broken or dislocated shoulder.

- Poor posture. Awkward sleeping positions. Sleeping on a soft mattress.

- Pinched nerve. Pain from a pinched nerve usually runs down one side of the arm.

- *Frozen shoulder.* This can result from lack of use due to pain from an injury. At first, pain occurs with movement. Over time, the pain gets better, but stiffness remains.

- *Torn rotator cuff.* This is a tear in a ligament that holds the shoulder in place. Symptoms are pain at the top and outer sides of the shoulders, especially when you raise or extend your arm. You may also feel or hear a click when the shoulder is moved.

- *Tendinitis.* This is swelling of a tendon (tissue that connects a muscle to bone). Left untreated, tendinitis can turn into "frozen shoulder." "Wry" neck is a similar problem.

- *Bursitis.* This is swelling of the sac (bursa) that surrounds the shoulder joint. Bursitis can be caused by injury, infection, overuse, arthritis, or gout.

- A whiplash injury.

- **Osteoarthritis.** (See page 182.)

- Infections that cause swollen lymph nodes in the neck.

Questions to Ask

With shoulder pain or neck pain, do you have any of these problems?
- A serious head or neck injury.
- Any **heart attack warning sign** listed on page 387.
- Any **symptom of meningitis** listed on page 101.

YES → Get Medical Care Fast

NO ↓

After an injury to the neck or shoulder, do you have any of these problems?
- The shoulder popped out of place and back into place.
- A burning, shooting pain or weakness is felt in the shoulders.
- The shoulder looks misshaped.
- The pain is very severe.
- Your arm is numb and can't be moved at all.

YES → Get Medical Care Fast

NO ↓

Flowchart continued on next page

Shoulder Pain & Neck Pain, Continued

Treatment

Treatment for shoulder pain and/or neck pain depends on the cause. Emergency medical care is needed for:

- A serious injury.

- A broken bone.

- A heart attack.

- **Meningitis.** This is an infection of the membranes that surround the brain.

Self-care can treat less serious causes of shoulder pain and/or neck pain.

Do you have any of these problems?
- Severe or persistent pain, swelling, or spasms in a shoulder.
- Painful and stiff shoulder that is very hard to move at all.
- Pain, tenderness, and limited motion in the shoulder.

YES → See Doctor

NO ↓

Do you have any of these problems?
- Throbbing shoulder pain or numbness that goes down the shoulder into the arm.
- A possible whiplash injury after being hit from behind.
- Fever and redness or swelling around the shoulder.

YES → See Doctor

NO ↓

Do you have both of these **signs of a gallbladder attack**?
- Pain in the right shoulder.
- Pain in the right upper abdomen.

YES → See Doctor

NO ↓

Is your neck pain or shoulder pain severe enough to interfere with sleep? Or, does the pain not get better after using self-care for 7 days?

YES → See Doctor

NO ↓

Use Self-Care

Self-Care / Prevention

For Pain

- Take an over-the-counter medicine for pain and/or swelling.

- To relieve tension and improve circulation, take walks. Start with 3 to 5 walks a day, each lasting 5 to 10 minutes. Gradually increase walking times.

For Bursitis, Tendinitis, or an Injury That Does Not Appear Serious

- Use **R.I.C.E.** (See page 197.)

- Try liniments and balms. These provide a cooling or warming sensation, but only mask the pain. They do not promote healing.

Get more information from:

HealthyLearn®
www.HealthyLearn.com
Click on MedlinePlus®

National Institute of Arthritis and Musculoskeletal and Skin Diseases (NIAMS)
www.nih.gov/niams

Shoulder Pain & Neck Pain, Continued

To Treat Neck Pain from a Whiplash Injury or Pinched Nerve

See a doctor anytime your motor vehicle is hit from the rear because the accident can cause a whiplash injury. After first checking with your doctor, do these things to ease neck discomfort:

- Rest as much as you can by lying on your back.

- Use cold and hot packs.

- Improve your posture. When you sit, use a chair with a straight back. Make sure your buttocks go all the way to the chair's back. When you stand, pull in your chin and stomach.

- Use a cervical (neck) pillow or a rolled hand towel under your neck.

- Avoid activities that may aggravate your injury.

- Cover your neck with a scarf if you go outside when the weather is cold.

Ways to Prevent Shoulder Pain & Neck Pain

- Avoid repeated activities that twist or put strain on the neck and shoulders. When you do repeated tasks, use proper posture, equipment, and techniques.

- Wear seat belts in vehicles. Use protective gear when you take part in sporting events.

- If you are out of condition, strengthen your muscles gradually.

- Don't sleep on your stomach. You may twist your neck in this position. Use a firm polyester pillow, a neck (cervical) pillow, or a rolled towel under your neck.

- Practice good posture. Stand straight. Don't let your shoulders slump, your head droop, or your lower back slouch.

- When you carry things, such as a shoulder bag, switch from one shoulder to the other.

- Don't prop a telephone between your ear and shoulder.

- Stretch and warm up before activities that require joint movement, such as sports.

- Do exercises to keep the muscles in your shoulder and neck strong and flexible. For example:

  - Sit straight in a chair. Flex your neck slowly forward and try to touch your chin to your chest. Hold for 10 seconds. Go back to the starting position. Repeat 5 times.

  - Look straight ahead. Slowly tilt your head to the right trying to touch your right ear to your right shoulder. Do not raise your shoulder to meet your ear. Hold for 10 seconds and straighten your head. Repeat 5 times on this side and then on your left side.

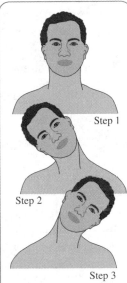

Step 1

Step 2

Step 3

Lateral bend of the neck. Do this exercise to keep your neck muscles strong and flexible.

Chapter 15

General Health Conditions

Allergies

Causes

- **Allergic rhinitis.** This is caused by breathing allergens from animal dander; dust; grass, weed and tree pollen; mold spores, etc.

- Asthma.

- Food allergies. Common ones are milk, fish, nuts, wheat, corn, and eggs.

- Skin allergies.

Anaphylaxis is a sudden and severe allergic reaction. It occurs within minutes of exposure. It worsens very fast. It can lead to anaphylactic shock and death within 15 minutes if emergency medical care is not received.

Insect stings, nuts, penicillin, and shellfish are common causes of a severe allergic reaction.

An allergy is an immune system problem to a substance (allergen) that is normally harmless. An allergen can be inhaled, swallowed, or come in contact with the skin.

Signs & Symptoms

For Common Allergies

- Sneezing. Watery eyes. Cold symptoms that last longer than 10 days without a fever. Dark circles under the eyes.

- Frequent throat clearing. Hoarseness. Coughing or wheezing.

- Skin rash.

- Loss of smell or taste.

- Ear and sinus infections occur again and again.

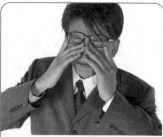

Allergy symptoms usually affect the breathing passages, eyes, or skin.

Signs of a Severe Allergic Reaction

- Shortness of breath. A hard time breathing or swallowing. Wheezing.

- Severe swelling all over, or of the face, lips, tongue, and/or throat.

- Feeling dizzy, weak, and/or numb.

- Pale or bluish lips, skin, and/or fingernails.

- Cool, moist skin or sudden onset of pale skin and sweating.

- Fainting. Decreasing level of awareness.

Treatment

How are allergies treated? Avoid the allergen(s). Skin tests can identify allergens. Allergy shots may be prescribed. Medications can prevent and relieve symptoms. Persons who have had a sudden, severe allergic reaction may be prescribed medicine, such as an EpiPen. This is used for a severe reaction **before** getting emergency medical care.

Allergies, Continued

Questions to Ask

Do you have any of these problems?
- **Signs of a severe allergic reaction** listed on page 208.
- Chest pain or tightening.
- Seizures.
- Cough that doesn't let up and a hard time breathing.

YES → Get Medical Care Fast

NO ↓

Do you have any of these problems?
- Flushing, redness all over the body.
- Severe hives.
- Hoarseness.
- Feeling restless. Anxiety. Trembling.
- Enlarged pupils.
- A severe reaction occurred in the past after exposure to a like substance.

YES → Get Medical Care Fast

NO ↓

Do you have any of these problems?
- Fever, fatigue, headache, or a rash that persists.
- New onset of joint pain.
- New onset of swelling in the limbs.
- Mild symptoms improve after taking an antihistamine, but come back or don't go away completely.

YES → See Doctor

NO ↓

Use Self-Care

Self-Care / Prevention

For a Severe Allergic Reaction
- Take prescribed medicine, such as an EpiPen, as advised. Then get emergency care!

- Wear a medical ID alert tag for things that cause a severe allergic reaction.
- Avoid things you are allergic to.

For Other Allergic Reactions
- If mild symptoms occur after you take a medicine, call your doctor for advice.
- For hives and itching, take an OTC antihistamine, such as Benadryl. Take it as prescribed by your doctor or as directed on the label.
- Don't use hot water for baths, showers, or to wash rash areas. Heat worsens most rashes and makes them itch more.
- For itching, use an oatmeal bath or calamine (not Caladryl) lotion. You can also use a paste made with 3 teaspoons of baking soda and 1 teaspoon of water.
- Avoid things you are allergic to.
- Read food labels. Don't eat foods that have things you are allergic to. When you eat out, find out if menu items have things you are allergic to before you order them.

(See **Self-Care / Prevention** for **Hay Fever** on page 84 and **Self-Care** for **Skin Rashes** on pages 136 to 143.)

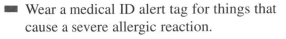

Get more information from:

HealthyLearn®
www.HealthyLearn.com
Click on MedlinePlus®

Asthma and Allergy Foundation of America
800.7.ASTHMA (727.8462) • www.aafa.org

Alzheimer's Disease (AD)

Signs & Symptoms

About 5.3 million persons in the U.S. have Alzheimer's disease (AD). It is the most common cause of dementia – a broad term that means cognitive function declines enough to interfere with daily life activities. Nearly half of people age 85 and older may have AD, but it is not a normal part of aging.

Causes

With AD, certain protein deposits (plaques) and twisted fibers (tangles) build up in the brain. Over time, this causes large numbers of nerve cells in the brain to die.

Risk factors for AD are getting older and a family history of the disease. Having heart disease, diabetes, high blood pressure, a stroke, or a brain injury may increase the risk. Staying physically and mentally active and eating healthy throughout life may lower the risk for AD.

Alzheimer's disease has a gradual onset. How quickly signs and symptoms occur and progress varies from person to person. The average time span is about 3 to 6 years after symptoms start. Survival can be as long as 20 years.

The Alzheimer's Association gives these 10 symptoms for AD:

- *Memory changes that disrupt daily life.* Persons with AD forget important dates, events, and/or information. They may also ask the same question over and over.

- *Problems doing familiar tasks.* Persons with AD may have a hard time fixing a meal or driving to a familiar place.

- *New problems speaking or writing.* Persons with AD often forget simple words or phrases or use unusual words for things. An example is calling a toothbrush "that thing for my mouth."

- *Problems with visual images and spatial relationships.* Persons may have problems with reading, color and contrast, and judging distance.

- *Problems with planning and/or solving problems.* Persons with AD have trouble making and following plans. They have trouble working with numbers, such as balancing a checkbook.

- *Problems with awareness of time and place.* Persons with AD may forget where they are, how they got there, and how to get back home. They may lose track of dates and seasons.

- *Poor or decreased judgment.* Persons with AD neglect daily grooming and may not dress right for the weather. They show poor judgment about money.

- *Misplacing things.* Persons with AD lose things and can not retrace their steps to find them. They put things in unusual places, such as a wristwatch in a sugar bowl.

- *Changes in mood or personality.* Persons with AD can get very confused, depressed, fearful, and worried. They rely on someone else to make decisions for them.

- *Withdrawal from social activities and work.* Persons with AD get less involved with hobbies, social events, sports, and work.

Alzheimer's Disease (AD), Continued

Treatment

A medical diagnosis suggests (or rules out) Alzheimer's disease. Other conditions, such as depression, a severe lack of vitamin B$_{12}$, and blood clots in the brain can cause symptoms like AD. So can side effects of some medicines.

There is no known cure for Alzheimer's disease. Prescribed medicines may help some persons with mild to moderate AD.

Questions to Ask

Is the person suddenly confused or disoriented? Is he or she not able to reason or communicate at all?

YES → Get Medical Care Fast

NO ↓

Are any of the **signs and symptoms of Alzheimer's disease** listed on page 210 present?

YES → See Doctor

NO ↓

Are any of these conditions present?
• Symptoms in a person with Alzheimer's disease worsen.
• The caretaker of the person with Alzheimer's disease needs care or guidance.

YES → Call Doctor

NO ↓

 Use Self-Care

Self-Care / Prevention

There is no known prevention. Studies are being done to find out ways to lower the risk of AD and delay the onset of symptoms. Some studies suggest to do things that keep the mind active. This includes crossword puzzles and reading.

Good planning, medical care, and social management help both the person and caregivers cope with symptoms and maintain the quality of life for as long as possible. An **Advance Directive** (see page 38) should be done in the early stages of AD to allow for the person's wishes. It's very helpful to put structure in the life of the person in the early stages of AD. To do this:

- Maintain daily routines.

- See that the person with AD eats well-balanced meals and stays as active as he or she can. Activities like going for walks with others are good.

- Post safety signs like "Don't touch." Make "to do" lists of daily tasks.

- Put things in their proper places after use. This helps the person find things when he or she needs them.

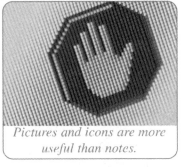

Pictures and icons are more useful than notes.

- Make sure the person carries identification or wears a medical ID bracelet.

Get more information from:

HealthyLearn®
www.HealthyLearn.com
Click on MedlinePlus®

Alzheimer's Disease Education & Referral (ADEAR) Center
800.438.4380 • www.nia.nih.gov/alzheimers

Alzheimer's Association
800.272.3900 • www.alz.org

Anemia

Anemia means that red blood cells or the amount of hemoglobin in red blood cells is low. Hemoglobin is a protein that carries oxygen in red blood cells.

Common types of anemia are low amounts of iron, folic acid (a B-vitamin), and vitamin B_{12}.

Causes

- Anemia from low iron. Often, the cause is blood loss from menstruation in females, peptic ulcers, and other medical problems.

- Anemia from low folic-acid. The cause is lack of folic acid in the diet.

- Anemia from low vitamin B_{12}. This usually results when the body doesn't absorb vitamin B_{12} from food, not a lack of vitamin B_{12} in the diet.

Signs & Symptoms

- Tiredness.

- Weakness.

- Paleness. This could be pale skin or paleness around the gums, nailbeds, or the linings of the lower eyelids.

- Shortness of breath.

- Heart palpitations or rapid heartbeat.

- Cravings for unusual things, such as laundry starch or dirt.

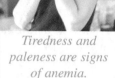

Tiredness and paleness are signs of anemia.

When folic acid is low, extra symptoms can occur. These include: Appetite loss and weight loss; nausea and diarrhea, swollen abdomen, and a sore, red tongue that looks glazed. When vitamin B_{12} is low, extra symptoms include: Chest pain on exertion; appetite loss and weight loss; nausea and diarrhea, a hard time concentrating, and a sore, red tongue that looks glazed. If vitamin B_{12} is very low, nervous system problems occur. These include: Numbness and tingling of the hands and feet; walking and balance problems; memory loss, confusion, dementia, or psychosis. This is known as pernicious anemia.

Treatment

Anemia shares symptoms with many health problems. It needs to be diagnosed by a doctor. Treatment for it depends on the type and what caused it. This includes:

- Treating the problem that caused it.

- Proper diet and vitamin and/or mineral supplements, as prescribed. {*Note:* Don't take iron supplements on your own. Persons with a genetic illness called **hemochromatosis** (iron overload disease) can be harmed with iron supplements.}

- Vitamin B_{12} shots, if needed.

Persons with severe anemia may need one or more blood transfusions.

Anemia, Continued

Questions to Ask

{*Note:* See, also, **Questions to Ask** in **Menstrual Bleeding Problems** on page 317.}

Do you feel very weak and do you have any of these problems?
- Palpitations. Fast or irregular heartbeat.
- You feel faint and breathless.
- Chest pain on exertion.
- Memory loss. Confusion.
- Dementia. Psychosis.

YES → Get Medical Care Fast

NO ↓

With blood in the stools or urine, black, tarlike stools, or heavy vaginal bleeding, do you feel lightheaded, weak, short of breath, and/or do you have severe abdominal pain?

YES → Get Medical Care Fast

NO ↓

Do you feel weak and do you have any of these problems?
- You feel dizzy with exertion or when you stand up.
- Red dots of bleeding under the skin.
- Ulcers in the mouth, throat, or rectum.
- Bruising that occurs without reason.
- Ringing in the ears.

YES → See Doctor

NO ↓

Do you feel tired and weak longer than 2 weeks after using self-care measures?

YES → Call Doctor

NO ↓

Use Self-Care

See Self-Care / Prevention in next column

Self-Care / Prevention

- Follow your doctor's treatment plan.

To Get and Absorb Iron

- Eat foods that are good sources of iron: Lean, red meats; green, leafy vegetables; beef liver; poultry; fish; wheat germ; oysters; dried fruit; and iron-fortified cereals.

- Eat foods high in vitamin C, such as citrus fruits, tomatoes, and strawberries. Vitamin C helps your body absorb iron from plant foods.

- Take the supplements your doctor advises.

- If you drink tea, drink it between meals. Tannins in tea block iron absorption. Or, add milk to tea. The calcium in milk binds with the tannins. (Herbal tea does not have tannins.)

- Avoid antacids, the food additive EDTA, and phosphates (found in soft drinks, beer, ice cream, etc.). These block iron absorption.

To Get and Absorb Folic Acid

- Eat good food sources of folate every day. Examples are asparagus, brussels sprouts, spinach, collard greens, broccoli, peas, oranges, cantaloupe, oatmeal, and whole-grain cereals.

- Eat fresh, raw fruits and vegetables often. Don't overcook food. Heat destroys folic acid.

- Take the supplement your doctor advises.

- Don't smoke. Don't drink alcohol.

For Getting B$_{12}$

- Eat animal sources of food. Good choices are lean meats, fish, poultry, nonfat or low-fat dairy products, and cereals with added vitamin B$_{12}$.

- Strict vegetarians (vegans) who eat no animal sources of food may need a vitamin B$_{12}$ supplement or foods fortified with it.

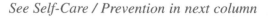

Cancer

With **cancer**, body cells become abnormal, grow out of control, and are or become malignant (harmful). Cancer is a leading cause of death in the U.S. About 1 in 4 of all deaths in the U.S. is due to cancer.

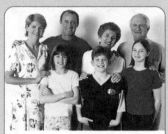

Genes for some cancers run in families.

Get more information from:

HealthyLearn®
www.HealthyLearn.com
Click on MedlinePlus®

Cancer Information Service
800.4.CANCER
    (422.6237)
www.cancer.gov

For information on clinical trials, access:
www.cancertrials.nci.nih.gov

Signs & Symptoms

Cancer can be present without any signs or symptoms. As different types of cancers grow, warning signs (see below) may occur. These could be due to problems other than cancer, too. See your doctor to find out. Pain does not usually occur in early stages of cancer.

For Bladder Cancer
- Blood in the urine. The color of the urine can be deep red or it can be a faint rust or smokey color.

- Pain when passing urine. The need to urinate often or urgently.

For Colon and Rectal Cancers
- A change in bowel habits.

- Constipation. Having stools more often and/or loose stools. Stools that are more narrow than usual. A feeling that the bowel does not empty all the way.

- Blood in or on the stool. This can be bright red or very dark in color.

- Stomach bloating, fullness, and/or cramps. Frequent gas pains.

- Weight loss for no known reason. Constant tiredness.

For Kidney Cancer
- Blood in the urine.

- A dull ache or pain in the back or side. A lump or mass that can be felt in the kidney area (mid back).

- An unexplained cough for more than 3 weeks.

For Lung Cancer
- A cough that doesn't go away. This could be a "smoker's cough" that gets worse. Coughing up blood.

- Constant chest pain. Back pain in some persons.

- Hoarseness. Shortness of breath and wheezing.

- Recurring pneumonia or bronchitis.

- Fatigue, appetite loss, and weight loss.

- Weakness in a shoulder, an arm, or a hand.

Cancer, Continued

For Throat Cancer

- Hoarseness or other changes in the voice.

- A lump on the neck or feeling of a lump in the throat.

- A cough that doesn't go away.

- A hard time swallowing. A feeling of fullness, pressure, or burning when swallowing.

- Repeated indigestion and heartburn. Frequent vomiting or choking on food.

- Pain behind the breastbone or in the throat.

For **Breast Cancer**, see page 304; for **Cervical Cancer**, see page 308; for **Ovarian Cancer**, see page 320; for **Prostate Cancer**, see page 294; for **Skin Cancer**, see page 134; and for **Cancer of a Testicle**, see page 297.

When cancer spreads to other parts of the body, it is called **metastasis**.

Causes

Cancer could result from a mix of: Viruses, a person's genetic makeup and immune status, and other risk factors. These include:

- Exposure to the sun's ultraviolet (UV) rays, nuclear radiation, X-rays, and radon.

- Use of tobacco and/or alcohol.

- Polluted air and water.

- Dietary factors, such as a high-fat diet, the use of nitrates and nitrites in cured meats, etc.

- Exposure to certain chemicals, such as asbestos, benzenes, vinyl chloride, etc.

Treatment

In many cases, cancer can be cured, especially when it is found and treated early.

Cancer treatment depends on the type of cancer, the stage it is in, and the body's response to treatment. In general, this includes: Surgery; radiation; and/or chemotherapy. Biological therapy, hormonal therapy, and stem cell or bone marrow transplants may be used to treat some cancers.

Questions to Ask

Is any **cancer warning sign** listed on pages 134, 214, 215, and 348 present?

Self-Care / Prevention

- Medical treatment, not self-care, is needed to treat cancer. Follow your doctor's guidelines.

- Do regular self-exams as advised.

- Get routine tests that can help detect early signs of cancer. (See **Tests & What They Are For** on page 21.)

- Do not smoke or use tobacco products. Avoid secondhand smoke. Limit exposure to asbestos, radon, pesticides, and herbicides.

- Have X-rays only when necessary. Limit exposure to the sun's ultraviolet (UV) rays. (See page 135.)

- Eat plenty of fruits, vegetables, and whole-grain breads and cereals.

- Consume salt-cured, salt-pickled, and smoked foods only in moderation.

- Drink alcoholic beverages only in moderation, if at all.

- Reduce stress. Emotional stress may weaken the immune system which fights off stray cancer cells.

Chest Pain

Signs & Symptoms	What It Could Be	What To Do
• Chest pressure, squeezing, burning, tightness, or pain (may spread to the arm, neck, back, tooth, or jaw). • Chest discomfort with: Shortness of breath; sweating; nausea; fast or uneven pulse; lightheadedness; fainting. Other **Heart Attack Warning Signs** listed on page 387. • Chest pain that does not respond to medicine for a person with angina or heart problems.	**Heart Attack.**	**Call 9-1-1!** See **Heart Attack** on page 387.
• Severe chest pain with extreme pain felt across the upper back (not just on one side) that came on within 15 minutes without an injury, back strain, etc. The pain can spread to the abdomen. • A knife-like sensation from front to back. • Dizziness and fainting.	**Dissecting aortic aneurysm.** This is a tear in the main artery from the heart.	**Call 9-1-1** or go to the emergency department of a hospital! Do not take aspirin.
Chest pain that gets worse when taking deep breaths and occurs with any of these conditions: • Sudden shortness of breath and severe problems breathing. • Rapid heartbeat. • Cough with bloody sputum. • Sudden onset of chest pain with calf pain. • Recent surgery or illness with prolonged bed rest.	**Blood clot(s) to the lungs.**	**Call 9-1-1** or go to the emergency department of a hospital!
• Sudden and sharp chest pain or tightness with breathing. • Increasing shortness of breath.	**Collapsed lung.** Trauma to the chest is the main cause.	**Call 9-1-1** or go to the emergency department of a hospital!
Squeezing, pressure, indigestion feeling, or pain (often dull) in the chest. The pain may spread to the arm, neck, jaw, or back. Symptoms come on or are made worse by stress or physical exertion. They ease with rest.	**Angina.**	See **Angina** on page 232.

Chest Pain, Continued

Signs & Symptoms	What It Could Be	What To Do
The pain is on only one side of the chest and is not affected by breathing. A burning feeling and a skin rash are at the site of the pain.	**Shingles.**	See **Shingles** on page 132.
Vague pain in the chest (if any). Shortness of breath; chronic fatigue; cough with phlegm or blood; night sweats; appetite and weight loss; and fever.	**Tuberculosis (TB).** Chronic lung infection with a certain bacteria.	See doctor.
Burning feeling in the chest or just above the stomach that comes and goes before, during, or after eating. It gets worse when you bend over or lie down.	**Heartburn** or **hiatal hernia.** {*Note:* This could also signal a heart attack.}	See **Heart Attack** on page 387, **Heartburn & Indigestion** on page 161, **Hiatal Hernia** on page 167, and **Peptic Ulcers** on page 171.
Chest pain that worsens with deep breaths, coughing, or touching the chest or ribs.	**Pleurisy.** The membrane that surrounds the lungs is inflamed. **Muscle strain or rib injury.**	See doctor for diagnosis. See, also, **Sprains, Strains & Sports Injuries** on page 404.
Chest pain with fever and coughing up green, yellow, or gray mucus.	**Flu**, **pneumonia**, **bronchitis**, or other upper respiratory infection.	See doctor. See **Colds & Flu** on page 100, **Pneumonia** on page 109, and **Bronchitis** on page 98.
Sudden, sharp pain below the left nipple that lasts less than a minute or so.	**Precordial catch syndrome.** This harmless, recurrent problem usually occurs in young adults.	See doctor for diagnosis. Try daily stretching exercises to reduce getting these pains.
Pain and tender feeling in the upper part of the chest. The pain gets worse when pressure is applied to the area. It can get worse with deep breaths, too.	**Costochondritis.** This is inflammation where the ribs attach to the breastbone.	See doctor for diagnosis. Take an OTC medicine for pain and swelling. Apply a heating pad set on low or a hot water bottle to the area of pain.

Chronic Pain

Chronic pain is pain that persists. It can last for weeks, months, or even years.

Signs & Symptoms

Symptoms vary due to the cause of the pain, the kind of pain, how severe it is, and the person's response to it. With the physical feeling of pain, symptoms often include:

- Anxiety.
- Depression.
- Fatigue.
- Irritability.
- Sleep problems.
- Stress.

Chronic pain can cause a person to be less active or not active at all. It can overwhelm a person's life.

Causes

Common causes of chronic pain include:

- Arthritis.
- Fibromyalgia.
- Headaches.
- Low back pain.
- Chronic illnesses, such as cancer.
- Damage to the nervous system. An infection, injury, or chronic disease, such as diabetes can cause this.
- Nervous system disorders. One is **trigeminal neuralgia.** This affects a large nerve in the head that sends impulses from areas of the face to the brain. With this, a sudden and severe pain is felt on one side of the cheek or jaw. Another one is **postherpetic neuralgia (PHN)**. This can occur after having shingles.

Often, more than one factor causes chronic pain. Sometimes, the cause is not found.

Treatment

Treatment depends on the cause and type of pain and the person's response to it. The first step is to find the cause. Early treatment for some causes, such as shingles, can prevent or lessen chronic pain. Treatment for chronic pain includes:

- Self-care measures. (See page 219.)
- Medications. These include over-the-counter and prescribed pain medicines, antidepressants, and medications to treat the illness that causes the pain.
- Acupuncture.
- Meditation. Yoga. Massage therapy.
- Brain or local electrical stimulation.

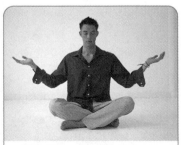

Meditate to help relieve chronic pain.

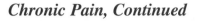

Chronic Pain, Continued

- Physical and occupational therapy.
- Counseling. Behavior changes.
- Hypnosis.
- Biofeedback.
- Surgery.

Questions to Ask

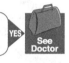

Does pain keep you from doing daily activities or getting proper sleep? **YES** → **See Doctor**

NO ↓

Does prescribed treatment for chronic pain not work? **YES** → **Call Doctor**

NO ↓

Use Self-Care

Self-Care / Prevention

- Get regular exercise. Follow your doctor's and/or physical therapist's advice. Aerobic exercise helps your body release endorphins. These are natural pain relievers.

- Maintain good health habits. Eat well, get regular sleep, etc.

- Take pain medication as prescribed by your doctor.

- Practice relaxation exercises. (See **Manage Stress** on page 53).

- Keep a pain log.
  - Record when, where, and how often you have pain.
  - Describe the type of pain and how intense it is.
  - List what makes the pain better or worse.
  - Discuss what you found out with your doctor or pain specialist.

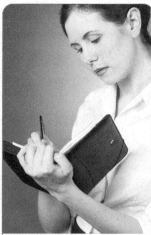

Keep a record of your pain. Discuss this with your doctor.

- Try to keep a positive outlook. Accept that life is not "pain-free." Focus on being in control of your pain. Alter activities that cause or increase the pain. Use aids to help you reach items, bathe, do chores, etc.

- Join a support group for persons with chronic pain.

Get more information from:

HealthyLearn®
www.HealthyLearn.com
Click on MedlinePlus®

American Chronic Pain Association (ACPA)
800.533.3231 • www.theacpa.org

American Pain Foundation
888.615.PAIN (615.7246)
www.painfoundation.org

Diabetes

Diabetes is having too much sugar (glucose) in the blood and not enough in the body's cells. Glucose needs to get into the cells to be used for energy. Insulin is needed for this to occur. Diabetes results when no insulin is made, not enough insulin is made, or the insulin is not used properly.

Signs & Symptoms

- Passing urine often.
- Excessive thirst.
- Extreme hunger.
- Unusual weight loss.
- Increased fatigue.
- Irritability.
- Blurry vision.

Diabetes can also be present without any of these symptoms.

Follow your doctor's advice for screening tests for diabetes. Persons with high blood pressure and/or high LDL-cholesterol should be screened. Fasting blood glucose tests help diagnose diabetes.

Fasting Plasma Glucose Test	
Plasma Glucose Result	**Diagnosis**
99 mg/dL and below	Normal
100 to 125 mg/dL	Pre-diabetes (impaired fasting glucose)
126 mg/dL and above	Diabetes*
*Confirmed by repeating the test on a different day	

Diabetes can be a very serious illness. If it is not treated, diabetes can lead to heart disease, stroke, kidney failure, and blindness.

Causes

For Four Types of Diabetes

Type 1. The pancreas gland makes no insulin or makes very small amounts. Most often, this occurs in children and young adults, but can happen at any age. In type 1 diabetes, symptoms tend to come on quickly.

Type 2. The body does not make enough insulin or does not use it the right way. Often, this occurs in persons who are over age 40, are overweight, and/or who don't exercise. In type 2 diabetes, symptoms tend to come on more slowly.

Pre-diabetes. With this type, blood glucose levels are higher than normal, but not high enough to be diabetes. Many people with pre-diabetes develop type 2 diabetes within 10 years. Modest weight loss and moderate physical activity can delay or prevent type 2 diabetes.

Gestational. This occurs during pregnancy. It usually ends when the pregnancy ends. It does, though, increase the risk for the mother to get diabetes in the future.

Diabetes, Continued

Questions to Ask

Do **signs of very low blood sugar (hypoglycemia)** occur, even after having a sugar source twice in the last 30 minutes?
- Blood sugar reading is <50 mg/dL.
- Weak, dizzy, or shaky feeling.
- Confusion.
- Numbness, tingling feeling of any part of the body, especially the hands, mouth, or lips.
- Sweating. Cold, clammy skin.
- Rapid pulse. Shallow breathing.
- Sudden blurred or double vision.
- Faintness. (May pass out.)

YES → Get Medical Care Fast

NO ↓

Do **signs of very high blood sugar (hyperglycemia)** occur?
- Tiredness. Weakness. Fatigue.
- Flushed skin. Weak, rapid pulse.
- Nausea and/or vomiting. Breath smells fruity.
- Hard time breathing. Usually short, deep breaths.
- Drunk-like behavior.
- Confusion. Dizziness. Can't be roused.

YES → Get Medical Care Fast

NO ↓

Do any of these problems occur?
- Sudden change of vision in one eye.
- **Signs and symptoms of dehydration** listed on page 372.
- Within hours to 2 days time, the skin on a foot turned grayish to black in color and sensation can't be felt in the foot.

YES → Get Medical Care Fast

NO ↓

Flowchart continued in next column

Does a person with diabetes have any of these problems?
- **Signs and symptoms of a urinary tract infection** listed on page 178.
- **Signs and symptoms of a skin infection** (e.g., redness, pain, pus, warm feeling at the site, and fever).
- A wound that does not heal. Any foot problem. Troublesome dry skin. A splinter that cannot be removed.
- Vomiting for more than 2 hours.
- Abdominal pain. Rectal problems.
- Loss of bladder control.
- For females, **signs and symptoms of a vaginal infection** on page 329.
- Fatigue that gets worse.

YES → See Doctor

NO ↓

Does a person without a diagnosis of diabetes have **signs and symptoms of diabetes** listed on page 220?

YES → See Doctor

NO ↓

Use Self-Care

Self-Care / Prevention

- ▪ Lose weight if you are overweight. Many cases of pre-diabetes and type 2 diabetes can be controlled by not being overweight.

- ▪ Do not smoke. If you smoke, quit!

- ▪ Follow the diet prescribed by your health care provider.

- ▪ Work with your doctor to develop an exercise program that works for you. When you exercise, carry something with you to eat or drink that has sugar. Examples are fruit juices, 6 or 7 hard candies, and 3 glucose tablets.

- ▪ Get a seasonal flu vaccine every year. Get other vaccines, as advised by your doctor.

Treatment

Treatment for diabetes depends on the type and how severe it is. Diabetes needs a treatment plan that maintains normal, steady blood sugar levels. This is done with:

- Proper diet.
- Weight loss, if needed.
- Exercise.
- Medicines:
  - Oral pills.
  - Insulin (through shots or an insulin pump device).
  - Medicines to treat other conditions.

Routine medical care and follow-up treatment are important to control blood sugar, blood pressure, and blood lipid levels and to prevent serious problems.

Get more information from:

HealthyLearn®
www.HealthyLearn.com
Click on MedlinePlus®

American Diabetes Association
800.232.3472
www.diabetes.org

Diabetes, Continued

- Find out if you should carry a glucagon emergency kit with you. Your doctor needs to prescribe this.

- Test your blood glucose with a home testing device. If told to, test your urine for ketones.

- Keep a journal of your blood glucose levels, your food intake, and the exercises you do. Share your journal with your doctor.

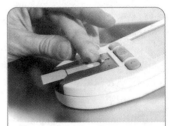
Test your blood sugar, as advised.

- Buy and wear a medical alert tag. Get one from a drug store or from: MedicAlert Foundation International 888.633.4298 or www.medicalert.org

- Take good care of your feet.
  - Keep your feet clean. Don't go barefoot.
  - Wear shoes and slippers that fit your feet well.
  - Cut toenails straight across. Do not cut them close to the skin. Have a foot doctor cut your toenails, if advised.

- Take good care of your skin and protect it from damage.
  - Keep your skin clean.
  - Avoid cuts, scrapes, punctures, etc. Treat any skin injury right away.
  - Don't get sunburned. Use sunscreen when in the sun.
  - Wear gloves in cold weather or when you do work that may injure your hands.

- Schedule eye exam(s) as advised.

- When you travel, plan, in advance, for your needs.
  - Before you leave home, locate one or more medical care facilities where you are going.
  - Take your medications; snacks and quick sugar sources; self-testing equipment; and glucagon emergency kit, if you have one.
  - If traveling by plane, ask for a special meal at least 24 hours ahead of time and/or bring foods that fit your meal plan(s).

- If you get sick, follow the plans worked out ahead of time with your doctor. This includes: Self-testing of blood sugar and ketones; what to eat and drink; and how to adjust insulin or oral pills.

Fatigue

With **fatigue**, a person is tired, weary, and lacks energy. Often, fatigue is a symptom of another health problem.

Signs & Symptoms

- Feeling drained of energy.
- Feeling exhausted.
- Having a very hard time doing normal activities.
- Having low motivation.
- Feeling inadequate.
- Having little desire for sex.

Causes

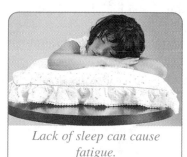

Lack of sleep can cause fatigue.

Causes that need medical care include anemia, depression, heart disease, low thyroid, lupus (the systemic type), and **chronic fatigue syndrome (CFS)**. (Find out more about CFS on page 224.)

Other physical causes include: Lack of sleep; poor diet; side effects of medicines; allergies; drug or alcohol problems; being in hot, humid conditions; and the flu.

Possible emotional causes are burnout, boredom, and a major life change, such as divorce or retirement.

Treatment

Treatment depends on the cause. Tell your doctor about any other symptoms that occur with the fatigue. He or she will explore both physical and emotional causes.

Questions to Ask

With fatigue, does any **heart attack warning sign** listed on page 387 occur? — **YES** ▸ Get Medical Care Fast

NO ▾

With fatigue, do you feel lightheaded; faint; or have a loss of balance or weakness, especially in one part or one side of the body? — **YES** ▸ Get Medical Care Fast

NO ▾

With fatigue, do these signs occur?
- The whites of your eyes and/or your skin looks yellow.
- Nausea and vomiting. Abdominal pain.
- Fever.
- Stools are pale and clay-colored.
- Dark-colored urine.

YES ▸ See Doctor

NO ▾

With extreme fatigue, do you have any of these signs?
- Fever, sore throat, and swollen lymph glands in the neck area.
- Muscle pain for more than 2 weeks, flu-like symptoms, insomnia, and headache.

YES ▸ See Doctor

NO ▾

With fatigue, do other **signs of depression** listed on page 275 occur? — **YES** ▸ See Doctor

NO ▾

Flowchart continued on next page

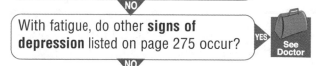

Fatigue, Continued

Chronic Fatigue Syndrome (CFS)

To be diagnosed with CFS, a person needs to have:

1. Severe chronic fatigue that lasts at least 6 months and no other medical cause could be diagnosed.

2. Four or more of these symptoms (and at the same time):

   - Problems with short-term memory or concentration.

   - Sore throat.

   - Tender lymph nodes.

   - Muscle pain.

   - Pain in joints without redness or swelling.

   - Unrefreshing sleep.

   - New type or pattern of headaches or headaches are more severe.

   - Relapse of symptoms after physical or mental exertion.

With fatigue, do any of these **signs and symptoms of lupus** occur?
- Joint pain for more than 3 months.
- Fingers that get pale, numb, or uncomfortable in the cold.
- Mouth sores for more than 2 weeks.
- Low blood counts from anemia, low white-cell count, or low platelet count.
- A "butterfly-shaped" rash on the cheeks for more than 1 month.
- Skin rash (raised patches with scaling) after being in the sun.
- Pain for more than 2 days when taking deep breaths.

YES → See Doctor

NO ↓

With fatigue, do you have any of these signs?
- Passing urine often.
- Increased thirst and hunger.
- Rapid weight loss or you gain a lot of weight.
- Extreme irritability or drowsiness.
- Itching and/or skin infections that don't clear up easily.
- Hair loss and dry, thick, flaky skin.
- Less tolerance to cold temperatures and numbness or tingling in the hands.
- Blurred vision, double vision, or the loss of vision in one eye.

YES → See Doctor

NO ↓

With fatigue and weakness, do **signs and symptoms of anemia** listed on page 212 occur?

YES → See Doctor

NO ↓

With daytime fatigue, do **signs and symptoms of sleep apnea** listed on page 257 occur?

YES → See Doctor

NO ↓

Flowchart continued on next page

Fatigue, Continued

Do any of these conditions describe the fatigue?
- It occurred for no apparent reason, lasted for more than 2 weeks, and has kept you from doing your usual activities.
- It started after taking medicine.
- For a female, it hits hard right before or after each monthly menstrual period.
- Pregnancy is possible.

YES → **See Doctor**

NO ↓

Use Self-Care

Self-Care / Prevention

- If fatigue is due to a medical problem, follow your doctor's or health care provider's guidelines for rest, diet, medication, etc.

- Get regular physical activity. Exercise can give you more energy, especially if you sit all day at work. Exercise can calm you, too.

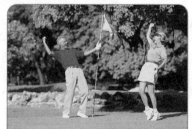

Doing physical activities you enjoy can help with fatigue.

- Cool off. Working or playing in hot weather can drag you down. Rest in a cool, dry place as often as you can. Drink plenty of water.

- Avoid too much caffeine and alcohol.

- Don't use illegal drugs.

- Lighten your work load. Assign tasks to others when you can, both at work and at home. Ask for help when you need it from family and friends. Hire help if you need to.

- Change your routine. Try to do something new and that you want to do every day.

- If you do too much, make time for some peace and quiet.

- Do something for yourself. Plan time to do things that meet only your needs, not just those of others.

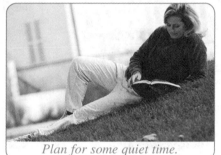

Plan for some quiet time.

Get more information from:

HealthyLearn®
www.HealthyLearn.com
Click on MedlinePlus®

Chronic Fatigue Syndrome & Fibromyalgia Information Exchange Forum (Co-Cure)
www.co-cure.org

Fever

Fever means that body temperature is above normal (about 98.6°F).

Signs & Symptoms

- A temperature higher than 99.5°F by mouth or ear or higher than 100.4°F by rectum.

- The skin feels warm.

Temperatures are more accurate when they are tested inside the body, such as by ear, mouth, or rectum. Rectal temperatures are advised for children under age 3 years old.

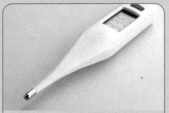

Use a digital thermometer to measure temperature. An ear thermometer is another option.

Don't use a glass mercury thermometer. If it breaks, droplets of toxic mercury can be released. If this happens, don't use a vacuum or broom to clean up the mercury. Call your local health or fire department to find out what to do.

Causes

Fever is usually a sign of another problem, such as an infection.

Body temperature changes during the day. It is usually lowest in the morning and highest in the late afternoon and evening. Other factors can increase body temperature. These include:

- Wearing too much clothing.

- Exercise.

- Hot, humid weather.

- Taking a temperature by mouth after drinking a hot liquid, like tea.

Treatment

Treatment includes self-care measures and treating the cause.

Questions to Ask

Does an infant or child up to 3 years old have any of these problems?
- Temperature of 100.4°F or higher in a baby less than 3 months old.
- Temperature of 104°F or higher in a child between 3 months and 3 years old.
- The child with a fever is crying and can't be consoled.

YES → Get Medical Care Fast

NO

With a fever, do any of these signs occur?
- Shortness of breath or a hard time breathing.
- Stiff neck; severe, headache that lasts; nausea or vomiting; and the person can't be roused.
- Acting very cranky.
- Confusion. Mental status changes.
- Severe pain in the abdomen.

YES → Get Medical Care Fast

NO

Flowchart continued on next page

Fever, Continued

With a fever, do any of these signs occur?
- Pain, redness, and swelling anywhere on the body.
- Ear pain that persists or pain in the sinuses (face).
- Pain in the chest with deep breaths.
- Sore throat.
- Green, yellow, or bloody-colored discharge from the nose, ears, or throat. A cough with colored phlegm.
- Pain or burning feeling when passing urine or passing urine often.
- Abnormal vaginal pain, discharge, or bleeding.

YES → See Doctor

NO ↓

Has the fever lasted longer than 3 days without getting better?

YES → See Doctor

NO ↓

Do any of these problems occur?
- Fever between 99.5°F and up to 100.4°F in an infant less than 3 months old.
- Fever of 102.2°F and up to 104°F in a child 3 months to 3 years old.
- Fever over 104°F in a person between 3 years old and 64 years old.
- Fever of 102°F or higher in a person age 65 or older or in a person whose immune system is lowered.

YES → See Doctor

NO ↓

Flowchart continued in next column

Has the person with the fever recently been in the hospital or had surgery? Or, does the person have a chronic illness, such as asthma, heart disease, lung disease, kidney disease, cancer, or diabetes?

YES →  Call Doctor

NO ↓

Do any of these statements apply?
- The fever went away for more than 24 hours, but came back.
- The fever came soon after a visit to another country.
- A fever <u>and</u> feeling dizzy came after having a DTaP or MMR vaccine.

YES → Call Doctor

NO ↓

 Use Self-Care

Self-Care / Prevention

- Drink lots of fluids, such as fruit juice, water, etc.

- Take a sponge bath with warm (about 70°F) water. Don't use cold or cool water. **Don't use rubbing alcohol.**

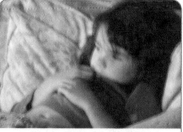
Rest when you have a fever.

- Take the right dose of an over-the-counter medicine to reduce fever.

- Rest.

- Don't do heavy exercise.

- Don't wear too many clothes. Don't use too many blankets.

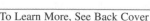

Headaches

Headaches are one of the most common health problems.

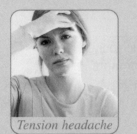

Tension headache

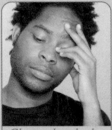

Cluster headache

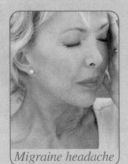

Migraine headache

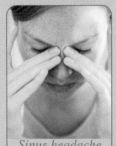

Sinus headache

Signs & Symptoms

For Tension or Muscular Headaches

- A dull ache in the forehead, above the ears, or at the back of the head.

- Pain in the neck or shoulders.

For Cluster Headaches

- Sharp, burning, and intense pain on one side of the head. The pain is so severe, you can't lie down or keep still.

- Pain in or on the sides of the eyes. The eyes water.

- Pupils look smaller. Eyelids droop.

Cluster headaches usually occur once or twice a year. They attack in groups, every day for a week or more at a time. Often, they start at night, but can start during the day, too. Cluster headaches can last from 15 minutes to 3 hours. They can interrupt sleep.

For Migraine Headaches

- One side of the head may hurt more than the other.

- Nausea or vomiting.

- Light hurts the eyes. Noise bothers you. The headache is worse with activity.

- After the headache, some people have a drained feeling with tired, aching muscles. Others feel great.

Migraines can occur with or without an aura. With an aura, spots or flashing lights or numbness occur 10 to 30 minutes before the headache. Ten percent of all migraines are this type; 90% occur without an aura.

For Sinus Headaches

- Pain in the forehead, cheekbones, and nose. The pain is worse in the morning.

- Increased pain when you bend over or touch your face.

- Stuffy nose.

Headaches, Continued

Causes

For Tension Headaches

Most headaches are this type. Common causes are tense or tight muscles in the face, neck, or scalp.

For Cluster Headaches

The cause is not known. These headaches are four times more common in men than in women. Heavy drinkers and smokers are at an increased risk for cluster headaches.

For Migraine Headaches

These headaches happen when blood vessels in the head open too wide or close too tight. They occur more often in females than in males. Migraines tend to run in families.

For people prone to migraine headaches, certain things trigger them.

- Menstruation in females.
- Caffeine and drinks with alcohol, such as red wine. Aged cheeses. Cured meats.
- Stress. Changes in sleeping patterns.
- Heavy exercise.

For Sinus Headaches

These occur when fluids in the nose aren't able to drain well. This builds up pressure in the sinuses. A cold, allergies, and airplane travel can cause a sinus headache.

Other Causes of Headaches

- Analgesic rebound from regular or repeated use of over-the-counter or prescribed pain relievers.

- Eating or drinking something very cold, such as ice cream. {*Note:* To prevent ice cream headaches, warm the ice cream for a few seconds in the front of the mouth.}
- Cigarette smoke, pollution, etc.
- Caffeine withdrawal.
- Uncorrected vision problems, such as nearsightedness.
- A symptom of a health problem. Examples are allergies, depression, high blood pressure, a pinched nerve in the neck, and dental problems.
- Low blood sugar. Hunger. Sensitivity to certain foods and drinks. (See box below.)

Foods & Drinks That May Cause Headaches
Alcoholic beverages, especially red wine.
Aspartame (the artificial sweetener in NutraSweet®).
Bananas (if more than ¹/₂ banana a day).
Caffeine from coffee, tea, cola, other soft drinks, chocolate, or some medications. Suddenly stopping caffeine intake.
Citrus fruits (if more than ¹/₂ cup a day).
Cured meats, such as frankfurters.
Food additives, such as MSG.
Hard cheeses like aged cheddar or provolone.
Nuts. Peanut butter.
Onions.
Sour cream.
Soy sauce.
Vinegar.

Less often, a headache is a symptom of a serious health problem that needs immediate care. Examples are acute glaucoma and stroke.

Headaches, Continued

Children's Headaches
- ■ Headaches tend to last less time than they do in adults.
- ■ Sometimes, an upset stomach and vomiting occur.
- ■ Headaches come in groups then are gone for months.

Treatment

Self-care can treat headaches caused by tension, fatigue, and/or stress. Certain over-the-counter medicines and prescribed medicines can treat migraine headaches.

Headaches that are symptoms of health problems are relieved when the condition is treated with success.

Children's headaches that come once in awhile can be treated with ibuprofen or acetaminophen. **Make sure to use the right type and dose for the child's weight.** Don't give aspirin to anyone younger than 19 years of age due to its link to Reye's Syndrome. If the child complains of head pain on a regular basis, take the child to his or her doctor.

Questions to Ask

Is the headache linked with any of these problems?
- A serious head injury or passing out.
- A blow to the head that causes severe pain, enlarged pupils, vomiting, or confusion.

YES → Get Medical Care Fast

NO

With a severe headache that lasts, do any other **symptoms of meningitis** listed on page 80 occur?

YES → Get Medical Care Fast

NO

Is the headache linked with any of these problems?
- Severe pain in and around one eye.
- Blurred vision or double vision.
- Slurring of speech.
- Mental confusion.
- Personality change.
- A problem moving the arms or legs.
- Unusual sleepiness.

YES → Get Medical Care Fast

NO

Has the headache come on fast and does it hurt much more than any headache in the past?

YES → Get Medical Care Fast

NO

Has the headache lasted more than 2 to 3 days and does the pain keep getting worse and last longer?

YES →  See Doctor

NO

Flowchart continued on next page

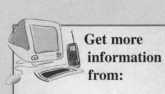

Get more information from:

HealthyLearn®
www.HealthyLearn.com
Click on MedlinePlus®

National Headache
Foundation
800.843.2256
www.headaches.org

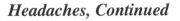

Headaches, Continued

Do you have nausea or vomiting with a headache that doesn't go away or that recurs? **YES** See Doctor

NO

Do you have **symptoms of a cluster headache** or **migraine headache** listed on page 228? **YES** See Doctor

NO

For pregnant females, does swelling of the legs, hands, and/or face also occur with the headache? **YES** See Doctor

NO

Is the headache not relieved by over-the-counter pain relievers and does it occur with any **signs and symptoms of a sinus infection** listed on page 90 or in a person with high blood pressure? **YES** See Doctor

NO

Do you have a headache at the same time of a day, week, or month, and do over-the-counter pain relievers not help the pain? **YES** See Doctor

NO

Do you take pain relievers more than 3 times a week for at least 3 weeks for headaches or did you get headaches only after taking a new medicine? **YES** See Doctor

NO

Use Self-Care

Self-Care / Prevention

- Don't smoke. If you smoke, quit.
- Try to stop the headache when it starts.

- Take an over-the-counter (OTC) medicine for pain as directed.

- Massage the back of your neck with your thumbs. Work from the ears toward the center of the back of your head. Also, rub gently along the sides of your eyes. Gently rub your shoulders, neck, and jaw. Get a massage.

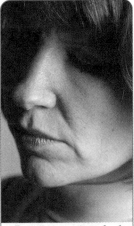

Rest in a quiet, dark room with your eyes closed.

- Take a warm bath or shower. Place a cold or warm washcloth or OTC hot or cold pack over the area that aches.

- Relax. Picture a calm scene in your head. Meditate or breathe deeply.

- Exercise on a regular basis. Get adequate rest.

- Try using a different pillow and/or sleep position.

- If you grind your teeth, tell your dentist or doctor.

- Keep a diary of when, where, and why headaches occur. Avoid items in **Foods & Drinks That May Cause Headaches** listed on page 229.

- To help prevent headaches and nausea caused by a hangover, try an OTC product, such as Chaser–Freedom From Hangovers.

- For a hangover: After drinking alcohol, take an OTC pain reliever. Eat solid foods. Rest or sleep. Have 2 or more glasses of water before you go to sleep. Drink 2 or more glasses of water when you wake up.

Heart Disease

Heart disease is a common term for **coronary artery disease (CAD)**. It is the number one cause of death in the U.S. in both men and women. With heart disease, arteries that supply blood to the heart become hardened and narrowed.

Heart disease can lead to these problems:

- **Angina.** With this, the heart muscle does not get as much blood and oxygen as it needs for a given level of work. A heart attack damages the heart muscle. Angina does not. It is a warning sign that a heart attack could occur, though.

- **Heart attack.** (See page 387.)

- **Heart failure (HF).** With this, the heart "fails" to supply the body with enough blood and oxygen for its needs. This develops slowly. It becomes chronic.

Signs & Symptoms

- Symptoms of angina are pain, discomfort, or a squeezing pressure in the chest. Aching in a tooth, jaw, or neck can also occur. Symptoms usually go away with rest and/or nitroglycerin. Angina attacks may occur with anger, excitement, or exertion, such as walking up a hill.

- Symptoms of a heart attack are listed on page 387.

- Symptoms of heart failure are: Shortness of breath; feeling very tired or weak; swelling in the lower legs, ankles, and feet; dry cough or one with pink, frothy mucus; rapid weight gain; and a fast heart beat.

Causes

Heart disease is caused by **atherosclerosis**. This is the buildup of plaque in the inner walls of the arteries. The plaque is made up of blood platelets, cholesterol, fibrous tissue, and sometimes calcium. The plaque narrows the arteries. This slows or blocks the flow of blood to the heart.

Some factors increase the risk of heart disease. The more risk factors; the higher the risk.

Risk Factors That Can't Be Changed

- A past heart attack or stroke.

- Family history of heart disease:
  - A father or brother had heart disease before age 55.
  - A mother or sister had heart disease before age 65.

- Being a male 45 years or older.

- Being a female 55 years or older.

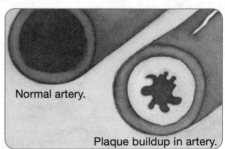

Normal artery.

Plaque buildup in artery.

Risk Factors That Can Be Controlled

- **High blood pressure.** (See page 238.)

- **High-risk blood cholesterol levels.** (See page 49.)

- Smoking. (See **Be Tobacco-Free** on page 50.)

- Being overweight or obese.

Heart Disease, Continued

- Lack of physical activity.
- Having diabetes and high blood cholesterol.
- Using cocaine or amphetamines.
- **Metabolic syndrome**. (See page 234.)

Other Factors that May Play a Role in Heart Disease

- Waist measurement > 40 inches for men; > 35 inches for women.
- C-reactive protein (CRP) in the blood. Levels of CRP rise when there is inflammation in the body.
- Elevated blood homocysteine levels.
- Infections, such as *chlamydia pneumoniae*.
- Elevated blood lipoprotein (a).
- Elevated blood triglycerides.

Treatment

The goals of treatment are to relieve symptoms, control or reduce risk factors, stop or slow further damage to the arteries, and prevent and treat cardiac events. Treatment includes:

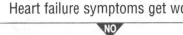
Take medicines as prescribed.

- **Self-Care / Prevention** measures on page 234.
- Medications.
- Procedures to open blocked or narrowed arteries or bypass them.
- Cardiac rehabilitation (rehab).

Questions to Ask

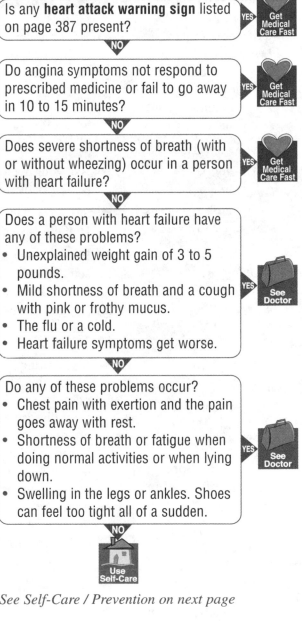

Is any **heart attack warning sign** listed on page 387 present?
→ YES: Get Medical Care Fast
↓ NO

Do angina symptoms not respond to prescribed medicine or fail to go away in 10 to 15 minutes?
→ YES: Get Medical Care Fast
↓ NO

Does severe shortness of breath (with or without wheezing) occur in a person with heart failure?
→ YES: Get Medical Care Fast
↓ NO

Does a person with heart failure have any of these problems?
- Unexplained weight gain of 3 to 5 pounds.
- Mild shortness of breath and a cough with pink or frothy mucus.
- The flu or a cold.
- Heart failure symptoms get worse.
→ YES: See Doctor
↓ NO

Do any of these problems occur?
- Chest pain with exertion and the pain goes away with rest.
- Shortness of breath or fatigue when doing normal activities or when lying down.
- Swelling in the legs or ankles. Shoes can feel too tight all of a sudden.
→ YES: See Doctor
↓ NO

Use Self-Care

See Self-Care / Prevention on next page

Metabolic Syndrome is having at least three of these five conditions:

1. *Abdominal obesity.* Waist measurement for this varies according to sex and ethnic group. Ask your doctor.

2. High triglycerides:*
   ≥ 150 mg/dL

3. *Low HDL-cholesterol:*
   < 40 mg/dL for males;
   < 50 mg/dL for females

4. *High blood pressure:*
   ≤ 130 mm Hg systolic and/or
   ≤ 85 mm Hg diastolic

5. *High fasting glucose:*
   ≥ 100 mg/dL

   * Or taking medication to treat this condition.

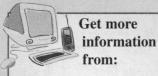

Get more information from:

The American Heart Association
800.242.8721
www.americanheart.org

National Heart, Lung, and Blood Institute (NHLBI)
www.nhlbi.nih.gov

Heart Disease, Continued

Self-Care / Prevention

■ Have regular medical checkups. Get your blood pressure checked at each office visit or at least every 2 years. Get your blood cholesterol tested regularly, as advised by your doctor.

■ Don't smoke. If you smoke, quit.

■ Get to or stay at a healthy weight.

■ Take all medications as prescribed.

■ Ask your doctor about the benefits and harms of aspirin therapy (e.g., 1 baby aspirin daily).

■ See your doctor if you have any of the **Signs & Symptoms** of **Diabetes** listed on page 220.

■ Follow a diet low in saturated fats, *trans* fats, and cholesterol. Limit sodium to 1,500 to 2,400 milligrams per day. Follow the **DASH Eating Plan.** (See page 46.)

■ Get regular exercise. Follow your doctor's advice.

■ Manage stress. Practice relaxation techniques.

■ If you drink alcohol, do so in moderation. Too much alcohol can raise the risk for high blood pressure, heart disease, stroke, and other health problems. Moderate drinking, may be linked to a lower risk of coronary heart disease in some persons. Moderation means no more than 2 drinks a day for men; 1 drink a day for women and persons age 65 and older. One drink = 4-5 oz. of wine; 12 oz. of beer; or 1¹/₂ oz. of 80-proof liquor.

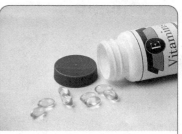

Get your doctor's advice on taking vitamins and other supplements.

■ Ask your doctor how much, if any, alcohol you should drink.

■ Get your doctor's advice about taking vitamins, minerals, and herbal products.

Heart Palpitations

Signs & Symptoms

Palpitations can be felt in the chest, throat, or neck. With them, it feels like the heart is pounding, racing, and/or fluttering. It can feel like the heart has skipped a beat.

Causes

Most of the time, palpitations are not a serious problem. Common causes include:

- Anxiety. Fear. Stress. Hyperventilation.
- Caffeine. Diet pills. Nicotine. Drugs.
- Exercise.
- Medicines. Examples are beta-blockers, some asthma and cold medicines, and thyroid pills.

Other causes are:

- An **arrhythmia** (heart rate or rhythm disorder).
- **Mitral valve prolapse (MVP)**. This is a heart valve problem. It may be treated with medicine. It is not usually a serious condition.
- **Anemia.** (See page 212.)
- **Hyperthyroidism.** (See page 260.)
- Low blood sugar.

Treatment

Treatment depends on the cause.

Questions to Ask

With palpitations, is any **heart attack warning** sign listed on page 387 present?

YES Get Medical Care Fast

NO

Flowchart continued in next column

To Learn More, See Back Cover

Do any of these problems occur?
- Fainting. Feeling faint or dizzy. Cool, clammy skin.
- Pulse of 150 or more beats per minute.
- New onset of a very irregular heartbeat and a history of a heart condition.
- Within 24 hours, palpitations occur 3 or more times. Each one lasts at least 10 minutes.

YES Get Medical Care Fast

NO

With palpitations, are any of these problems present?
- **Signs of hyperthyroidism** on page 260.
- Symptoms persist for hours or days.
- **Heart disease risk factors** on pages 232 and 233.
- A person with an arrhythmia has new or worse symptoms.

YES See Doctor

NO

 Use Self-Care

Self-Care / Prevention

- If palpitations occur with exercise, stop the activity. Rest. When you exercise again, gradually increase how long and how intense you do the activity.
- To relieve stress and anxiety, do relaxation exercises.
- Limit or avoid caffeine, nicotine, and alcohol.
- Don't take cold/allergy medicines. Don't take appetite suppressants.
- Call your doctor if rest doesn't help or if palpitations occur again and again.

Hepatitis

Hepatitis is liver inflammation. With hepatitis, the liver has trouble screening poisons from the blood. Also, the liver can't regulate bile. This is a liquid that helps digest fats.

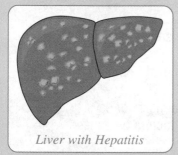

Liver with Hepatitis

Signs & Symptoms

Signs and symptoms depend on the cause. Some persons have no symptoms. When symptoms first occur, they include fatigue, fever, appetite loss, nausea and vomiting, and joint pain.

Later, symptoms are dark urine, pale, clay-colored stools, and **jaundice**. This is a yellow color to the whites of the eyes and/or the skin.

Causes

One or More Types of Viral Hepatitis

- *Hepatitis A.* This is spread through food or water contaminated by the feces of an infected person that has the virus.

- *Hepatitis B.* This is caused by contact with infected blood or bodily fluids from an infected person. Examples are sharing drug needles or having sex. A mother can pass this virus to her baby during childbirth, too.

- *Hepatitis C.* Most often, the cause is contact with infected blood on needles, razors, toothbrushes, etc. Blood transfusions given before July, 1992 could be the cause, if the blood had the virus. Sexual contact may spread the virus, too.

- *Hepatitis D.* Sharing drug needles or having sexual contact with an infected person can cause this type, but only in persons who already have hepatitis B. It is not common in the U.S.

- *Hepatitis E.* This is caused by contact with food, water, or something contaminated with the feces of an infected person. This type is not common in the U.S. It is more common in Africa and India.

Non-Viral Causes of Hepatitis

- Some immune system disorders, such as **Wilson's disease**. With this, too much copper is stored in the liver and other body organs.

- Chronic alcohol or drug use.

- Reaction to certain medicines. One example is long-term use or an overdose of acetaminophen. Heavy drinkers are more prone to this.

- Some herbs may cause hepatitis. Examples are kava and chaparral.

In some cases, the cause is not known.

Treatment

Treatment depends on the type of hepatitis and how severe it is. For non-viral forms, this includes treating the disorder or stopping the use of the substance that caused it. For viral forms, treatment includes self-care measures and medications.

Hepatitis, Continued

Questions to Ask

Is the person with hepatitis unable to be roused or is he or she confused or very, very sleepy?

YES → Get Medical Care Fast

NO ↓

Do any of these problems occur?
- Yellow skin or the whites of the eyes look yellow.
- Dark urine. Pale, clay-colored stools.
- Symptoms return after recovering from hepatitis.

YES → See Doctor

NO ↓

Do you have 2 or more of these symptoms, especially after being exposed to someone with hepatitis?
- Unexplained fatigue.
- Fever.
- Appetite loss.
- Nausea and vomiting.
- Joint pain.

YES → See Doctor

NO ↓

Use Self-Care

Self-Care / Prevention

To Help Prevent Hepatitis A and E

- Get a hepatitis A vaccine if advised by your doctor or health department. (See **Immunization Schedule** on page 23.) There is no vaccine for hepatitis E.

- When you travel to countries where the virus is widespread, wash your hands often. Drink boiled water. Don't eat unpeeled or uncooked fruits or foods rinsed with water. Don't use ice.

- If exposed to hepatitis A, contact your doctor to get immune globulin (IG) within 2 weeks of exposure.

To Help Prevent Hepatitis B, C, and D

- Get 3 doses of hepatitis B vaccine if advised by your doctor. (See **Immunization Schedule** on page 23.) There is no vaccine for hepatitis C.

- Practice **Safer Sex**. (See page 252.)

- Don't share IV drug needles.

- Don't share razors or toothbrushes. See that sterilized items are used for ear piercing, etc.

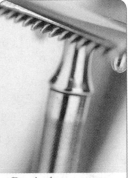
Don't share razors.

To Help Prevent Non-Viral Forms

- Use alcohol in moderation, if at all.

- Don't combine alcohol and acetaminophen. Take products that contain acetaminophen, such as Tylenol, as directed. Heed warnings listed on the label.

To Treat Hepatitis

- Follow your doctor's advice for medicines, etc.

- Rest.

- Drink at least 8 glasses of fluids a day.

- Avoid alcohol and any drugs or medicines that affect the liver, such as acetaminophen.

- Follow a healthy diet. Take vitamins and minerals as advised by your doctor.

Get more information from:

HealthyLearn® • www.HealthyLearn.com
Click on MedlinePlus®

National Center for HIV/AIDS, Viral Hepatitis, STD, and TB Prevention
800.CDC.INFO (232.4636)
www.cdc.gov/nchhstp

To Learn More, See Back Cover

High Blood Pressure

High blood pressure (HBP) is when blood moves through the arteries at a higher pressure than normal. The heart strains to pump blood through the arteries.

Blood pressure is measured with a blood pressure cuff placed on the arm. The first (higher) number measures systolic pressure. This is the maximum pressure against the artery walls while the heart beats. The second (lower) number measures diastolic pressure. This is the pressure between heartbeats, when the heart refills. The results are given as systolic/diastolic pressure, such as 120/80 mm Hg.

Blood Pressure Category (ages 18+)	Systolic (mm Hg)	Diastolic (mm Hg)
Normal	<120	and <80
Prehypertension	120–139	or 80–89
Stage 1 hypertension	140–159	or 90–99
Stage 2 hypertension	≥160	or ≥100

For persons with HBP, blood pressure goal is <140/90 mm Hg. For African Americans and persons with diabetes or kidney disease, the goal is <130/80 mm Hg.

Signs & Symptoms

There are usually no signs or symptoms. Only 2 out of 3 people with HBP know that they have it.

Causes

The exact cause is not known. Risk factors include:

- Family history of HBP.
- Aging.
- Smoking cigarettes.

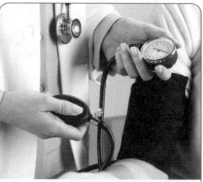

Get your blood pressure checked at each office visit, at least every 2 years, or as advised.

- Race. HBP is more common in African Americans than in Caucasians.
- Gender. HBP is more common in men than in women.
- Being inactive. Obesity. Sleep apnea.
- Emotional distress.
- Too much sodium intake in some persons.

Treatment

When self-care measures are not enough, one or more medicines may be prescribed. If it is not treated, HBP can lead to heart, kidney, eye problems, and stroke.

High Blood Pressure, *Continued*

Questions to Ask

Does a person with high blood pressure have any of these problems?
- Chest pain.
- Trouble breathing.
- Severe headache.
- Palpitations.
- Feeling dizzy.
- Numbness or tingling in the hands or feet.
- Confusion.

YES  Get Medical Care Fast

NO

Do medicine(s) for high blood pressure make you dizzy or cause other problems?

YES  Call Doctor

NO

Do you have any risk factor for high blood pressure and have you not had your blood pressure checked within 2 years?

YES Call Doctor

NO

 Use Self-Care

Self-Care / Prevention

To Help Prevent High Blood Pressure
- Get to and/or stay at a healthy weight.
- Don't smoke. If you smoke, quit.
- Limit alcohol to 2 drinks or less a day for males; 1 drink or less a day for females and persons age 65 and older.
- Do regular exercise.
- Manage stress.
- Follow the **DASH Eating Plan**. (See page 46.)

- Limit total sodium from table salt and salt and sodium in foods. Try to get no more than 1,500 to 2,400 milligrams per day. This is the amount in about $^2/_3$rds to 1 teaspoon of salt. Read food labels for sodium content.

To Treat High Blood Pressure
- Follow tips to prevent HBP.

- Take medicine as prescribed. {*Note:* Most persons need more than one medicine to treat high blood pressure.} Tell your doctor about side effects. Are you dizzy? Do you feel faint? Do you have a dry cough without a cold?

- Limit caffeine.

- Discuss all prescribed and over-the-counter medicines with your doctor before you take them. Find out about drug and food interactions, too. You may

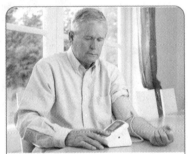

Check your blood pressure at home, as advised by your doctor.

be told not to have grapefruit juice if you take certain medicines. Your pharmacist can answer questions, too.

Get more information from:

HealthyLearn® • www.HealthyLearn.com
Click on MedlinePlus®

The American Heart Association
800.242.8721 or www.americanheart.org

National Heart, Lung, and Blood Institute
(NHLBI) • www.nhlbi.nih.gov

HIV / AIDS

HIV stands for **human immunodeficiency virus**. **AIDS** is **acquired immune deficiency syndrome**. It is caused by HIV. The virus destroys the body's immune system. This leaves a person unable to fight off diseases. The virus also attacks the central nervous system causing mental problems.

One million people in the U.S. have HIV, but about 25% of them do not know they have it. This is one reason the Centers for Disease Control and Prevention (CDC) advise testing for HIV as a routine part of medical care.

Signs & Symptoms

Many people have no symptoms when first infected with HIV. Within a month or two, some people have flu-like symptoms. These include fever, fatigue, headache, and swollen glands in the neck and groin. These symptoms usually go away within a week to a month. They are often mistaken for other infections.

In adults, symptoms of HIV may take a few months to 10 or more years to appear. In children born with HIV, symptoms appear within 2 years.

Symptoms of HIV Before the Onset of AIDS
- Swollen glands.
- Fatigue. Weight loss.
- Fever and sweating that occur often.
- Skin rashes that persist. Flaky skin.
- Infections. These include herpes, shingles, and yeast infection.
- Short-term memory loss.
- Getting sick often. Slow growth in children.

AIDS is the most advanced stage of HIV. With AIDS, a low level of cells in the blood called T4 cells occurs. Persons with AIDS get many illnesses. These include skin infections, pneumonia, and cancer.

Symptoms of AIDS
- Extreme fatigue. Weight loss.
- Severe and chronic diarrhea.
- Fever. Severe headaches.
- Shortness of breath. Coughing. A hard time swallowing.
- Abdominal cramps. Nausea. Vomiting.
- Lack of coordination. Vision loss.
- Mental status changes. Seizures. Coma.

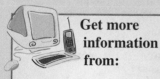

Get more information from:

HealthyLearn®
www.HealthyLearn.com
Click on MedlinePlus®

AIDSinfo
800.HIV.0440 (448.0440)
www.aidsinfo.nih.gov

HIV / AIDS, Continued

Causes

HIV is spread when body fluids, such as semen and blood, pass from an infected person to another person. This includes having unprotected sexual contact and/or sharing drug needles.

Infected females can give HIV to their babies during pregnancy, birth, or breast-feeding. The risk of the baby getting HIV is lowered a great deal if the female takes antiviral medicines during the pregnancy and delivery. The baby takes medicine the first six weeks of life, too.

HIV is *not* spread from donating blood, touching, hugging, or (dry) kissing a person with HIV. A cough, a sneeze, tears, sweat, or using a hot tub, or public restroom *does not* spread HIV either.

Treatment

A rapid oral HIV test and blood tests detect antibodies to HIV. There is no cure for AIDS, but treatment helps the immune system fight HIV, infections, and cancers that can occur with it. Treatment includes medications (often used in multidrug combinations) and treating infections.

Questions to Ask

Have you tested positive for HIV? **YES** See Doctor

NO

Do you have any of these conditions?
- A sexually transmitted infection (STI).
- Persistent yeast infections in the mouth (thrush) or vagina.
- Unprotected sex with a current or past sexual partner that has HIV.

YES See Doctor

NO

Flowchart continued in next column

Do you do high risk activities for getting infected with HIV listed on this page? Or, do you want to get tested for HIV for "peace of mind"? **YES** See Doctor or Health Department for HIV testing

NO

Use Self-Care

Self-Care / Prevention

- Take medication as prescribed.

- Take steps to reduce the risk of getting infections and diseases. Get enough rest. Eat healthy foods. Take vitamins and minerals as advised by your doctor.

- Get emotional support. Join a support group for persons infected with HIV. Let your family and friends know how they can help you.

To Reduce the Risk for HIV
- Follow **Safer Sex**. (See page 252.)

- Don't have sex with people who are at high risk for HIV:
  - Persons with multiple sex partners or who inject illegal drugs.
  - Partners of persons infected or exposed to HIV.
  - Persons who have had multiple blood transfusions, especially before 1985, unless tested negative for HIV.

- Don't share needles with anyone. Don't have sex with people who use or have injected illegal drugs.

- Don't share personal items that have blood on them, such as razors.

Memory Loss

With **short-term memory loss**, you can't recall things learned in the past seconds to minutes. With **long-term memory loss**, you forget things learned in the distant past, such as in childhood. It is normal to have some memory loss as you age. It is common to forget where you put your eyeglasses or keys. You may have a hard time recalling the name of a person or place, and say, "It is on the tip of my tongue." This memory loss is temporary and not severe. When it persists or interferes with your daily life, it can be a sign of a problem.

Signs & Symptoms

Signs and symptoms of serious memory loss, such as amnesia, depend on the cause. The memory loss can be partial or complete. It can occur for a short time or persist. It can also come on suddenly or slowly.

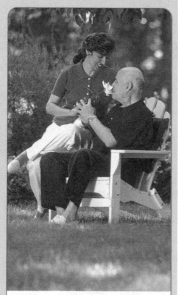

Signs and symptoms may be noticed by the person's relatives and friends who can tell when memory lapses worsen.

Causes

Other than the normal memory loss that comes with aging, causes include:

- **Depression.** (See page 275.)

- Excess alcohol. Drug use.

- Side effects of some medicines.

- Alzheimer's disease and other forms of **dementia**. Dementias result in a decline of all areas of mental ability. This includes learning, problem solving, language, behaviors, and memory loss.

- **Mild cognitive impairment**. This is a medical illness. With this, people have abnormal memory for their age and education. They have a harder time learning new information or recalling things.

- **Posttraumatic stress disorder.** (See page 284.)

- Seizures. Head trauma.

- Stroke.

- Brain infections or tumors.

Treatment

Memory loss that persists, is severe, or that interferes with daily life needs a medical diagnosis. When another problem is the cause and is treated with success, memory loss improves. For other causes, such as Alzheimer's disease, there is no cure. The goal is to treat symptoms and provide safety and comfort.

Memory Loss, Continued

Questions to Ask

Is the person suddenly very confused or not aware of time, place, persons, and things?

YES **Get Medical Care Fast**

NO

Are these **signs and symptoms of dementia** present?
- Poor memory of recent events, etc.
- Making up stories to explain memory loss.
- Getting lost in familiar places.
- Not being able to finish tasks.
- Social withdrawal or depression.
- General confusion.
- Behaviors that are paranoid, anxious, irritating, childlike, or rigid.
- No interest in personal hygiene, grooming, or getting dressed.
- Unclear speech.

YES **See Doctor**

NO

Are any of these problems present?
- **Signs and symptoms of Alzheimer's disease** listed on page 210.
- **Signs and symptoms of depression** listed on page 275.
- Memory loss that can't be explained.

YES **See Doctor**

NO

 Use Self-Care

Self-Care / Prevention

To Help Prevent Memory Loss
- Keep the brain active. Read, do puzzles, etc.
- Eat a balanced diet. Take vitamins and minerals, as advised by your doctor.

- Get regular exercise.
- Protect the head from injury.
- Follow tips under **Prevention** for **Stroke (Brain Attack)** listed on page 407.
- Don't smoke or use illegal drugs. Limit alcohol.
- Manage stress.
- Get regular eye exams. Get your hearing checked. If needed, wear eyeglasses and/or a hearing aid.

To Help Remember Things
- Follow a routine for daily and weekly activities.
- Listen carefully. Link newly learned things to past memories.
- Repeat what you want to remember out loud. Write it down if you need to.
- Keep track of important things to do, phone numbers, etc. Use a calendar, planner, PDA, etc.
- Set up a system to remind you of daily medications to take, bills to pay, appointments to keep, etc.
- Put your keys, eyeglasses, etc. in the same place.

See also **Self-Care / Prevention** for **Alzheimer's Disease** on page 211.

Get more information from:

HealthyLearn® • www.HealthyLearn.com
Click on MedlinePlus®

Multiple Sclerosis

Multiple Sclerosis (MS) is a chronic disease of the brain and spinal cord. With MS, a covering that protects nerves (myelin) and the nerves are damaged or destroyed. Over time, scar tissue forms along the damaged myelin. Nerves can't send signals like they should. As a result, movement, sensation, etc. are impaired or lost.

Signs & Symptoms

- Fatigue.
- Feelings of pins and needles. Numbness. Leg stiffness.
- Poor coordination. Unsteady gait. Impaired movement.
- Bladder problems.
- Blurred vision. Double vision. Loss of vision in one eye.
- Depression. Mild problems with memory, learning, etc.
- Swallowing problems.

Early signs and symptoms may be mild and present for years before MS is diagnosed.

Symptoms vary from person to person. They may last for hours or weeks. They can vary from day to day and can come and go with no set pattern.

Some persons have only a few symptoms over the course of the disease. For others, symptoms continue and/or worsen with time. Most persons with MS get symptom flare-ups (relapses) that are followed by partial or complete recoveries (remissions).

Causes

The exact cause of MS is not known. It may be due to a number of factors. These include: A virus, genetics, and an immune system problem. Toxins, trauma, poor nutrition, and other factors may also play a role.

Persons more likely to develop MS are: White adults between the ages of 20 and 50; women; residents of North America, Europe, and Southern Australia; and first-degree relatives of persons with MS.

Things known to come before the onset of MS include: Overwork; fatigue; the postpartum period for women; acute infections; and fevers.

Get more information from:

HealthyLearn®
www.HealthyLearn.com
Click on MedlinePlus®

Multiple Sclerosis Foundation
888.MS.FOCUS
(673.6287)
www.msfocus.org

National Multiple Sclerosis Society
www.nationalmssociety.org

Multiple Sclerosis, Continued

Treatment

There is no cure yet for MS, but most people with it live a normal life span. Treatment for MS includes:

- Prescribed medication to lessen the number and severity of flare-ups and to slow the progression of the disease. Research favors early treatment with this type of medicine.

- Short-term courses of IV or oral corticosteroids. These reduce inflammation during MS flare-ups.

- Medications to control and treat MS symptoms. Treating infections, when present.

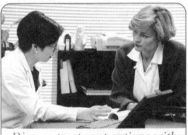
Discuss treatment options with your doctor.

- Physical and occupational therapy.

- Counseling. Support groups.

- Clinical trails. Access www.clinicaltrials.gov.

Questions to Ask

Does a person with multiple sclerosis have any of these problems?
- New or worsening symptoms.
- **Signs and symptoms of depression** listed on page 275.
- **Signs of a urinary tract infection** listed on page 178 or of a **skin infection** listed on page 120.

YES → See Doctor

NO ↓

Flowchart continued in next column

Does a person have one or more of these problems?
- Gradual onset of vision loss (especially in one eye), blurred vision, or double vision.
- Fatigue, weakness, numbness, or tingling in the arms or legs.
- A tingling feeling that spreads down the spine and into the legs when bending the neck forward.

YES → See Doctor

NO ↓

Use Self-Care

Self-Care / Prevention

- Follow your doctor's guidelines for home care.

- Maintain a normal routine at work and at home. Avoid activities that lead to fatigue or put too much physical stress on the body. Get plenty of rest.

- Manage emotional stress.

- Avoid the heat and sun. Don't take hot showers or baths. Increased body temperature can cause symptoms. Cool baths or swimming in a pool may improve symptoms by lowering body temperature.

- Treat a fever as soon as it occurs.

- Get regular exercise. Physical therapy may be helpful.

- Have body massages to help maintain muscle tone.

- Get counseling, if needed.

- Get a seasonal flu shot every year and other vaccines as advised.

To Learn More, See Back Cover

Parkinson's Disease

Parkinson's disease (PD) affects the nervous system. It occurs equally in men and women of all races and ethnic groups. It most often affects people over the age of 50. The average age of onset is 60 years.

Signs & Symptoms

Early symptoms can be subtle. They occur gradually and include:

- Feeling a little shaky. A person's handwriting can look spidery.
- Being tired. Speaking too softly.
- Losing track of a word or thought.
- Having no facial expression.
- Feeling irritable or depressed for no known reason.

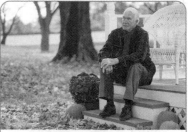

Movement can be difficult for persons with Parkinson's disease.

The Four Main Symptoms

- Tremor. This usually starts in the head, but can start in a foot or in the jaw. {*Note:* About 30% of people with Parkinson's disease do not shake or tremble or rarely do so.}
- Stiffness of the limbs and trunk.
- Slow movement. Less natural movement. The person may not be able to wash or dress quickly or easily.
- Loss of balance and coordination. This can lead to a stooped posture, a shuffling gait, and falls.

Other Symptoms

- Problems with chewing and swallowing.
- Having a hard time changing positions.
- Depression. Anxiety.
- Speech changes. The person may speak too softly or in a monotone. The person may slur or repeat words, or speak too fast.
- Bladder or bowel problems, such as constipation.
- Skin that is too oily or too dry.
- Restless sleep. Being drowsy during the day. Having a harder time staying asleep at night.
- Dementia (in advanced stages).

Get more information from:

HealthyLearn®
www.HealthyLearn.com
Click on MedlinePlus®

American Parkinson's Disease Association
800.223.2732
www.apdaparkinson.com

National Parkinson Foundation
800.327.4545
www.parkinson.org

Parkinson's Disease, Continued

Causes

The exact cause of Parkinson's disease is not known. What is known, though, is that certain cells in the lower part of the brain can't produce dopamine. Nerves need this to coordinate body movement.

{*Note:* Some medicines can bring on symptoms like ones of Parkinson's disease. Examples are strong tranquilizers and Reglan, a drug used for some digestive problems.}

Risk Factors

- Family history of the disease.

- Aging. For some persons, the neurons that produce dopamine wear away with aging.

- Rarely, repeated trauma to the head. This can happen to boxers. Muhammad Ali has this condition.

- Damage to nerve cells through a chemical process called oxidation.

- Toxins in the environment.

Treatment

Parkinson's disease is not yet curable. Symptoms can be relieved or controlled. Treatment includes:

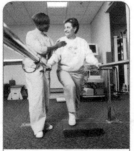

Exercise and physical therapy help a person who has Parkinson's disease with movement and balance.

- Medicines, such as levodopa, selegiline, and apomorphine.

- Physical therapy. Speech therapy.

- Direct electrical brain stimulation.

- Neurosurgery.

Questions to Ask

Are one or more **signs and symptoms of Parkinson's disease** listed on page 246 present?

YES → See Doctor

NO ↓

Does a person with Parkinson's disease have either of these problems?
- Bothersome side effects from medicines.
- New, unexpected symptoms occur during treatment.

YES → See Doctor

NO ↓

 Use Self-Care

Self-Care / Prevention

- Follow your treatment plan.

- Plan and maintain safety in the home. Replace razor blades with electric shavers. Use nonskid rugs and handrails to prevent falls, etc.

- Make tasks easy to do. Wear loafers, not tie shoes. Wear clothes that can be pulled on. Use items with snaps or Velcro closures instead of buttons.

- Prevent constipation. (See **Self-Care / Prevention** for **Constipation** on page 153.)

- Stay as active as you can. Do the activities and exercises advised by your doctor and/or physical therapist.

- Take warm baths. Get massages to help with rigid muscles.

- Eat healthy foods. If you take levodopa, limit the protein in your diet, as advised by your doctor. A high protein diet can lessen the effects of levodopa.

Sexually Transmitted Infections (STIs)

Sexually transmitted infections (STIs) are ones that pass from one person to another through sexual contact. This can be from vaginal, anal, or oral sex, and from genital-to-genital contact. STIs are also called **sexually transmitted diseases (STDs)**.

Common STIs in the U.S. are:

- Chlamydia.
- Genital herpes.
- Gonorrhea.
- Hepatitis B.
- HIV/AIDS.
- Human papillomavirus (HPV). This causes genital warts.
- Trichomoniasis.
- Syphilis.

Information for these STIs is given below and on the next 5 pages. See pages 236 and 237 for information on **Hepatitis B**. See pages 240 and 241 for information on **HIV/AIDS**.

Chlamydia

Signs & Symptoms

For Females

75% of females have few or no symptoms, but can still transmit the infection. When present, symptoms show up 2 to 4 weeks after infection. They include:

- Slight yellowish-green vaginal discharge. Abnormal vaginal bleeding.
- Vaginal irritation or pain.
- Need to urinate often and pain or burning feeling when passing urine.
- Pain in the abdomen.

In females, chlamydia can cause **pelvic inflammatory disease (PID)**. This can cause infertility.

For Males

25% of males have few or no symptoms. When present, symptoms show up 2 to 4 weeks after infection. They include:

- Watery, mucous discharge from the penis.
- Burning or discomfort when passing urine.
- Pain in the scrotum.

Causes

A specific bacterial infection.

Treatment

- Oral antibiotics for the infected person and his or her partner(s).
- Avoiding sex until treatment is finished in the infected person and his or her partner(s).

Sexually Transmitted Infections (STIs), Continued

Genital Herpes

Signs & Symptoms

For Females and Males

- Painful sores and/or blisters on the genital area, anus, thighs, and/or buttocks.

- Itching, irritation, and tingling can occur 1 to 2 days before the outbreak of the blisters.

- Outbreaks may be triggered by stress, other illnesses, and vigorous sexual intercourse.

After a few days, the blisters break open and leave painful, shallow ulcers. These can last from 5 days to 3 weeks.

With outbreaks, especially the first one, there may be flu-like symptoms (swollen glands, fever, body aches). Outbreaks that follow are usually milder and shorter. Once infected, the virus lives in nerve cells. New outbreaks can occur even without contact.

Causes

- Herpes simplex virus (HSV-1 or HSV-2). HSV-2 is the common cause. HSV-1 most often affects the oral area as **cold sores**.

- The virus is spread by direct skin-to-skin contact from the site of infection to the contact site. It can be spread when no symptoms are noticed. Oral sex can spread herpes from the mouth to the genital area and from the genital area to the mouth.

Treatment

- There is no cure. Antiviral medicines can help prevent and shorten outbreaks. During delivery, an infant may need protection from infection if the mother has active herpes.

- Self-care measures. (See tips under **For Genital Herpes** on page 253.)

Gonorrhea

Signs & Symptoms

For Females

Sixty to 80% of females have no symptoms. If present, they appear in 2 to 10 days and include:

- Mild vaginal itching and burning. Thick, yellow-green vaginal discharge.

- Burning when passing urine.

- Severe pain in the lower abdomen.

For Males

Males may have no symptoms, but usually have:

- Pain at the tip of the penis. Thick, yellow, cloudy, penile discharge.

- Pain and burning when passing urine.

Causes

A specific bacterial infection. If it is not treated, it can spread to joints, tendons, or the heart. In females, it can cause **pelvic inflammatory disease (PID)**. This can cause infertility.

Treatment

- Antibiotics.

- Pain relievers.

- Treating sexual partner(s) to avoid getting infected again.

- Follow-up test to find out if the treatment worked.

Sexually Transmitted Infections (STIs), Continued

Human Papillomavirus (HPV)

Signs & Symptoms

In Females and Males

Often, there are no visible signs or symptoms. Genital warts can appear several weeks after being infected or may not show up for months or even years. This makes it hard to know when the virus was acquired and which partner was the carrier. Genital warts:

- Can be soft or hard; pink, red, or yellow-gray in color.

- Are inside the vagina, on the lips of the vagina, or around the anus in females.

- Are on the penis, inside the head of the penis, on the scrotum, or around the anus in males.

Causes

HPV is spread by direct skin-to-skin contact during vaginal, anal, or (rarely) oral sex with an infected partner. Genital warts are not caused by touching warts on the feet, hands, etc.

Treatment

- HPV vaccine can prevent cervical cancer and genital warts due to HPV. It is advised for girls 11 to 12 years of age, but can be given to females from age 9 to age 26.

- Genital warts can be treated with topical creams or a gel prescribed by a doctor. You apply these yourself. Medical treatments can remove genital warts.

- See also, **Cervical Cancer** on pages 308 to 309.

Syphilis

Signs & Symptoms

- *Primary stage.* A large, painless, ulcer-like sore (chancre) appears around the area of sexual contact in 2 to 6 weeks.

- *Secondary stage.* A month later, a widespread skin rash appears on the palms of the hands, soles of the feet, and sometimes around the mouth and nose. The rash has small, red, scaly bumps that do not itch. Other types of rashes, swollen lymph nodes, fever, and flu-like symptoms may also occur. Small patches of hair may fall out of the scalp, beard, eyelashes, and eyebrows.

- *Latent stage.* The infection may go unnoticed for years, but damages the heart, muscles, and other organs and tissues.

Causes

A specific bacterial infection. It can lead to heart failure, blindness, dementia, or death if not treated. {*Note:* An elderly person with signs of dementia should be evaluated for syphilis.}

Treatment

- Antibiotics (usually Penicillin-G given by a shot into the muscle). All persons who have syphilis should be tested for HIV, as advised.

- After treatment, follow-up blood tests are needed in 6 and 12 (and possibly 3) months.

- Once treatment is complete, you're no longer contagious, but you can get infected again.

Sexually Transmitted Infections (STIs), Continued

Trichomoniasis

Signs & Symptoms

For Females

Symptoms may not be present for years. If they do occur, symptoms include:

- Vaginal itching and burning.

- A yellow-green or gray vaginal discharge with an odor.

- Burning or pain when passing urine.

- Pain during sex.

For Males

Symptoms are not usually present. Males can infect their sexual partners and not know it.

When present, symptoms in males include:

- Discomfort when passing urine.

- Pain during sex.

- Irritation and itching of the penis.

Causes

A protozoan.

Treatment

- The oral medication metronidazole (Flagyl).

- Treating sexual partners to prevent spreading the infection and getting it again.

Questions to Ask

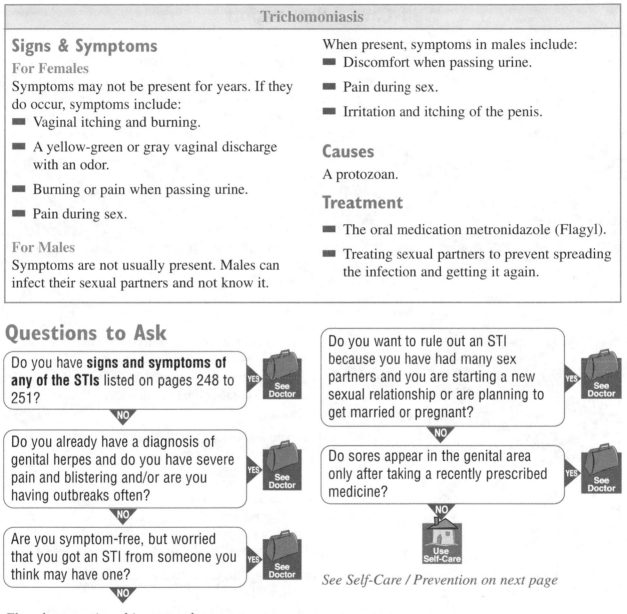

Do you have **signs and symptoms of any of the STIs** listed on pages 248 to 251? **YES** → See Doctor

NO ↓

Do you already have a diagnosis of genital herpes and do you have severe pain and blistering and/or are you having outbreaks often? **YES** → See Doctor

NO ↓

Are you symptom-free, but worried that you got an STI from someone you think may have one? **YES** → See Doctor

NO ↓

Flowchart continued in next column

Do you want to rule out an STI because you have had many sex partners and you are starting a new sexual relationship or are planning to get married or pregnant? **YES** → See Doctor

NO ↓

Do sores appear in the genital area only after taking a recently prescribed medicine? **YES** → See Doctor

NO ↓ Use Self-Care

See Self-Care / Prevention on next page

Sexually Transmitted Infections (STIs), Continued

Self-Care / Prevention

Safer Sex To Help Prevent STIs

- The only sure way to avoid STIs is not having sex. This includes intercourse, oral sex, anal sex, and genital-to-genital contact. Caressing, hugging, dry kissing, and masturbation are no risk or extremely low-risk practices. So is limiting your sexual contact to one person your entire life. This is if your partner does not have an STI and has sex only with you.

- Latex and polyurethane condoms can help reduce the risk of spreading HIV and other STIs (i.e., chlamydia, gonorrhea, and trichomoniasis). To do this, they must be used the right way for every sex act. They do not get rid of the risk entirely. Barriers made of natural membranes, such as from lamb, do not give good protection against STIs.

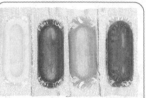

Condoms reduce the risk of HIV and some STIs.

- Females and males should use latex or polyurethane condoms every time they have genital-to-genital contact and/or oral sex. Use polyurethane condoms if either partner is allergic to latex. You don't need condoms to prevent STIs if you have sex only with one partner and neither of you has an STI.

- For oral-vaginal sex and oral-anal sex, use latex dams ("doilies"). These are latex squares.

- Latex condoms with spermicides, such as nonoxynol-9 (N–9) are no better than other lubricated condoms for preventing HIV/STIs. Spermicides with N–9 do not prevent chlamydia, cervical gonorrhea, or HIV. Don't use spermicides alone to prevent HIV/STIs. Using spermicides with N–9 often has been linked with genital lesions which may increase the risk of spreading HIV. Also, N–9 may increase the risk of spreading HIV during anal intercourse.

- Use water-based lubricants, such as K-Y Brand Jelly. *Don't use oil-based or "petroleum" ones, such as Vaseline. They can damage latex barriers.*

Get more information from:

HealthyLearn®
www.HealthyLearn.com
Click on MedlinePlus®

American Social Health Association (ASHA)
www.ashastd.org

CDC-Info
800.CDC.INFO
(232.4636)
www.cdc.gov/STD

Sexually Transmitted Infections (STIs), Continued

- To lower your risk for HPV, use latex or polyurethane condoms. These work best at covering areas of the body that HPV is most likely to affect. A diaphragm does not prevent the spread of HPV.

- Don't have sex while under the influence of drugs or alcohol. You are less likely to use "safer sex" measures.

- Limit sexual partners. Sexual contact with many persons increases the risk for STIs, especially if no protection is used.

- Discuss a new partner's sexual history with him or her before you start having sex. Know that persons are not always honest about their sexual past.

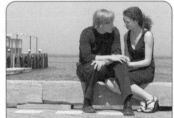

*Discuss "safer sex" with a partner **before** having sex.*

- Avoid sexual contact with persons whose health status and health practices are not known.

- Follow your doctor's advice to check for STIs.

To Treat STIs

Medical care is needed for STIs. With medical care, do the self-care measures that follow.

For Genital Herpes

- If prescribed an oral antiviral medicine, take it as advised.

- Bathe the affected area twice a day with mild soap and water. Pat dry with a towel or use a hair dryer set on warm. Using a colloidal oatmeal soap or bath may be soothing.

- Use a sitz bath to soak the affected area. You can buy a sitz bath basin from a medical supply or drug store.

- Apply ice packs on the affected genital area for 5 to 10 minutes to relieve itching and swelling.

- Wear loose-fitting pants or skirts. Don't wear pantyhose. Wear cotton (not nylon) underwear.

- If pain is made worse when you urinate, squirt tepid water near the urinary opening while you pass urine. Or, urinate while using a sitz bath.

- Take a mild pain reliever as directed.

- Ask your doctor about using a local anesthetic ointment, such as lidocaine, during the most painful part of an outbreak.

- Wash your hands if you touch the blisters or sores. Don't touch your eyes during an outbreak. Doing this could spread the virus to your eyes.

- To help avoid spreading the virus to others, use latex barriers during sex and skin-to-skin contact.

For HPV

- If you are female, don't smoke. If you smoke, quit.

- A vaccine for HPV is advised for girls 11 to 12 years of age, but can be given to females from age 9 to age 26.

For Trichomoniasis

- Don't drink alcohol for 24 hours before, during, and 24 hours after taking metronidazole. The combination causes vomiting, dizziness, and headaches.

See also **Self-Care / Prevention** for **Hepatitis B** on page 237 and for **HIV/AIDS** on page 241.

Sickle Cell Anemia

Signs & Symptoms

Red blood cells are normally round. In **sickle cell anemia**, the red blood cells take on a sickle shape. This makes the blood thicker and doesn't let oxygen get to the body's tissues like it should.

When sickled cells get stuck in the blood vessels, they cut off the blood supply. With no oxygen, pain occurs. The result is a "Sickle Cell Crisis."

- Bone and joint pain. This is the most common complaint. The pain can also be in the chest, back, or abdomen.
- Shortness of breath and a hard time breathing.
- Swollen hands and feet.
- Jaundice. The whites of the eyes and/or the skin looks yellow.
- Paleness.
- Repeated infections, especially pneumonia or meningitis.
- Kidney problems. Leg ulcers. Gallstones (at an early age). Gout.
- Seizures.
- Strokes (at an early age).

Treatment

Medical treatment is needed. Painful episodes are treated with painkillers, fluids, and oxygen. Persons over the age of 2 should get a pneumonia vaccine. All persons with sickle cell disease should get *H. influenzae* type b vaccines and a yearly flu shot.

The average life span with proper medical care is between the ages of 40 and 50. About half of persons with sickle cell anemia live past 50 years.

Causes

Sickle cell anemia is inherited. In the U.S., it mostly affects African Americans, but can occur in other ethnic groups. Examples are persons whose ancestors are from Cuba, Central and South America, Greece, Italy, Turkey, and Saudi Arabia. About 1 in 12 African Americans carries the gene for the sickle cell trait. If both parents carry the trait, the chance of having a child with sickle cell anemia is 1 out of 4. About 1 in 375 African Americans and about 1 in every 1,000 Latin Americans are born with sickle cell anemia. Signs of the disease aren't noticed until the end of the infant's first year. All hospitals in the U.S. screen newborns for sickle cell disease.

To prevent sickle cell anemia in offspring, couples, especially African American couples, should have a blood test to see if they are carriers for the sickle cell trait. Genetic counseling can help them decide what to do.

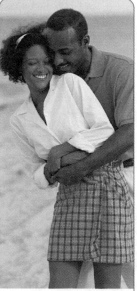

Sickle cell anemia mostly affects African Americans.

Sickle Cell Anemia, Continued

Questions to Ask

Does any **stroke warning sign** listed on page 407 occur?

NO ↓

Do any of these problems occur?
- Severe shortness of breath or chest pain with rapid breathing.
- Severe abdominal pain.
- Constant vomiting.
- Chest pain with or without a cough.
- Fainting. Seizure.
- Severe pain in a bone or joint.

NO ↓

Does the person with sickle cell anemia have any of these problems?
- Swelling of the feet and hands and shortness of breath.
- Increased yellow color to the skin or the whites of the eyes.
- Redness, swelling, pus, fever, or a sore that does not heal.
- Bloody or cloudy urine.
- Increased paleness.
- A new onset of weakness.
- Leg sores.
- Mild symptoms after exposure to high altitudes or cold temperatures.

NO ↓

Does an infant have any of these signs?
- Nosebleeds.
- Frequent respiratory infections.
- Paleness. Fatigue. Acting very cranky.
- Yellow color to the skin or the whites of the eyes.
- Feeding poorly.

NO ↓

Flowchart continued in next column

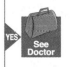 YES → **See Doctor**

YES → **Get Medical Care Fast**

Does an adolescent or young adult with sickle cell anemia have severe joint pain, anemia that worsens, leg sores, or gum disease?

YES → **See Doctor**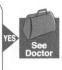

NO ↓

Use Self-Care

Self-Care / Prevention

- Follow your doctor's treatment plan. Wear a medical alert tag.

- Avoid physical stress and high altitudes.

- Discuss airplane travel with your doctor.

- Ask your doctor what over-the-counter medicines you can use *before* you try any.

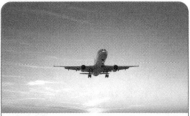

When you travel by air, travel only in large commercial airplanes with pressurized cabins.

- Drink at least 8 glasses of water a day. Get the rest you need.

- Follow a balanced diet. Have at least 5 servings of fruits and vegetables a day. Take folic acid (a B vitamin) supplements and other vitamins and minerals, as advised by your doctor.

- Don't wear tight clothing.

- If at home and in a "sickle cell crisis:"
  - Stay warm. Apply warm compresses to painful parts of your body.
  - Rest in bed.
  - Take pain medication, as prescribed.

To Learn More, See Back Cover

Sleep Disorders & Snoring

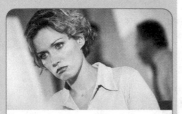

Lack of sleep makes it hard to focus and to make decisions.

Not getting enough sleep can cause you to be sleepy during the day. It can make you less able to function. Snoring and sleep disorders can cause these problems, too. Information on common sleep disorders and snoring is given below and on the next 3 pages.

Insomnia

Signs & Symptoms
- Having trouble falling asleep. Waking up in the middle of the night. Waking up too early and not being able to get back to sleep.
- Feeling like you didn't get enough sleep.

Causes
- Too much caffeine. Drinking alcohol and/or smoking before bedtime.
- Too much noise when falling asleep.
- Emotional stress. Depression. Anxiety. The manic phase of bipolar disorder.
- **Fibromyalgia.** (See page 188.)
- Over active thyroid gland.

- Any condition, illness, injury, or surgery that causes enough pain or discomfort to interrupt sleep. Heart or lung conditions that cause shortness of breath when lying down. Side effects of some medicines, such as over-the-counter diet pills or decongestants.
- Changes in sleep/wake schedules, such as with work shift changes and jet lag.
- In children, nightmares or bed-wetting.

Treatment
- Self-care and prevention tips. (See pages 258 and 259.)
- Treating the problem.
- Prescribed short-acting sleeping pills.

Restless Leg Syndrome (RLS) and Periodic Limb Movements in Sleep (PLMS)

Signs & Symptoms
- Creeping, crawling, pulling and/or painful feelings in one or both legs.
- Jerking or bending leg movements that you can't control during sleep.

Causes
The cause is not known. These factors play a role:
- Family history of RLS.

- The last months of a pregnancy.
- Chronic diseases, such as kidney failure, diabetes, and rheumatoid arthritis.

Treatment
- Self-care and prevention tips.
- Prescribed medicines to control symptoms.
- A type of electric nerve stimulation.

Sleep Disorders & Snoring, Continued

Sleep Apnea

Signs & Symptoms

- Loud snoring and snorting sounds while sleeping on the back.

- Repeated periods when breathing stops 10 or more seconds during sleep.

- Waking up many times during the night. Excessive daytime sleepiness.

- Exhaustion. Hard time concentrating. Acting very cranky. Depression or other mental changes.

- Early morning headaches.

Causes

- Too much muscle tissue is in the airway or the tissue relaxes and sags. These things narrow or block the airway. Persons who snore loudly and are overweight are more prone to these problems.

- A physical problem in the nose or upper airway.

Treatment

The goal is to keep the airway open during sleep. This is done with self-care measures and one of these treatments:

- A mouth guard dental device custom made by a dentist. This is worn during sleep. It pushes the lower jaw forward to open the air passage behind the tongue.

- A nasal **continuous positive airway pressure (CPAP)** device. Pressure from an air blower forces air through the nasal passages using a mask worn over the nose during sleep.

- Surgery to correct the cause of the airway obstruction.

Snoring

Signs & Symptoms

- Loud sounds. Harsh breathing. Snorting sounds. These occur during sleep.

Causes

- Sleeping on the back. The tongue falls back toward the throat and partly closes the airway.

- Nasal congestion from allergies or colds. Smoking. Drinking alcohol. Taking sedatives. Overeating (especially before bedtime).

- Sleep apnea or chronic respiratory disease.

- An obstructed airway. This can be due to enlarged tonsils or being overweight.

- Changes in hormones, such as during menopause or the last month of pregnancy.

Treatment

Self-care treats most cases. Other options are:
- Wearing a dental device to keep the tongue from falling back.

- Surgery, if needed, to correct the problem.

- Treatment for sleep apnea, if needed.

Sleep Disorders & Snoring, Continued

How Much Sleep is Needed?

- Adults need between 7 and 9 hours of sleep each night.

- Teens need at least 8½ to 9¼ hours of sleep each night.

- After 6 months of age, most children sleep between 9 and 12 hours at night. Up to age 5, children may also take daytime naps for a total of ½ to 2 hours a day.

Get more information from:

HealthyLearn®
www.HealthyLearn.com
Click on MedlinePlus®

National Center on Sleep Disorders Research (NCSDR)
301.435.0199
www.nhlbi.nih.gov/about/ncsdr

National Sleep Foundation
www.sleepfoundation.org

Questions to Ask

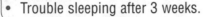

Do **signs and symptoms of sleep apnea** listed on page 257 occur?

YES → See Doctor

NO ↓

Are any of these conditions present?
- Trouble falling or staying asleep due to pain or discomfort from an illness or injury or the need to wake up often to use the bathroom.
- Disturbed sleep since taking medication. Or, side effects from taking prescribed sleeping pills. Examples are feeling dizzy or confused or hallucinating.
- Trouble sleeping after 3 weeks.

YES → Call Doctor

NO ↓

Do any of these problems occur?
- Snoring keeps you or your sleep partner from getting enough, restful sleep.
- Snoring persists despite using self-care measures.
- You think you're getting enough sleep, but still feel sleepy during the day.

YES → Call Doctor

NO ↓

Use Self-Care

Self-Care / Prevention

For Insomnia

- Avoid caffeine for 8 hours before bedtime.

- Avoid long naps during the day.

- Have no more than 1 alcoholic drink with or after dinner.

- Before you go to bed, have food items rich in the amino acid L-tryptophan (milk, turkey, tuna fish) or foods with carbohydrates (cereal, bread, fruit).

- Avoid nicotine. Don't smoke. Stay away from secondhand smoke.

- Get regular exercise, but not within a few hours of going to bed.

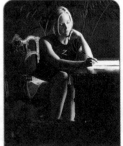

An hour or two before going to bed, dim the lights.

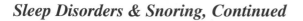

Sleep Disorders & Snoring, Continued

- Before bedtime, take a warm bath or read a book, etc. Avoid things that hold your attention, such as watching a suspense movie.

- Keep your bedroom quiet, dark, and comfortable.

- Follow a bedtime routine. Lock or check doors and windows, brush your teeth, etc.

- Count sheep! Picture a repeated image. Doing this may bore you to sleep.

- Listen to recordings that help promote sleep.

- Take over-the-counter sleep aids, (e.g., melatonin, Tylenol PM,

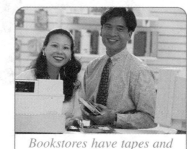

Bookstores have tapes and CDs that promote sleep.

etc.) as advised by your doctor. Don't take anyone else's sleeping pills.

- If you wake up and can't get back to sleep or can't fall asleep, after 30 minutes, get out of bed. Read a relaxing book or sit quietly in the dark. In about 20 minutes, go back to bed. Do this as many times as needed.

For Restless Leg Syndrome (RLS)

- Take medications as prescribed. Let your doctor know if the medicine no longer helps.

- For relief, move the legs. Walk, rub, or massage them or do knee bends.

- Limit or avoid caffeine.

- Take a warm bath before bedtime.

For Sleep Apnea

- Lose weight, if you are overweight.

- Don't drink alcohol. Don't use tobacco products.

- Don't take sleeping pills or sedatives.

- Use methods, such as those listed under **Self-Care / Prevention – For Snoring** (see below) to keep from sleeping on your back.

For Snoring

- Sleep on your side. Prop an extra pillow behind your back so you won't roll over. Sleep on a narrow sofa for a few nights to get used to staying on your side.

- Sew a large marble or tennis ball into a pocket on the back of your pajamas. This can help you stay on your side when you sleep.

- If you must sleep on your back, raise the head of the bed 6 inches on bricks or blocks. Or buy a wedge that is made to be placed between the mattress and box spring to elevate the head section.

- Lose weight, if you are overweight. Excess fatty tissue in the throat can cause snoring. Losing 10% of your body weight will help.

- Don't smoke. If you do, quit. Limit or don't have alcohol, sedatives, or a heavy meal within 3 hours of bedtime.

- To relieve nasal congestion, try a decongestant before you go to bed. {*Note:* See information for **Decongestant** use on page 28.}

- Get rid of allergens in the bedroom. These include dust, down-filled (feathered) pillows, and down-filled bed linen.

- Try over-the-counter "nasal strips." These keep the nostrils open and lift them up. This helps lessen congestion in nasal passages.

Thyroid Problems

The thyroid is a small, butterfly-shaped gland in the lower front of the neck, below the voice box (larynx), and above the collarbone. It makes hormones that help convert food to energy. It regulates growth and fertility. It also maintains body temperature.

Treatment

Medical care is needed for thyroid problems.

Hypothyroidism is treated with iodine and/or thyroid medicine.

Hyperthyroidism treatment varies. It includes radioactive iodine, medication, and surgery, if needed.

Some treatments result in the need to continue to take thyroid medicine.

Follow-up care is needed for both of these thyroid problems.

Signs & Symptoms

Hypothyroidism occurs when the thyroid gland does not make enough thyroid hormone. Body functions slow down. Signs and symptoms are:

- Fatigue. Sleeping too much.
- Depression.
- Dry, pale skin. Dry hair that tends to fall out.
- The voice deepens.
- Weight gain for no reason.
- Feeling cold often.
- Heavy and/or irregular menstrual periods in females.
- Poor memory.
- Constipation.

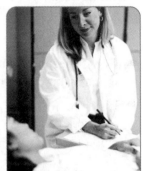

A physical exam and blood tests diagnose thyroid problems.

Hyperthyroidism occurs when the thyroid makes too much thyroid hormone. Body functions speed up. Two common forms are **Graves' disease** and **multinodular goiter**. Signs and symptoms are:

- Swelling in the front of the neck. The thyroid gland gets larger. This is called goiter.
- One or both eyes bulge. Tremors. Feeling nervous.
- Mood swings.
- Weakness.
- Frequent bowel movements.
- Heat intolerance.
- Shortened menstrual periods in females.
- Weight loss for no reason.
- Fine hair or hair loss.
- Rapid pulse. Heart palpitations.

{*Note:* In elderly persons, symptoms for this can be more like ones for hypothyroidism.}

Thyroid Problems, Continued

Causes

For Hypothyroidism

- Immune system problems.

- Removal of the thyroid gland.

- Treating the thyroid gland with radioactive iodine for hyperthyroidism.

- Too much or too little iodine in the diet.

Risk factors for hypothyroidism include: A family history of the disease; having diabetes; and taking certain medicines, such as lithium.

For Hyperthyroidism

- Immune system problems.

- Family history of the illness.

- Taking too much thyroid hormones from pills.

Questions to Ask

Do you notice a lump in your neck (between your Adam's apple and collarbone)?

YES → **See Doctor**

NO ↓

Do you have **signs and symptoms of hypothyroidism or hyperthyroidism** listed on page 260? Or, are you being treated for a thyroid problem and do symptoms return or get worse?

YES → **See Doctor**

NO ↓

Are you being treated for a thyroid problem and do you need to schedule follow-up testing?

YES → **Call Doctor**

NO ↓

Use Self-Care

See Self-Care / Prevention in next column

Self-Care / Prevention

- Take medication as directed.

- Tell your doctor if symptoms come back or still bother you.

- Follow your doctor's advice for self-care measures.

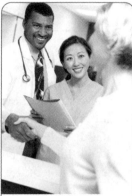

Schedule and keep follow-up visits to monitor treatment.

Neck Check

To see if you have a lump on your thyroid gland or if it is enlarged, the American Association of Clinical Endocrinologists recommends this quick self-test:

1. Tilt your chin up slightly and swallow a glass of water in front of a mirror.

2. Look at your neck as you swallow.

3. Check for any bulges or protrusions between your Adam's apple and collarbone. If you see any, contact your doctor.

Get more information from:

HealthyLearn®
www.HealthyLearn.com
Click on MedlinePlus®

American Thyroid Association
www.thyroid.org

Chapter 16

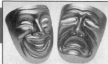

Mental Health Conditions

Mental Health

Every year, one in every 4 adults in the U.S. has a mental disorder. Less than one-third of them receive treatment. Less than one-half of children with a mental disease get treatment in any given year.

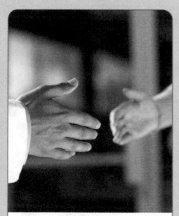

Seeking help is a sign of strength, not weakness.

People who are mentally healthy feel good about themselves. They feel comfortable with others, too. They are also able to deal with the demands and changes in everyday life.

People feel down, angry, or anxious in response to many things. Feelings like these can come and go quite often. These feelings may signal the need for professional help when:

- They are disturbing.
- They interfere with daily life.
- They linger for weeks or months.

Many people do not seek help because of the "stigma" of having an "emotional" problem. This view keeps them from getting the care they need.

Mental Health Facts

- About 27% of the people who seek medical help for physical problems have emotional problems.
- Depression and anxiety are the most common reasons people seek mental health treatment.
- Eight to 14 million persons in the U.S. suffer from depression.
- 80 to 90% of mental disorders can be treated with medication and other therapies.
- About 10% of persons in the U.S. have phobias.
- 18.6 million persons in the U.S. need treatment for a serious alcohol problem. 22 million people in the U.S. abuse drugs.
- Nearly 25% of the elderly who are thought to be senile have some form of mental illness that can be treated.
- Therapy does not have to take a long time. Almost 50% of the people who enter therapy will complete it in 7 or less sessions.

Alcohol & Drug Problems

Alcohol and drug problems are abuse or dependence on these substances.

Signs & Symptoms

For Alcohol or Drug Abuse

- Failure to fulfill work or home duties.
- Legal problems, such as getting arrested for drunk driving, etc.
- Physical harm from car accidents, etc.
- Relationship problems.

For Alcohol or Drug Dependence

- *Cravings.* There are strong needs for the substance.
- *Loss of control.* The person is unable to limit taking the substance.
- *Physical dependence.* Withdrawal symptoms occur when the substance is stopped after a period of using it.
- *Tolerance.* Greater amounts of the substance is needed in order to "get high" or have the desired effects.

Causes

- Increased use and tolerance of alcohol or drugs.
- Mental health problems, such as depression and anxiety.

- Family history of alcohol abuse. A person is about 4 times more likely to be an alcoholic if one parent is; and 10 times more likely if both parents are.
- Prolonged fatigue or stress.
- Prolonged use of prescribed pain pills.
- Ongoing problems with family, money, etc.
- Events that result in change. Examples are retirement, failing health, and the death of a friend or loved one. At first, having a drink or taking a drug brings relief. Later it turns into a problem.
- Being with people who use drugs or drink a lot.
- Having problems dealing with others.

Treatment

For Alcohol Problems

Alcoholism is a disease that needs treatment. Treatment includes:

- Self-help groups, such as Alcoholics Anonymous (AA).
- "Rehab" centers. Alcohol treatment programs.
- Counseling.
- Nutrition therapy.
- Medication.

If you suspect a drinking problem in you, a family member, or a friend, seek advice.

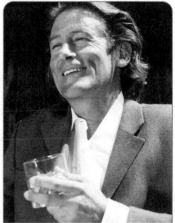

Most alcoholics deny or don't see that they have a disease.

Alcohol & Drug Problems, Continued

For Drug Problems

Treatment varies. It depends on the substance being used and the person's needs. Types of treatment include:

- Emergency medical care for overdoses or for violent behaviors, etc.
- Medical treatment for physical problems due to the drug use and/or for drug withdrawal.
- Counseling.
- Nutrition therapy.
- Support groups, such as Narcotics Anonymous (NA) and Cocaine Anonymous (CA).

Questions to Ask

With a suspected drug overdose, do any of these problems occur?
- Loss of or decreasing level of consciousness.
- Severe shortness of breath. Wheezing.
- Hallucinations. Confusion. Convulsions.
- Slow and/or shallow breaths (10 or fewer breaths per minute and/or time lapses of more than 8 seconds between breaths).
- Pulse rate of 40 or fewer beats per minute.

NO

Is the person suddenly hostile, violent, and aggressive?
{***Note:*** Use caution. Protect yourself. Do not turn your back to the person or move suddenly in front of him or her. If you can, see that the person does not harm you, himself or herself. Call the police for help if you cannot handle the situation.}

NO

Without symptoms, do you suspect that a person has taken a drug overdose (e.g., pill containers are emptied, etc.) or tried to commit suicide?

NO

Call Poison
Control Center
800.222.1222

Flowchart continued on next page

Alcohol & Drug Problems, Continued

Does drinking or drug abuse cause memory lapses or blackouts?

YES → See Doctor or See Counselor

NO ↓

Have 3 or more of the problems listed below occurred in the last 12 months?

- More of the substance is needed to get drunk or reach a desired effect.
- If the substance is stopped or less is taken, withdrawal symptoms occur. These include:
  - Shaking.
  - Acting very cranky.
  - Not being able to sleep.
  - Depression.
  - Headaches.
  - Anxiety.
  - Hallucinations.
- The substance or one like it is taken to relieve or avoid withdrawal symptoms.
- The substance is taken in larger amounts often or over a longer period of time than intended.
- Being unable to cut down or control the use of the substance, even if desired.
- A lot of time is spent doing things needed to get the substance, use it, or to recover from its effects.
- Important social, work, or leisure activities are stopped or done less often to use the substance.
- The substance is still taken even though it causes or worsens physical or emotional problems.

YES → See Doctor or See Counselor

NO ↓

Flowchart continued in next column

Does an alcohol user answer "Yes" to one or more of these "**CAGE**" questions?
- Have you ever felt you should **C**ut down on your drinking?
- Have people **A**nnoyed you by criticizing your drinking?
- Have you ever felt bad or **G**uilty about your drinking?
- Have you ever had a drink to steady your nerves or to get rid of a hangover (**E**ye opener)?

YES → See Doctor or See Counselor

NO ↓

Has alcohol or drug abuse led to any of the following in the last 12 months?
- Failure to fulfill major duties at work, school, or home.
- Doing things that could cause physical harm while under the influence of the substance, such as driving, operating a machine, or having unsafe sex.
- Legal problems, such as getting arrested for drunk driving.
- Problems with others, such as physical fights, arguments, etc.

YES → See Doctor or See Counselor

NO ↓

Use Self-Care

Self-Care / Prevention

- Avoid places, such as certain parties, where you can get drugs.

- Learn how to relax without alcohol or drugs. Listen to calm music. Do deep breathing exercises, etc.

Alcohol & Drug Problems, Continued

To Prevent Problems with Alcohol and Illegal Drugs

- Seek help for a mental health problem, such as depression, before it leads to drug or alcohol problems.

- Learn as much as you can about the harmful effects of alcohol and drugs. Visit a self-help meeting for drug users, such as Alcoholics Anonymous (AA) or Cocaine Anonymous (CA). See first hand the problems that drugs have caused others.

- Talk to your doctor or the contact person for your Employee Assistance Program (EAP) at work. He or she can evaluate your risk level and help you get treatment.

To Prevent Problems with Prescribed Medicines

- Use medicines only as prescribed. Don't increase the dosage or take it more often than your doctor tells you to. Consult your doctor first.

- Don't use medicine prescribed for someone else.

- Ask your doctor about the risks of addiction when he or she prescribes sleeping pills, tranquilizers, and/or strong pain relievers. Find out how long you should take these medicines. Ask if there are ways to treat your problem without them.

- Find out how to gradually use less of a medicine to avoid harmful side effects.

- Don't mix medications, such as Vicodin or Xanax with alcohol to enhance the "buzz." Don't use Adderall to pull an all-nighter.

Self-Care for Wise Alcohol Use

- Follow the tips in **Use Alcohol Wisely** on page 51.

Other Tips

- Some prescribed drugs and alcohol do not mix. Some mixtures can be fatal. Don't have alcohol with prescribed drugs if the drug's label or your doctor or pharmacist tells you not to. Ask your doctor how much, if any, alcohol you can have if you take any prescribed drugs.

- Eat when you drink. Food helps to slow alcohol absorption.

- Know your limit and stick to it. You may decide it is better not to drink at all.

- Don't drink and drive. Choose a driver who will not be drinking.

Get more information from:

HealthyLearn®
www.HealthyLearn.com
Click on MedlinePlus®

Alcoholics Anonymous (AA)
www.aa.org

Al-Anon/Alateen
888.4AL.ANON
(425.2666)
www.al-anon.alateen.org

Center for Substance Abuse Treatment (CSAT)
800.662.HELP
(662.4357)
www.findtreatment.samhsa.gov

Anger

Anger is a natural response to frustration and/or events that cause displeasure. Too much or pent up anger can play a role in mental and physical problems. Chronic anger can lead to illnesses, drug and alcohol problems, headaches, domestic violence, etc. Anger turned inward can result in depression. Anger can also be a symptom of depression. See **Depression** on page 275.

Studies have found that anger and depression can increase the risk for heart disease, high blood pressure, and stroke.

Angry outbursts can cause relationship problems with others. On the other hand, learning to manage anger and frustration can enhance emotional well-being and lead to a healthier, happier life.

Signs & Symptoms

Anger can range from mild displeasure to outright rage. Symptoms of anger include:

- Feeling restless.
- Teeth clenching. Trembling of the lips or hands.
- Increased heart rate and blood pressure.
- Yelling, slamming doors, etc.
- Being less productive.
- Sleeping problems.
- Violent outbursts.

Causes

Unmet expectations can cause anger. So can feeling frustrated and disrespect from others. Physical pain and discomfort from heat, noise, crowds, etc., can provoke an anger response. Low blood sugar can do this, too.

Questions to Ask

Did anger become a problem after a stroke, head injury, or head surgery? **YES → See Doctor**

NO

With outbursts of anger do you have any of these problems?
- Memory loss or confusion.
- You are less able to figure things out or remain alert.
- You can't perform routine tasks.

YES → See Doctor or See Counselor

NO

Does anger result in any of these problems?
- Physical or emotional harm.
- Destruction of property.
- Anger can't be controlled when drinking or taking a drug.
- Long term anger causes a lot of stress or a feeling of having no power.

YES → See Doctor or See Counselor

NO

Do any of these problems occur?
- Sudden fits of anger occur when not eating for several hours, especially in a diabetic.
- In females, anger leads to aggression 10 to 14 days before menstrual periods.
- Anger interferes with day-to-day life.

YES → Call Doctor

NO

Use Self-Care

See Self-Care / Prevention on next page

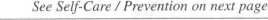

Anger, Continued

Treatment

Self-care measures can help in most cases. When these are not enough, an evaluation from a doctor or mental health care provider may be needed. Treatment will depend on the cause.

Self-Care / Prevention

■ Don't ignore anger. Express it in a healthy way.

- Share your angry feelings with a person you trust and feel safe with, such as a friend, partner, teacher, etc.

- Get the anger "off your chest." Do this calmly and without being cruel. Tell persons you feel angry with how they have upset you. You will likely start to feel better.

- If you can't express your anger out loud, write it down.

■ Express your wants, needs, and feelings, in ways that do not offend others. Doing so can keep you from feeling that you were taken advantage of and getting angry as a result. Use "*I*" rather than "*you*" statements. For example, say "*I* get angry when *I* feel put down by your comments in front of our friends." Don't say, "*You* make me angry when *you* put me down in front of our friends."

■ List reasons and times when you have too much anger. Note if there are any patterns to your anger and if they can be changed.

■ Channel the energy from anger into something positive or creative. Clean out drawers. Take a short walk or do other exercises. Paint, write poems, etc.

■ Distract yourself. If you're stuck in traffic, try to accept the delay and that it is beyond your control. Instead of clenching the steering wheel, play pleasant music on the radio or listen to tapes or CDs that are calming.

■ To lessen anger outbursts, think of what will happen as a result of your anger.

■ Find humor in situations that result in anger.

■ Practice learning to lighten up.

■ Use stress management techniques on a routine basis. (See **Self-Care / Prevention** for **Stress** on pages 285 and 286.)

■ Think before you act or speak. Try to understand your anger. Plan how you want to react or respond.

■ Eat healthy foods. Eat at regular times.

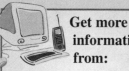

Get more information from:

HealthyLearn®
www.HealthyLearn.com
Click on MedlinePlus®

Mental Health America
(MHA)
800.969.6642
www.mentalhealth
america.net

Anxiety & Panic Attacks

Anxiety is a feeling of dread, fear, or distress. This can be from a real threat or one that exists in the mind.

A **panic attack** is a brief period of acute anxiety that comes on all of a sudden. It occurs when there is no real danger. It comes without warning.

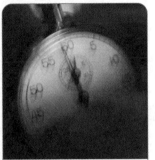

A panic attack lasts only a few minutes, but seems to last for hours.

Signs & Symptoms

- Rapid pulse and/or breathing rate. Racing or pounding heart.

- Dry mouth. Sweating. Trembling.

- Shortness of breath. Faintness.

- Numbness and tingling of the hands, feet, or other body part.

- Feeling of a "lump in the throat."

- Stomach problems.

- Sleep problems.

Persons having a panic attack may rush to an emergency room. Why? They think they are having a heart attack. They feel like they are going crazy or going to die.

Persons who have repeated panic attacks begin to avoid places they link with past attacks. If the person had the panic attack in a grocery store and had to leave the store to feel safe, the person avoids going to the grocery store. This can lead to a phobia called **agoraphobia**.

A person who has 4 or more panic attacks in any 4 week period could have **panic disorder**. The disorder can also be present if the person has less than 4 panic attacks in 4 weeks, but fears having another one.

Causes

Some anxiety is normal. It can alert you to seek safety from physical danger. Anxiety is not normal, though, when it overwhelms you and interferes with day-to-day life.

Anxiety can be a symptom of many conditions. These include:

- Having too much caffeine. Withdrawal reaction from nicotine, alcohol, caffeine, drugs, or medicines, such as sleeping pills.

- A side effect of some medicines.

- Low blood sugar.

- An overactive thyroid gland.

- **Cushing's Syndrome**. With this, the glands above the kidneys called the adrenal glands, make too much of a hormone.

- **A heart attack.** (See page 387.)

Anxiety & Panic Attacks, Continued

Anxiety disorders are common problems. They often respond to treatment.

Anxiety can also be a symptom of illnesses known as anxiety disorders. These include:

- Phobias.

- Panic disorder.

- **Obsessive-compulsive disorder (OCD)**. With this, a person has persistent, involuntary thoughts or images (obsessions). The person also does ritualistic acts, such as washing the hands, according to certain self-imposed rules (compulsions).

- **Posttraumatic stress disorder (PTSD)**. (See page 284.)

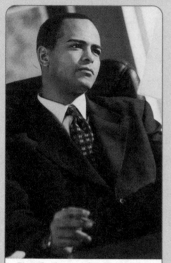

Psychological counseling is one method of treatment for anxiety.

Treatment

When anxiety is mild and/or does not interfere with daily living, it can be dealt with using self-care measures (see page 271). Treatment also includes:

- Treating any medical condition which causes the anxiety or panic attacks.

- Medication.

- Counseling.

- Self-help groups for anxiety disorders.

Questions to Ask

With anxiety, do you have any of these problems?
- Any **heart attack warning sign** listed on page 387.
- Extreme shortness of breath without chest pain.
- Feeling lightheaded. Passing out.
- Suicide attempts or plans.

YES → Get Medical Care Fast

NO ↓

With the anxiety, do you have these problems?
- Excessive hair growth.
- Round face and puffy eyes.
- Skin reddens, thins, and has stretch marks.
- High blood pressure.

YES → See Doctor

NO ↓

Flowchart continued on next page

Anxiety & Panic Attacks, *Continued*

With the anxiety, do you have **signs and symptoms of hyperthyroidism** listed on page 260 or of **posttraumatic stress disorder** listed on pages 284 and 285?

YES →  See Doctor

↓ **NO**

Do you have anxiety only at these times?
- When you don't eat or when you do too much physically, especially if you are a diabetic.
- During the 2 weeks before your menstrual period, if you are female.

YES → Call Doctor

↓ **NO**

Do you get anxiety only after taking an over-the-counter or prescribed medicine or after withdrawing from medication, nicotine, alcohol, or drugs?

YES → Call Doctor

↓ **NO**

Does anxiety keep you from doing the things you need and like to do every day?

YES → Call Doctor

↓ **NO**

Have you had any of these problems?
- Panic attacks and you have had fears of getting another one for 1 month or longer.
- Worry about what would happen with another panic attack.
- A change in what you do related to panic attacks. You avoid places, are not able to leave the house, or are afraid to be left alone.

YES → Call Doctor *or* Call Counselor

↓ **NO**

Flowchart continued in next column

Do any of the following keep you from doing daily activities?
- You check something over and over again, such as seeing if you've locked the door, even though it is locked.
- Repeated, unwanted thoughts, such as worrying you could harm someone.
- Repeated, senseless acts, such as washing your hands over and over again.

YES → Call Doctor *or* Call Counselor

↓ **NO**

Use Self-Care

Self-Care / Prevention

- Look for the cause of the stress that results in anxiety. Deal with it. Use stress management techniques. Do deep breathing exercises. Meditate.

- Lessen your exposure to things that cause you distress.

- Talk about your fears and anxieties with someone you trust, such as a friend, partner, teacher, etc.

- Exercise regularly (e.g., 30 minutes to 1 hour, 5 times a week).

- Eat healthy foods. Eat at regular times. Don't skip meals.

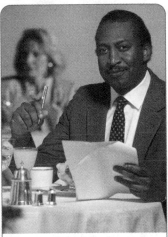

Eat meals at regular times.

Anxiety & Panic Attacks, Continued

- If you are prone to low blood sugar episodes, eat 5 to 6 small meals per day instead of 3 larger ones. Avoid sweets on a regular basis, but carry a source of sugar with you at all times, such as a small can of orange juice. This will give you a quick source of sugar in the event that you get a low blood sugar reaction.

- Limit or avoid caffeine intake after noon.

- Avoid nicotine and alcohol.

- Avoid medicines that stimulate. Examples are over-the-counter diet pills and pills to keep you awake.

- Do some form of relaxation exercise daily. Examples are meditation and deep breathing.

- Plan your schedule for what you can handle both physically and mentally.

- Rehearse for planned events that have made you feel anxious in the past or that you think will cause anxiety. Imagine yourself feeling calm and in control during the event. Do this several times before it really occurs.

- Face the fear. Accept it, don't fight it. (This may need outside help.)

- Be prepared to deal with symptoms of anxiety. For example, if you have hyperventilated in the past, carry a paper bag with you. If you do hyperventilate, cover your mouth and nose with the paper bag. Breathe into the paper bag slowly and rebreathe the air. Do this in and out at least 10 times. Remove the bag and breathe normally a few minutes. Repeat breathing in and out of the paper bag as needed.

- Help others. The positive feelings from this can help relieve some of your anxiety.

- Read self-help books on anxiety, panic attacks, etc.

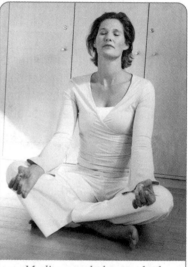

Meditate to help you deal with anxiety.

Get more information from:

HealthyLearn®
www.HealthyLearn.com
Click on MedlinePlus®

Agoraphobics in Motion (AIM)
www.aim-hq.org

Anxiety Disorders Assoication of America
www.adaa.org

Mental Health America (MHA)
800.969.6642
www.mentalhealth america.net

Codependency

Codependency describes someone who becomes the "caretaker" of an addicted or troubled person. The person can be addicted to alcohol, drugs, or gambling. He or she can be troubled by a physical or mental illness. A codependent can be the person's spouse, lover, child, parent, sibling, coworker, or friend.

Signs & Symptoms

A codependent does these things:

- Enables or allows the person to continue his or her destructive course and denies that the person has a problem.
- Rescues or makes excuses for the person's behavior.
- Takes care of all household chores, money matters, etc.
- Rationalizes that the person's behavior is normal by simply letting it take place. The codependent may take part in the same behavior as the addicted or troubled person.
- Acts like a hero or becomes the "super person" to maintain the family image.
- Blames the person and makes him or her the scapegoat for all problems.
- Withdraws from the family and acts like he or she doesn't care.

Causes

A person is more likely to become codependent if he or she:

- Puts other people's wants and needs before his or her own.

- Is afraid of being hurt and/or rejected by others. Is afraid of hurting others' feelings.
- Has low self-esteem or has a self-esteem tied to what is done for others.
- Expects too much of himself or herself and others.
- Feels overly responsible for others' behaviors and feelings.
- Does not think it is okay to ask for help.

Questions to Ask

> Do you do 3 or more of these things?
> - You think more about another person's behavior and problems than about your own life.
> - You feel anxious about the addicted or troubled person's behavior and constantly check on him or her.
> - You worry that trying to stop controlling the other person could cause him or her to fall apart.
> - You blame yourself for the person's problems.
> - You cover up or "rescue" the person when caught in a lie or other embarrassing situation related to the addiction or other problem.
> - You deny that the person has a "real" problem with drugs, alcohol, etc. and get angry and/or defensive when others suggest that a problem exists.

YES See Counselor

NO Use Self-Care

See Self-Care / Prevention on next page

Codependency, Continued

Treatment

Most codependents do not realize they have a problem. They think they are helping the troubled person, but they are not.

The first step in treatment is to admit to the problem. Self-care and counseling treat codependency. For many people, self-care is not easy to do without the help of a counselor.

Self-Care / Prevention

■ Read books and online information on codependency. You may find you identify with what you read and gain understanding.

■ Focus on these 3 <u>C</u>s:

• You did not <u>c</u>ause the other person's problem.

• You can't <u>c</u>ontrol the other person.

• You can't <u>c</u>ure the problem.

■ Don't lie or make excuses. Don't cover up for the person's drinking or other problem. Admit that this way of living is not normal. Accept that the troubled person has a real problem and needs professional help.

■ Refuse to come to the person's aid. Every time you bail the person out of trouble, you reinforce their helplessness and your hopelessness.

■ Get help for physical, verbal, and/or sexual abuse. For information, contact: National Domestic Violence Hotline 800.799.SAFE (799.7233).

■ Join a support group for codependents. Examples are self-help groups for family and friends of substance abusers, such as Al-Anon and Alateen. For information, contact: AL-ANON / ALATEEN Family Group Headquarters, Inc., 888.4AL-ANON (425.2666) www.al-anon.org.

■ Continue with your normal family routines. For example, include a drinker when he/she is sober.

■ Focus on your own feelings, desires, and needs. Vent negative thoughts in healthy ways. Do what is good for your own well-being.

■ Set limits on what you will and won't do. Be firm and stick to your limits.

■ Explore new interests. Find diversions from your loved one's problem.

■ Be responsible for yourself and others in the family to live a better life. Do this whether your loved one recovers or not.

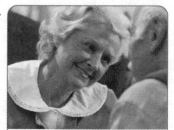

Allow others to express their feelings.

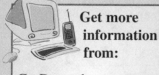

Get more information from:

Co-Dependents Anonymous
602.277.7991
www.codependents.org

Depression

Depression is a state of sadness and despair. Like diabetes, depression is a real medical illness.

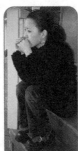

Depression makes a person less able to manage life.

Signs & Symptoms

- Feeling sad, hopeless, helpless, and/or worthless.
- Fatigue. Loss of interest in life.
- Having a hard time concentrating or making decisions.
- Changes in eating and sleeping patterns.
- Acting very cranky. Anger. Anxiety.
- Thoughts of suicide or death.

The number of symptoms and how severe they are vary from person to person.

Causes

Most likely, depression is caused by a mix of: A family history of the illness; brain chemical problems; emotional issues; and other factors, such as a medical illness or alcohol abuse.

Another cause is **seasonal affective disorder (SAD)**. With this, depression occurs between late fall and early spring due to a lack of natural sunlight.

In some persons, extreme stress, grief, etc. may bring on depression. In others, depression occurs even when life is going well.

Treatment

Treatment includes medication(s), counseling, and self-care measures. Persons who are depressed should see a doctor for diagnosis and treatment.

Questions to Ask

Have you just attempted suicide or written a suicide note? Are you making plans for suicide? Do you have thoughts of suicide or death over and over?

YES → Get Medical Care Fast

NO ↓

Have you had a lot less interest or pleasure in almost all activities most of the day, nearly every day for at least 2 weeks?

YES → See Doctor

NO ↓

Have you been depressed most of the day, nearly every day and had any of these problems for at least 2 weeks?
- Feeling hopeless, worthless, guilty, slowed down, or restless.
- Changes in appetite or weight.
- Problems concentrating, thinking, remembering, or making decisions.
- Feeling tired all the time. Trouble sleeping or sleeping too much.
- Headaches or other aches and pains.
- Stomach problems.
- Sexual problems.
- Feeling worried or anxious.
- Thoughts of death or suicide.

YES → See Doctor or See Counselor

NO ↓

Has depression kept you from doing daily tasks for more than 2 weeks and caused you to withdraw from normal activities?

YES → See Doctor or See Counselor

NO ↓

Flowchart continued on next page

Depression, Continued

FYI
Antidepressant medicines can increase the risk for suicidal thoughts and behaviors, especially in children and adolescents. This risk may be higher within the first days to a month after starting the medicine. Persons who take antidepressants should be closely monitored.

Has the depression occurred with any of the following?
- Recent delivery of a baby.
- A medical problem.
- Taking an over-the-counter or prescribed medicine. This includes antidepressants.
- Abusing alcohol or drugs.
- Dark, cloudy weather or winter months.

YES ▶ See Doctor

NO

Do you feel depressed and do any of the following apply?
- You had depression in the past and it was not treated.
- You were treated for depression in the past and it has returned.
- You took medication for depression in the past.
- A close relative has a history of depression.

YES ▶ See Doctor **or** See Counselor

NO

Use Self-Care

Self-Care / Prevention

■ Take medications as prescribed. Get your doctor's advice before you take over-the-counter herbs, such as St. John's Wort, especially if you take other medications.

■ Don't use illegal drugs. Limit alcohol. These can cause or worsen depression. Drugs and alcohol can also make medicines for depression work less. Harmful side effects can happen when alcohol and/or drugs are mixed with medicine.

■ Eat healthy foods. Eat at regular times. Get regular exercise.

■ Try not to isolate yourself. Be with people you trust and feel safe with, even though you feel down.

■ Do something you enjoy.

■ Keep an emergency number handy (e.g., crisis hotline, trusted friend's number, etc.) in case you feel desperate.

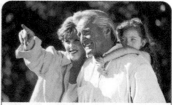
Spend time with persons you like to be with.

■ If you have thoughts of suicide, remove any weapons, pills, etc. that could be used for suicide and get medical help.

Get more information from:

HealthyLearn®
www.HealthyLearn.com
Click on MedlinePlus®

Mental Health America (MHA)
800.969.6642
www.mentalhealth america.net

Depression-screening.org
www.depression-screening.org. (This Web site has a depression screening test.)

Eating Disorders

Common eating disorders are **anorexia nervosa, binge eating disorder, and bulimia nervosa**. With these, persons are obsessed with food and/or body weight. Eating disorders are a way to cope. They are serious health problems.

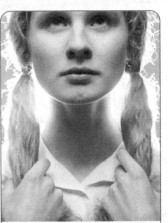

Eating disorders affect mental and physical health.

Signs & Symptoms

For Anorexia Nervosa

- Loss of a lot of weight in a short time.

- Intense, irrational fear of weight gain and/or of looking fat. Obsession with fat, calories, and weight.

- Distorted body image. Despite being below a normal weight for height and age, the person sees himself or herself as fat.

- A need to be perfect or in control in one area of life.

- Marked physical signs. These include loss of hair, slowed heart rate, and low blood pressure. The person feels cold due to a lowered body temperature. In females, menstrual periods can stop.

For Binge Eating Disorder

- Periods of nonstop eating that are not related to hunger.

- Impulsive binging on food without purging.

- Dieting and/or fasting over and over.

- Weight can range from normal weight to mild, moderate, or severe obesity.

For Bulimia Nervosa

- Repeated acts of binge eating and purging. Purging can be through vomiting; taking laxatives, water pills, and/or diet pills; fasting; and exercising a lot to "undo" the binge.

- Excessive concern about body weight.

- Being overweight, underweight, or normal weight.

- Dieting often.

- Dental problems. Mouth sores. Chronic sore throat.

- Spending a lot of time in bathrooms.

- Because of binge-purge cycles, severe health problems can occur. These include an irregular heartbeat and damage to the stomach, kidneys and bones.

Causes

An exact cause has not been found. Persons from all backgrounds, ages, and genders are affected.

Risk Factors for Eating Disorders

- A family history of eating disorders.

- Pressure from society to be thin.

- Personal and family pressures.

- Sexual, physical, or alcohol abuse in the past.

- Fear of starting puberty. Fear of having sex.

- Pressure for athletes to lose weight or to be thin for competitive sports.

- Chronic dieting.

To Learn More, See Back Cover

Eating Disorders, Continued

Treatment

- Counseling. This can be individual, family, group, and/or behavioral therapy.

- Support groups.

- Medication.

- Nutrition therapy.

- Outpatient treatment programs.

- Hospitalization, if needed.

Questions to Ask

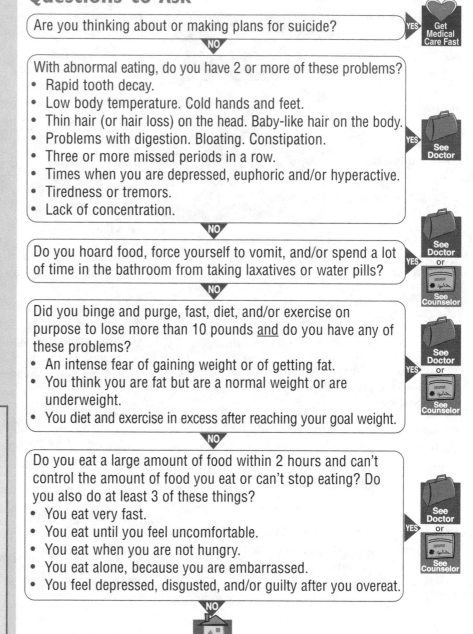

Are you thinking about or making plans for suicide?

YES → Get Medical Care Fast

NO

With abnormal eating, do you have 2 or more of these problems?
- Rapid tooth decay.
- Low body temperature. Cold hands and feet.
- Thin hair (or hair loss) on the head. Baby-like hair on the body.
- Problems with digestion. Bloating. Constipation.
- Three or more missed periods in a row.
- Times when you are depressed, euphoric and/or hyperactive.
- Tiredness or tremors.
- Lack of concentration.

YES → See Doctor

NO

Do you hoard food, force yourself to vomit, and/or spend a lot of time in the bathroom from taking laxatives or water pills?

YES → See Doctor or See Counselor

NO

Did you binge and purge, fast, diet, and/or exercise on purpose to lose more than 10 pounds <u>and</u> do you have any of these problems?
- An intense fear of gaining weight or of getting fat.
- You think you are fat but are a normal weight or are underweight.
- You diet and exercise in excess after reaching your goal weight.

YES → See Doctor or See Counselor

NO

Do you eat a large amount of food within 2 hours and can't control the amount of food you eat or can't stop eating? Do you also do at least 3 of these things?
- You eat very fast.
- You eat until you feel uncomfortable.
- You eat when you are not hungry.
- You eat alone, because you are embarrassed.
- You feel depressed, disgusted, and/or guilty after you overeat.

YES → See Doctor or See Counselor

NO

Use Self-Care

See Self-Care / Prevention on next page

Get more information from:

HealthyLearn®
www.HealthyLearn.com
Click on MedlinePlus®

National Eating Disorders Association Information and Referral Helpline
800.931.2237
www.nationaleating disorders.org

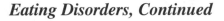

Eating Disorders, Continued

Self-Care / Prevention

Eating disorders need professional treatment.

To Help Prevent an Eating Disorder

■ Learn to accept yourself and your body. You don't need to be or look like anyone else. Spend time with people who accept you as you are, not people who focus on "thinness."

■ Know that self-esteem does not have to depend on body weight.

■ Eat nutritious foods. Focus on whole grains, beans, fresh fruits and vegetables, low-fat dairy foods, and low-fat meats.

■ Commit to a goal of normal eating. Realize that this will take time. It will also take courage to fight fears of gaining weight.

■ Don't skip meals. If you do, you are more likely to binge when you eat.

■ Avoid white flour, sugar and foods high in sugar and fat, such as cakes, cookies, and pastries. Bulimics tend to binge on junk food. The more they eat, the more they want.

■ Find success in things that you do.

■ Get regular moderate exercise 3 to 4 times a week. If you exercise more than your doctor advises, do non-exercise activities with friends and family.

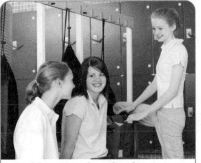

Hobbies, work, school, etc. can promote self-esteem.

■ Learn as much as you can about eating disorders from books and places that deal with them.

■ To help their children avoid eating disorders, parents should promote a balance between their child's competing needs for independence and family involvement.

To Treat an Eating Disorder

■ Follow your treatment plan.

■ Attend counseling sessions and/or support group meetings as scheduled.

■ Identify feelings before, during, and after you overeat, binge, purge, or restrict food intake. What is it that you are hoping the food will do?

■ Set small goals that you can easily reach. Congratulate yourself for every success. This is a process. Accept setbacks. Learn from them.

■ Talk to someone instead of turning to food.

■ Learn to express your rights. You have the right to say "no" and the right to express your feelings and your opinions. You have the right to ask that your needs are met.

■ Keep a journal of your progress, feelings, thoughts, etc., but not about what you eat. The journal is just for you, not for others to read or judge. This is a safe place to be honest with yourself. The journal can also help you identify your "triggers" so that you can deal with them in the future.

■ Don't let the scale run your life. Better yet, throw out the scale!

Gambling Problems

Signs & Symptoms

For most people, gambling is a social event done responsibly. For as much as 4% of all adults, though, gambling can disrupt their lives. About 2 million (1%) of adults in the U.S. meet the criteria for **pathological gambling**. (See Signs & Symptoms at right.)

Another 4 to 8 million persons (2–3%) are **problem gamblers**. They are not pathological gamblers, but have problems due to gambling.

Treatment

Problem gambling is an illness. It needs professional treatment.

For Pathological Gambling

Pathological gamblers are addicted to gambling. They do 5 or more of these things:

- They are pre-occupied with gambling. They dwell on past gambling events, plan future gambling bouts, and/or think about ways to get money to gamble with.

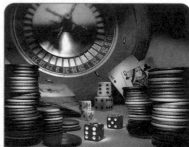

Problem gambling disrupts a person's life.

- They need to increase the amount of money to gamble with to get a desired level of excitement.

- They have tried to control, limit, or stop gambling without success.

- They are restless or very cranky when they try to limit or stop gambling.

- They gamble to escape problems or to relieve negative feelings.

- They gamble to get even for past gambling losses.

- They lie to others to hide how much they are involved with gambling.

- They have stolen or done another illegal act to get money for gambling.

- They have lost a job, a relationship, etc., due to gambling.

- They rely on others to bail them out from money problems due to gambling.

Other Problems Pathological Gamblers Have

- They abuse alcohol or drugs.

- They sleep poorly.

- They are prone to stress-related conditions, such as high blood pressure, headaches, and mood disorders, such as depression.

Gambling Problems, *Continued*

- They have thoughts of suicide.
- They gamble constantly.
- They want to have wealth and material goods without working hard to get them.
- They think that money is both the cause of and solution to all of their problems.
- They feel important or "in control" and over-confident while betting.

Causes

Problem gambling occurs when gambling can't be controlled. It may follow years of social gambling, but then may be set into motion by a stressful event or greater exposure to gambling.

Problem gamblers report that one or both parents had a drinking and/or gambling problem.

Questions to Ask

Do you have one or more **signs & symptoms for pathological gambling** listed on page 280? **YES** See Counselor

NO

Do you gamble only when your mood is abnormally and constantly elevated? **YES** See Counselor

NO

Use Self-Care

See Self-Care / Prevention in next column

Self-Care / Prevention

Along with professional treatment:
- Learn all you can about gambling and its effects.
- Contact Gamblers Anonymous (GA) listed below.
- Ask your family and friends to help you take part in non-gambling activities.
- When you feel compelled to gamble, do something else. Exercise. Take a warm bath or shower. Spend time on a hobby.
- Get involved in school, church, and community activities. These can help distract you from gambling.

Get more information from:

HealthyLearn® • www.HealthyLearn.com
Click on MedlinePlus®

Gamblers Anonymous
888.GA.HELPS (424.3577)
www.gamblersanonymous.org

National Council on Problem Gambling
Helpline Network
800.522.4700
www.ncpgambling.org

Grief / Bereavement

Grief is a deep sadness or sorrow that results from a loss. The loss can be a major or minor one. It can result from something positive or negative.

Bereavement is grieving most often linked with the death of a loved one.

Treatment

Understanding the normal stages of grief, the passage of time, and self-care measures treat most cases of grief. When these are not enough, counseling can help.

Get more information from:

HealthyLearn®
www.HealthyLearn.com
Click on MedlinePlus®

AARP Grief Support
www.aarp.org/family/
lifeafterloss

Signs & Symptoms

Stages of Grief

1. *Shock.* You feel dazed or numb.
2. *Denial and searching.*
   - You are in a state of disbelief.
   - You ask questions, such as, "Why did this happen?" or "Why didn't I prevent this?"
   - You look for ways to keep your loved one or loss with you.
   - You think you see or hear the deceased person.
   - You begin to feel that the loss is real.

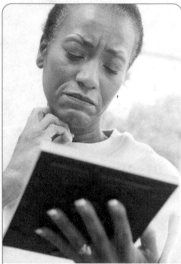

It is normal to feel sad after a loss.

3. *Suffering and disorganization.*
   - You feel guilty, anxious, depressed, lonely, afraid, etc.
   - You may place blame on everyone and everything.
   - You may get physical symptoms. These include headaches, stomachaches, constant fatigue, and/or shortness of breath.
   - You withdraw from routine and social contacts.

4. *Recovery and acceptance.*
   - You begin to look at the future instead of dwelling on the past.
   - You adjust to the reality of the loss.
   - You develop new relationships.
   - You develop a positive attitude.

Grieving the loss of a loved one can last weeks, months, or years.

Grief / Bereavement, Continued

Causes

- A new or lost job, a promotion, demotion, or retirement.

- Relationship changes, such as getting divorced or having a child leave home.

- An illness, injury, and/or disability.

- The death of a family member or friend. Loss of property. Moving to a new place.

Factors that shape a person's response to a loss, such as death include:

- Age, gender, and health.

- How sudden the loss was.

- Cultural background. Religious beliefs.

- Finances.

- Social network.

- History of other losses or traumatic events.

Each of these factors can add to or reduce the pain of grieving.

Questions to Ask

Have you just attempted suicide? Have you written a suicide note? Are you making plans for suicide or having repeated thoughts of suicide or death?

YES → Get Medical Care Fast

NO

Do you overuse medication and/or alcohol to feel better or to cope or "numb" the pain?

YES → See Doctor or See Counselor

NO

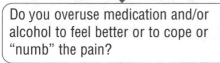

Flowchart continued in next column

Do you have any of these problems?
- Extreme stress with your marriage and/or children.
- You can't cope day to day.
- You have ongoing problems with insomnia. You cry too much. You are depressed, feel guilty, or eat too much or too little.
- You refuse to sort through the deceased's belongings after time passes.

YES → See Doctor or See Counselor

NO → Use Self-Care

Self-Care / Prevention

- Eat regular meals.

- Get regular physical activity.

- Allow friends and family to help you. Don't hold your feelings inside. State how you really feel. Visit them, especially during the holidays, if you would otherwise be alone. Travel during the holidays if this helps.

- Share and maintain memories of a lost loved one. Being reminded of the past can help with the process of coming to grips with a loss.

- Try not to make major life changes, such as moving during the first year of grieving.

- Join a support group for the bereaved. People and places to contact include your EAP representative, your student counseling center, churches or synagogues, funeral homes, and hospice centers.

- Adopt a pet.

- Read self-help books about grief and death.

Stress & Posttraumatic Stress Disorder

Stress is the body's response to changes and increased demands. It is a natural part of life. Stress means different things to different people. Usually, it is linked with negative feelings.

Left unchecked, stress can lead to or worsen health problems. These include headaches, back or neck pain, and high blood pressure.

Posttraumatic stress disorder (PTSD) is a severe stress reaction from living through or seeing an event that threatens life. With PTSD, symptoms (see next column) usually begin within 6 weeks to 3 months of the event. Symptoms of PTSD can begin years later, though. When symptoms do occur, they must last for at least one month for a diagnosis of PTSD to be made. PTSD is a medical diagnosis made by a mental health professional.

Signs & Symptoms

Physical symptoms of stress are: Increased heart rate and blood pressure; rapid breathing; and tense muscles.

Emotional reactions include being angry and having a lack of concentration.

Signs & Symptoms of PTSD in Adults
"Avoidance" Symptoms
▬ You avoid people, places, and activities that recall the event.
▬ You avoid thoughts, feelings, or mention of the event.
▬ You have much less interest in doing necessary activities.
▬ You feel detached or estranged from others.
▬ You forget an important aspect of the event.
"Increased Arousal" Symptoms
▬ You are very easily startled.
▬ You have a hard time concentrating.
▬ You have a hard time falling or staying asleep.
▬ You are very cranky.
"Re-experiencing the Event" Symptoms
▬ You have recurring, intrusive thoughts of the event that cause distress.
▬ You have nightmares.
▬ You have flashbacks of the event.

Stress & Posttraumatic Stress Disorder, *Continued*

Signs & Symptoms of PTSD in Children
Crying.
Headaches and other physical complaints.
Thumb sucking.
Depression. Being inactive.
Bathroom accidents.
Fear of being alone. Clinging to others.
Nightmares. The child may not be able to recall the dream's contents.
Fear of weather.
Being irritable. Being confused.
Not being able to concentrate.
Aggressive behavior.
Withdrawal.
Expressing things or parts of the event in repeated play.

Other symptoms of PTSD are intense fear or horror and feeling helpless, in a "daze," detached, etc.

Causes

Marriage or divorce, job loss or the threat of being fired, all create stress. So do countless other things.

Living through or seeing an event that threatens life can cause PTSD. Events include combat exposure, sexual or physical assault, and a serious accident. A past unhealed trauma increases the risk for PTSD. People with depression or other mental health conditions are also at greater risk.

Questions to Ask

Does stress result in any of these problems?
- Suicide attempts, plans for suicide, writing a suicide note, or recurrent thoughts of suicide or death.
- Impulses or plans to commit violence.

YES → **Get Medical Care Fast**

NO ↓

After being part of a traumatic event, are **signs and symptoms of PTSD** listed on page 284 or on this page present?

YES → **See Doctor** or **See Counselor**

NO ↓

Do you need alcohol and/or drugs to deal with stress?

YES → **See Doctor** or **See Counselor**

NO ↓

Are you often anxious or nervous, and/or confused about how to handle a problem?

YES → **See Doctor** or **See Counselor**

NO ↓

Does stress result in any of these problems?
- You withdraw from others.
- You can't do daily activities.
- You neglect to take care of your health.

YES → **Call Doctor** or **Call Counselor**

NO ↓

Use Self-Care

Self-Care / Prevention

- Maintain good health habits. Eat healthy foods. Get enough sleep.

Stress & Posttraumatic Stress Disorder, Continued

Treatment

Self-care measures deal with most cases of stress. When these are not enough, counseling and/or medical care may be needed.

Professional treatment is needed for PTSD. Left untreated, PTSD will not go away and can greatly affect a person's life.

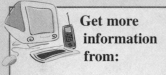

Get more information from:

HealthyLearn®
www.HealthyLearn.com
Click on MedlinePlus®

National Center for Posttraumatic Stress Disorder (PTSD)
www.ptsd.va.gov

The National Institute for Occupational Safety and Health (NIOSH)
800.CDC.INFO
    (232.4636)
www.cdc.gov/niosh/
topics/stress

- Limit caffeine. It causes anxiety and increases the stress response.

- If you drink alcohol, do so wisely. (See **Use Alcohol Wisely** on page 51.)

- Get regular exercise.

- Check with your doctor about taking vitamins and minerals. This is especially true for ones labeled "stress tablets" or "stress formulas."

- Don't let your emotions get "bottled up inside." Share your feelings with others.

- Do a "stress rehearsal." Imagine yourself feeling calm and handling the stressful situation.

- Balance work and personal life. Do things you enjoy and look forward to. Escape for a little while. See a movie, visit a friend, etc.

- Be with cheerful people. Help others.

- Reduce or manage exposure to things that cause stress.

- Rank order daily tasks. Don't commit to doing too much.

- Studies show that having a pet, such as a dog or cat, appears to buffer the effects of stress on health.

- View changes as positive challenges.

- Laugh a lot. Keep a sense of humor.

- Take a bath or shower with warm water. Listen to music that is calming.

- Reward yourself with little things that make you feel good. Give yourself some "me" time.

- Count to 10 when you're so upset you want to scream. This helps to calm you down. Avoid unnecessary arguments.

- Have a warm cup of herbal tea.

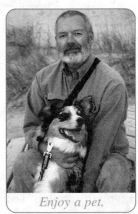

Enjoy a pet.

- Do relaxation exercises daily. Imagine a soothing, restful scene. Do deep muscle relaxation. (Tense and relax muscle fibers.) Meditate. Do deep breathing.

- Remember that it is not an event that causes stress, but how you react to it. Change your thoughts about an event to help manage stress.

Suicidal Thoughts

A lot of people think about suicide. They may say things like "I wish I was dead," at times of great stress. Casual thoughts of suicide that don't last may not be a sign of a problem.

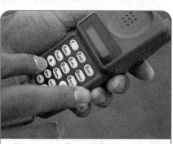

Let your doctor know if you have thoughts of suicide.

For most people, they are a way to express anger and other strong feelings. The signs and symptoms that follow need medical care.

Signs & Symptoms

- Writing a suicide note.
- Suicidal threats, gestures, or attempts.
- Thoughts of suicide that don't go away or occur often.

Causes

- Depression. Bipolar disorder. Schizophrenia.
- Grief. Loss of a loved one.
- A side effect of some medicines. One is isotretinoin. This is prescribed for severe acne. Some antidepressants have this effect, too. This is more of a risk in the first days to the first month they are taken.
- A family history of suicide or depression.
- Money and relationship problems.

Questions to Ask

(*Note:* In some suicides, no warning signs are shown or noticed.)

Are any of these problems present?
- Suicide attempts or gestures. Does the person stand on the edge of a bridge, cut his or her wrists, etc.?
- Plans are being made for suicide. Has the person gotten a weapon or pills that could be used for suicide?
- Thoughts of suicide or death occur over and over. Suicide intent is stated. A suicide note is written.
- After being very depressed, the person suddenly felt better and stated something like "Now I know what I have to do," or "Now I see how to make everything better."

YES → 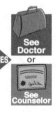 Get Medical Care Fast

NO ↓

Has the person recently done any of these things?
- Repeated statements that show thoughts of suicide, such as, "I want to be dead," or "I don't want to live anymore."
- Given away favorite things. Cleaned the house. Gotten legal matters in order.

YES → See Doctor or See Counselor

NO ↓

With thoughts of suicide or death, are any of these problems present?
- Depression or **symptoms of depression** listed on page 275.
- Bipolar disorder (manic-depression).
- Schizophrenia.
- Any other mental health or medical condition.

YES → 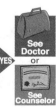 See Doctor or See Counselor

NO ↓

Flowchart continued on next page

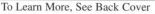

Treatment

- Emergency care.

- Treating the mental and/or physical problems that lead to thoughts and attempts of suicide. Examples are bipolar disorder and depression. (See **Depression** on page 275.)

- Counseling.

- Talking with family and friends often.

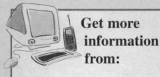

Get more information from:

HealthyLearn®
www.HealthyLearn.com
Click on MedlinePlus®

Mental Health America
(MHA)
800.969.6642
www.mentalhealth
america.net

National Suicide
Prevention Lifeline
800.273.TALK
    (273.8255)
www.suicideprevention
lifeline.org

Suicidal Thoughts, Continued

Have thoughts of suicide occurred after taking, stopping, or changing the dose of a prescribed medicine (this includes certain antidepressants) or using drugs and/or alcohol?

YES → See Doctor or See Counselor

NO

Does the person thinking about suicide have other blood relatives who died from or attempted suicide?

YES → See Doctor or See Counselor

NO

Use Self-Care

Self-Care / Prevention

For Suicidal Thoughts

- Call the National Suicide Prevention Lifeline at 800.273.8255.

- Let someone know. Talk to your doctor, a trusted family member, friend, or teacher. If it is hard for you to talk to someone, write your thoughts down. Let someone else read them.

To Help Prevent a Suicide

- Keep firearms, drugs, etc., away from persons at risk.

- Take courses that teach problem solving, coping skills, and suicide awareness.

- If you think the person is serious about suicide, get help. Watch and protect him or her until you get help. Keep the person talking. Ask questions such as, "Are you thinking about hurting or killing yourself?"

- Urge the person to call for help (e.g., his or her health care provider, a suicide prevention hotline, EMS, etc.) Make the call yourself if the person can't or won't.

- Express concern. The person needs to know that someone cares. Most suicidal persons feel alone. Tell the person how much he or she means to you and others. Talk about reasons to stay alive. Don't judge. The person needs someone to listen, not preach moral values.

- Tell the person that depression and thinking about suicide can be treated. Urge him or her to get professional care. Offer help in seeking care.

Violence & Abuse

Violence is the intended use or threat of force or power against one or more persons or even oneself. It results in physical or emotional harm, deprivation, or, too often, death. Worldwide, violence causes 44% of deaths among males; 7% among females.

Abuse is one form of violence. It can be emotional, physical, economic, and/or sexual.

Violence and abuse are law and order issues, as well as, personal and public health issues.

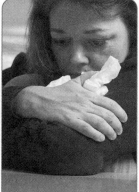

Violence and abuse are common and complex problems.

Signs & Symptoms

A person who commits violence and abuse does the things listed below. The signs often progress from ones that cause less harm to ones that can threaten life.

- Uses verbal abuse, such as name calling.
- Acts possessive and extremely jealous.
- Has a bad temper. Does violent acts in front of others, but doesn't harm them. An example is putting a fist through a wall.
- Gives threats.
- Acts cruel to animals.
- Pushes, slaps, and/or restrains others.
- Punches. Kicks. Bites. Sexually assaults.
- Chokes others. Breaks bones. Uses weapons.

Causes

Violence and abuse are ways to gain and keep control over others. Persons who commit violence or abuse come from all groups and backgrounds. Often, they have these problems:

- Poor skills to communicate.
- A family history of violence. They may have been abused in the past. They may have seen one parent beat the other.
- Alcohol or drug abuse.

Questions to Ask

Does violence cause any of these problems?
- The person is not responsive. The person has a serious injury or bleeds a lot.
- The person has severe problems breathing or has chest pain due to the abuse.

YES → Get Medical Care Fast

NO ↓

Do any of these problems occur?
- The person is being abused right now.
- A weapon is used during an assault.
- A child is threatened or neglected. A child is left alone in a car.
- The person has been raped.
- The person does not feel safe.
- The abused person is pregnant.

YES → Get Medical Care Fast
(Call Police.)

NO ↓

Is the person in an abusive relationship? Is a child suspected of being abused, mistreated, and/or neglected?

YES → 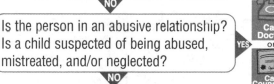 Call Doctor or Call Counselor

NO ↓

 Use Self-Care

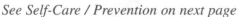

See Self-Care / Prevention on next page

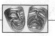

Violence & Abuse, Continued

Treatment

Treatment for the victim of abuse or violence depends on the situation and includes:

- Emergency medical care. Calling the police.

- Going to a safe place, such as a shelter for victims of abuse.

- Counseling.

- Training to be assertive.

In general, persons who abuse others or commit violence find it hard to change their behavior without professional help.

Get more information from:

National Center for Victims of Crime
800.FYI.CALL
(394.2255)
www.ncvc.org

National Domestic Violence Hotline
800.799.7233
www.ndvh.org

Self-Care / Prevention

To Handle Being in an Abusive Relationship
- Get help!

- Have a safety plan for times you feel unsafe or in danger.
  - Decide who you will call (e.g., police, neighbors, relatives, a shelter). Make a list of these telephone numbers. Memorize them, too.
  - Decide where you will go. If you have children and pets, develop safety plans. Practice the safety plans with your children. Have a plan for taking them with you. Have plans for where they should go if you can't get away.
  - Keep extra keys to your car and house in a safe place unknown to the person abusing you.
  - Put some cash in a safe place that you can get quickly in case you need money for transportation to a safe place.

To Manage Conflict Without Violence
- When you communicate, state your needs without putting others down.

- Learn to deal with frustration, rejection, ridicule, jealousy, and **anger** (see page 268).

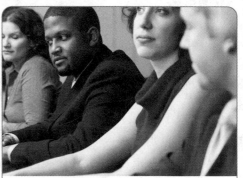

Accept differences in others.

- Accept differences in others. This includes sexual preferences, ethnic and religious backgrounds, etc. You do not need to change your beliefs, but don't expect other persons to change theirs, either.

- Be an active listener. Focus on what the other person is saying. Try to understand his or her point of view. Or, simply accept it as an opinion.

- Take a course that teaches skills to manage conflict.

- When you can't resolve a conflict on your own, get help.

Chapter 17

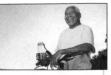

Men's Health Issues

Erectile Dysfunction (ED)

With, **erectile dysfunction (ED)**, a male can't get or keep an erection firm enough for sex in 25% or more of attempts. Sometimes, ED is called **impotence**. Impotence can be ED, but can also mean a lack of sexual desire and problems with orgasm.

Signs & Symptoms

- Not being able to get an erection at all.
- An erection is too brief, weak, or painful for satisfying sex.
- An erection loses strength with penetration.

Causes

Blood vessel diseases, diabetes, and other physical problems are the usual cause of ED. Other causes are smoking and a side effect of some medicines, such as beta-blockers and water pills. Only 10% to 20% of ED cases are due to emotional factors, such as stress and fear of not being able to perform. Suspect this cause if erections occur during sleep or when waking up.

Treatment

- Treatment for conditions that cause ED.
- Medication.
- A vacuum erection device.
- Self-injection therapy or a penile implant.

Questions to Ask

Did ED occur with prostate or other surgery, trauma to the pelvis, or after taking prescribed medicines? **YES** → See Doctor

NO ↓

Does ED cause a problem for you or your partner? **YES** → Call Doctor

NO ↓

Use Self-Care

Self-Care / Prevention

- Take medicine for ED as prescribed.
- Check with your doctor before you take herbs, etc. sold for ED. These include Actra-Rx, ginko biloba, yohimbe, Siberian ginseng, and Yilishen.
- If you have diabetes, follow your treatment plan.
- Don't smoke. Don't use street drugs.
- Don't have more than 2 alcoholic drinks a day.
- Relax. Manage stress. Get plenty of rest.
- Share your fears, needs, etc. with your partner.
- Don't focus just on performance. Find pleasure when you hug, kiss, and caress your partner.

Get more information from:

HealthyLearn® • www.HealthyLearn.com
Click on MedlinePlus®

Jock Itch

Jock itch is an infection of the skin on the groin and upper inner thigh areas.

Signs & Symptoms

- Redness.
- Itching.
- Raised red rash with borders. Center areas of the rash are dry with small scales.

Treatment

Over-the-counter antifungal creams treat most cases of jock itch. Stronger creams or an oral medicine can be prescribed, if needed.

Causes

Jock itch is usually caused by a fungus. It can also result from garments that irritate the skin and from taking antibiotics. Jock itch is more likely to occur in hot, humid conditions.

Questions to Ask

Does any liquid ooze from the rash? Or, do symptoms worsen or last longer than 2 weeks despite using self-care?

YES — See Doctor

NO — Use Self-Care

Self-Care / Prevention

To Treat Jock Itch

- Use over-the-counter antifungal cream, powder, or lotion for jock itch. Follow package directions.

To Prevent Jock Itch

- Don't wear tight, close-fitting clothing. Wear boxer shorts, not briefs. Change underwear often, especially after tasks that leave you hot and sweaty.

- Bathe or shower right away after a workout. Don't use antibacterial (deodorant) soaps. Dry the groin area well.

- Apply talc or other powder to the groin area to help keep it dry. If you sweat a lot or are very overweight, use a drying powder with miconazole nitrate.

- Wash workout clothes after each wearing. Don't store damp clothing in a locker or gym bag.

- Sleep in the nude or in a nightshirt.

- Don't share towels or clothes that have come in contact with the rash.

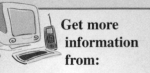
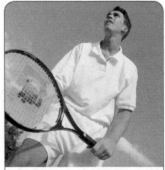

Wear loose-fitting clothes during exercise.

Premature Ejaculation

Releasing semen too soon is the most common sexual problem in males, especially young men.

Signs & Symptoms

With premature ejaculation, a man <u>often</u> releases semen before he and/or his partner wants this to occur.

Causes

Most likely, the cause is having a penis that is too sensitive and pelvic muscles that are very spastic. Stress, guilt, worry, etc. do not cause this problem.

Treatment

- Self-care measures.
- Medicine. A very low dose of a certain kind of antidepressant is prescribed. Taken 4 hours before sex, the medicine may prolong the release of semen by at least 5 to 10 minutes.

The things that follow are not cures or proven treatments, but may be helpful to some, but not all men.
- Using condoms.
- Masturbating often.
- Using a cream that numbs the head of the penis.

Questions to Ask

Does releasing semen too soon cause a problem for you or your partner?

YES → Call Doctor

NO → Use Self-Care

Self-Care / Prevention

- *The Squeeze Technique.* If a man feels he is about to release semen too soon, he firmly pinches the penis directly below the head. Using the

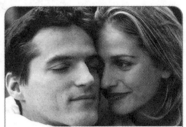

Just taking slow, deep breaths may help slow the release of semen.

thumb and first 2 fingers of one hand, he squeezes for 3 to 4 seconds. (This was developed by William H. Masters, M.D. and Virginia E. Johnson. They founded the Reproductive Biology Research Foundation.)

- *The Start/Stop Method.* The couple should not have sex for 2 weeks. The man then concentrates on the sensations in his penis as his partner touches his genitals and brings him to an erection. The man asks his partner to stop just before semen is released. After a few minutes, his partner continues to arouse him, then stops again. This sequence is repeated 2 more times. The fourth time semen is released. Then, each time the couple has sex, foreplay is prolonged.

Prostate Problems

Prostate problems are:

- **Prostatitis.** The prostate is inflamed or infected. This can be an acute or chronic problem.

- **Enlarged prostate – Benign prostatic hyperplasia (BPH).** This is not cancer.

- **Prostate cancer.**

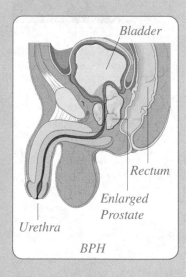

Bladder

Rectum

Enlarged Prostate

Urethra

BPH

The prostate gland is below the bladder and in front of the rectum. It surrounds the upper part of the urethra. (This tube empties urine from the bladder.)

Prostate problems more likely to occur in men age 50 and older. A digital rectal exam (DRE) and a prostate-specific antigen (PSA) blood test can help detect prostate cancer. Men over age 50 should talk to their doctors about the benefits and risks of having these tests. African American men and men with a family history of prostate cancer should do this starting at age 45.

Signs & Symptoms

For Prostatitis

- Pain and burning when you pass urine, have an erection, or ejaculate.

- Strong urge to urinate. You pass urine often, even at night.

- A hard time starting to urinate. You don't empty your bladder all the way.

- Pain in the lower back and/or between the scrotum and anus.

- Blood in the urine. Fever and/or chills.

For an Enlarged Prostate

- Increased urge to pass urine. You pass urine often, especially during the night.

- Delay in onset or decreased or slow stream when you pass urine.

- You don't empty your bladder all the way.

For Prostate Cancer

Prostate cancer may have no symptoms until it is advanced. When symptoms occur, they include:

- Symptoms of an enlarged prostate.

- Blood in the urine.

- Swollen lymph nodes in the groin area.

- **Erectile dysfunction.** (See page 291.)

- Pain in the hips, pelvis, ribs, or spine.

Prostate Problems, Continued

Causes

For Prostatitis

A bacterial infection is usually the cause. With the chronic form, the infection comes back again and again. Sometimes, urine tests may not show bacteria. A prostate exam can confirm an infection.

For an Enlarged Prostate

- Normal aging. More than half of men in their 60s have benign prostatic hyperplasia (BPH). Up to 80 percent of men in their 70s and 80s may have BPH.

- Prostate infections can increase the risk.

For Prostate Cancer

- Aging. The chances increase rapidly after age 50. About 80% of all cases occur in men over age 65.

- Race.

- Family history of prostate cancer.

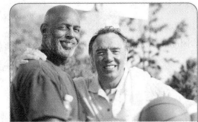

African American men are twice as likely to get prostate cancer as Caucasian American men.

- A diet high in fat and dairy products and low in fruits and vegetables may increase the risk. A low-fat diet may help lower the risk. Eating tomato products, such as spaghetti sauce and tomato soup, may help lower the risk, too. These foods are a great source of lycopene. This plant chemical gives tomatoes their red color. It is also found in pink grapefruit and watermelon.

Treatment

For Prostatitis

Treatment is antibiotics and self-care.

For an Enlarged Prostate

- When symptoms are minor, no treatment may be needed at that time. The BPH is monitored to see if it causes problems or gets worse. This is called "**watchful waiting.**"

- Medicine. One type helps relax the bladder neck muscle and the prostate. Another type causes the prostate to shrink.

- Surgery. There are many types and many new procedures.

For Prostate Cancer

Treatment depends on the man's age and health. It also depends on how slow the cancer is expected to grow or if it has spread beyond the prostate. Treatment includes:

- Watchful waiting. This means getting no treatment, but having tests at certain times to check for changes that may need treatment.

- Surgery. There are many types.

- Radioactive "seed" implants.

- Radiation therapy.

- Hormonal therapy.

{*Note:* Prostate surgery for BPH and prostate cancer can result in problems, such as impotence and/or incontinence. Discuss the benefits and risks of treatment options with your doctor. Most men who have surgery have no major problems.}

Prostate Problems, Continued

Questions to Ask

Do you have signs and symptoms of prostatitis, an enlarged prostate, or prostate cancer? Or, if you have been told you have prostate cancer or an enlarged prostate, do symptoms get worse or do you have new symptoms?

YES  See Doctor

NO

Do symptoms of prostatitis not improve after 3 days of treatment, get worse during treatment, or come back after treatment is done?

YES See Doctor

NO

 Use Self-Care

Self-Care / Prevention

For Prostatitis

- Take antibiotics as prescribed.

- Rest until fever and pain are gone.

- Take an over-the-counter medicine for pain and swelling, if needed. Take it as directed.

For an Enlarged Prostate

- Stay sexually active.

- Don't take over-the-counter (OTC) medications with antihistamines unless approved by your doctor.

- Discuss the use of the OTC plant extract saw palmetto with your doctor before you take it.

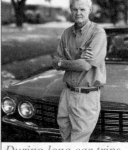
During long car trips, stop often to urinate.

For Both an Enlarged Prostate and Prostatitis

- Take warm baths.

- Don't let your bladder get too full. Urinate as soon as you get the urge. Relax when you urinate.

- Drink 8 or more glasses of water every day. Don't drink liquids before going to bed.

- Don't smoke.

- Reduce stress.

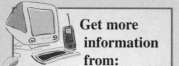

Get more information from:

HealthyLearn®
www.HealthyLearn.com
Click on MedlinePlus®

American Urological Association (AUA) Foundation
www.urologyhealth.org

Testicle Problems

The testicles (also called testes) are two oval shaped organs that make and store sperm. They also make male sex hormones. The testicles are inside the scrotum. This sac of skin hangs under the penis. The scrotum can swell or be painful without a testicle problem. An example of this is an inguinal hernia. (See **Hernias** on page 165.)

Problems that affect the testicles include: Injury, swelling and infection; torsion; undescended testicles; and cancer.

Signs & Symptoms

For Injury, Swelling, and/or Infection

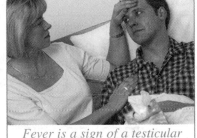

Fever is a sign of a testicular or other infection.

- Pain and swelling in the scrotum.

- Feeling of heaviness in the scrotum.

For Torsion of a Testicle

- Sudden and severe pain in the scrotum.

- Swelling. Most often, this occurs in one testicle.

- Fever.

- Abdominal pain. Nausea. Vomiting.

For Undescended Testicles

- In baby boys, testicles do not descend into the scrotum from the abdomen before birth or within months of birth like they should.

For Cancer of a Testicle

In the early stages, there may be no symptoms. When symptoms occur, they include:

- A lump on a testicle, epididymis, or vas deferens.

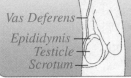

Vas Deferens
Epididymis
Testicle
Scrotum

- An enlarged testicle.

- A heavy feeling, pain or discomfort in the testicle or scrotum.

- A change in the way a testicle feels.

- A dull ache in the lower abdomen or groin.

- Enlarged or tender breasts.

- Sudden pooling of fluid in the scrotum.

Causes

For Injury, Swelling, and Infection

- Trauma to the testicles from being hit, kicked, struck, etc. Often, this occurs during sports. Though rare, trauma to the abdomen can cause the testicles to move outside the scrotum.

- **Orchitis**. With this, a testicle is inflamed. Often it is due to an infection, such as mumps or chlamydia. The epididymis can also be inflamed from an infection.

For Torsion of a Testicle

When the spermatic cord twists, a testicle rotates. This cuts off blood supply to and from the testicle.

- This usually occurs in males under age 30, most often between the ages of 12 and 18.

- Symptoms often occur after physical activity or during sleep.

- Symptoms may occur for no known reason.

Testicle Problems, Continued

For Undescended Testicles
Testicles fail to drop from inside the pelvic area down into the scrotum before birth or within a year of birth.

For Cancer of a Testicle
The cause is not known. Risk factors include:
- Undescended testicles that are not corrected in infants and young children. Parents should see that their infant boys are checked at birth for this problem.
- Having cancer of a testicle in the past.
- A family history of cancer of a testicle, especially in an identical twin.
- Injury to the scrotum.

Treatment

For Injury, Swelling, and/or Infection
- Pain from a minor injury to a testicle usually goes away on its own.
- Antibiotics treat bacterial infections. Untreated infections can cause infertility.

For Torsion of a Testicle
Emergency medical care is needed. The testicle may be untwisted by hand. If not, surgery is needed to restore blood flow to the testicle.

For Undescended Testicles
Surgery is done to bring the testicles down into the scrotum.

For Cancer of a Testicle
This kind of cancer is almost always curable if it is found and treated early. Surgery is done to remove the testicle. Other things can further treat the disease:
- Chemotherapy.
- Radiation therapy.
- If needed, lymph nodes are removed by surgery.

Questions to Ask

Do you have any of these problems all of a sudden?
- Severe pain in the scrotum or in one testicle.
- Tenderness and swelling in the scrotum (most often in one testicle) with fever, abdominal pain, nausea, and/or vomiting.
- A tender nodule in the upper and outer area of a testicle.
- A testicle is bluish in color.

YES → Get Medical Care Fast

NO ↓

Have you had an injury, trauma, or abuse (including sexual assault) to the genital area? Or, does bleeding come from the scrotum?

YES → Get Medical Care Fast

NO ↓

Do you get a fever and swelling and pain in the testicle(s) after having the mumps?

YES → Get Medical Care Fast

NO ↓

Are **signs and symptoms of cancer of a testicle** listed on page 297 present?

YES → See Doctor

NO ↓

Are **signs and symptoms of chlamydia** listed on page 248 present?

YES →  See Doctor

NO ↓

Flowchart continued on next page

Testicle Problems, *Continued*

Do you have any of these problems?
- Swelling in the scrotum that was soft and painless, but is now painful or very uncomfortable.
- Swelling in the scrotum and/or a change in the way the scrotum normally feels.

YES See Doctor

NO

In a baby boy, has a testicle not descended into the scrotum by one year of age?

YES See Doctor

NO

 Use Self-Care

Self-Care / Prevention

To Avoid Injury to the Scrotum
- Wear protective gear and clothing during exercise and sports.
- Wear an athletic cup to protect the testicles.

To Help Prevent Infections
- See that your children get vaccines for measles, mumps, and rubella (MMR) as advised by their doctor. (See **Immunization Schedule** on page 23.)
- To help prevent STDs, follow **"Safer Sex"** guidelines. (See page 252.)

To Treat Infections
- Take medication as prescribed.
- Take an over-the-counter medicine for pain and swelling, if needed. Follow directions.
- Rest.
- Apply cold compresses or an ice pack to painful, swollen area.

Testicular Self-Exam
Talk to your doctor about doing testicular self-exams (TSEs). If you choose to do TSEs, follow your doctor's advice.

The best time to do a TSE is after a warm bath or shower. This relaxes the scrotum, allows the testicles to drop down, and makes it easier to find anything unusual. Doing a TSE is easy and takes only a few minutes.

1. Stand in front of a mirror. Look for any swelling on the skin of the scrotum.

2. Examine each testicle with both hands. Place your index and middle fingers underneath the testicle and your thumbs on top. Gently roll one testicle then the other between your thumbs and fingers. One testicle may be larger.

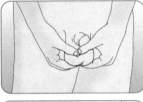

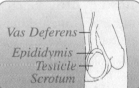

Vas Deferens
Epididymis
Testicle
Scrotum

This is normal. Examine each testicle for any lumps. These are usually painless and about the size of a pea.

3. Find the epididymis. This is the comma-shaped cord behind the testicle. It may be tender to the touch. Check it for lumps.

4. Examine the vas deferens. This is the tubelike structure at the back of each testicle. Check it for lumps.

 Get more information from:

HealthyLearn® • www.HealthyLearn.com
Click on MedlinePlus®

Cancer Information Service
800.4.CANCER (422.6237) • www.cancer.gov

 To Learn More, See Back Cover

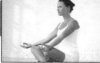

Chapter 18

Women's Health Issues

Birth Control

The chart on this page and the next 3 pages gives information on birth control methods. Discuss one(s) best suited for your needs with your doctor or health care provider. Ask for advice on more options. More than one birth control method may be needed to prevent getting pregnant <u>and</u> reduce the risk for sexually transmitted infections (STIs).

Method	Failure Rate*	Comments	HIV/STI Protection
Abstinence. No sexual intercourse between a female and a male.	0%	Has no medical or hormonal side effects.	Yes
Birth Control Patch. Hormones released from a skin patch worn on the skin weekly for 3 weeks; not worn the 4th week.	1%	Needs to be prescribed. Not a good method for females over 198 pounds. Increases the risk for blood clots and other serious problems.	No
Birth Control Pill. Hormones in pill form. Many types.	3%	Needs to be prescribed. Some medicines lessen the effects of the pill. Risk for blood clots, heart disease, and stroke, especially in women over 35 who smoke.	No
Cervical Cap. Plastic cap placed over the opening of cervix. Used with a spermicide.	16% if never gave birth; 32% if gave birth	Needs to be prescribed. Inserted before intercourse. Should be left in place for at least 6, but no more than 48 hours after last intercourse. Using this method can cause abnormal Pap tests.	No
Condom (Female). Polyurethane barrier placed inside the vagina.	21%	Can get over-the-counter. Should not be used at same time with a male condom. Can take time and patience to use the right way.	Yes

* Failure rate is the number of pregnancies expected per 100 females per year. If no method is used, the chance of pregnancy is between 85 and 90%.

Chart continued on next page

Birth Control, Continued

Method	Failure Rate*	Comments	HIV/STI Protection
Condom (Male). Latex or polyurethane sheath worn over an erect penis.	15%	Can get over-the-counter. Slight risk of breakage. Loses quality when exposed to ultraviolet light, heat, and oil-based lubricants and creams.	Yes
Depo-Provera. Hormone given through a shot every 3 months.	Less than 1%	Needs to be prescribed. May cause irregular periods, weight gain, fatigue, and headaches. Once stopped, it can take 4 to 18 months for a woman to be fertile again. Can cause bone loss if taken for more than 2 years.	No
Diaphragm. Reusable, thin, soft, rubber cap that covers the cervix. Used with a spermicide.	6–16%	Needs to be prescribed. Should be checked for leaks. Size may need to be changed with weight changes. May dislodge during intercourse. Should be left in place at least 6, but no more than 24 hours after last intercourse.	No
Emergency Contraception Pills. High-dose birth control pills that need to be started within 72 hours after unprotected intercourse. Called "Plan B."	11–25% – the sooner used, the more effective.	Can get over-the-counter if age 18 and older. Needs to be prescribed for women age 17 and younger. The pills are taken in 2 doses, 12 hours apart. Can cause nausea, vomiting, breast tenderness, infertility, and blood clots.	No
Emergency IUD Insertion. Needs to be done within 7 days of unprotected intercourse.	Less than 1%	Needs to be done by a health care professional.	No
FemCap. Silicone rubber device. Fits snugly over the cervix.	14% if never gave birth; 29% if gave birth	Needs a prescription. Should be left in place for at least 6, but no more than 48 hours after last intercourse.	No

* Failure rate is the number of pregnancies expected per 100 females per year. If no method is used, the chance of pregnancy is between 85 and 90%.

Chart continued on next page

Birth Control, Continued

Method	Failure Rate*	Comments	HIV/STI Protection
Implanon®. Thin plastic implant about the size of a match stick. Releases a low dose of the hormone progestin for up to 3 years.	Less than 1%	Needs to be inserted and removed by a health care professional. Can cause irregular menstrual bleeding, mostly fewer and lighter periods or no periods.	No
Intrauterine Device (IUD). ParaGard. Small copper device inserted into uterus. {*Note:* An IUD does not prevent an ectopic pregnancy. With this, an embryo starts to grow outside the uterus. Most often, this is in a fallopian tube.}	8%	Needs to be inserted and removed by health care professional. Can be left in place for up to 12 years. May become dislodged. Risk of infection and piercing of the uterus. Need to learn how to check for the 2 strings that hang from the bottom of the IUD to make sure it is in the right position.	No
Intrauterine System (IUS). Mirena®. T-shaped device placed in uterus. Releases low dose of hormones every day for 5 years.	Less than 1%	Needs to be inserted and removed by a health care professional. May lessen menstrual cramps. Needs to be replaced every 5 years.	No
Lea's Shield. Silicone cup with an air valve and a loop (aids in removal) that fits snugly over the cervix. Used with a spermicide.	15%	Needs to be prescribed. Should be left in place at least 8 hours after last intercourse, but no more than 48 hours total.	No
Natural Family Planning. Ovulation signs need to be checked for and kept track of.	20%	Sexual intercourse must be limited to "safe" days. Takes training, time, and record keeping to work right. Method for planning a pregnancy, too.	No
NuvaRing®. A soft, flexible ring that a female inserts deep into the vagina. Contains hormones.	1–5%	Needs to be prescribed. A new Ring is inserted once and kept in place for 3 weeks. It is removed the week of menstrual period. May cause increased risk for vaginal problems.	No

* Failure rate is the number of pregnancies expected per 100 females per year. If no method is used, the chance of pregnancy is between 85 and 90%.

Chart continued on next page

Birth Control, Continued

Method	Failure Rate*	Comments	HIV/STI Protection
Spermicides (Foams, Jellies, Creams, Suppositories). Chemicals inserted into the vagina kill sperm before it enters the uterus.	15–29%	Can get over-the-counter. More reliable when used with condoms, diaphragms, etc. Inserted between 5 and 90 minutes before intercourse. Need to reapply for repeated acts of intercourse.	No
Sponge. Today® Sponge polyurethene foam barrier that contains spermicide. It is moistened with water and inserted into the vagina. It does not have hormones.	9–19%	Can get over-the-counter. Works for full 24 hours for repeated acts of intercourse. Must be left in place for 6 hours after last intercourse. Should not be worn for more than 24 hours after sex.	Some
Sterilization (Female). One type is a Tubal Ligation (having tubes tied). This surgery burns, cuts, or ties off the fallopian tubes. Another type, tubal implants (Essure®), is not surgery. A device is inserted through the vagina and uterus into each fallopian tube. This causes scar tissue to grow and plug the tubes.	Less than 1%	Permanent form of birth control. Should be used only when no more children are desired. Surgery usually needs general anesthesia. Sterilization implants do not.	No
Sterilization (Male). Vasectomy. Cuts the tubes through which sperm travels from the testes.	Less than 1%	Permanent form of birth control. Done as outpatient with local anesthesia. Not effective right away. Sperm can still be present for 20 ejaculations.	No
Withdrawal. The penis is removed before ejaculation.	Up to 27%	Have to control ejaculation. Sperm can leak before this occurs.	No

* Failure rate is the number of pregnancies expected per 100 females per year.
 If no method is used, the chance of pregnancy is between 85 and 90%.

Get more information from:

HealthyLearn® • www.HealthyLearn.com • Click on MedlinePlus®

National Women's Health Information Center
800.994.9662 • www.womenshealth.gov

To Learn More, See Back Cover

Breast Lumps & Breast Cancer

Feeling a lump in a breast can be scary. For a lot of women, the first thought is cancer. The good news is that 80 to 90% of breast lumps are not cancer.

Treatment

Benign breast lumps may go away if you breast-feed for many months or take a low-dose birth control pill. Prescribed medicines can get rid of severe breast lumps. These have side effects, though.

For Breast Cancer
- Surgery.
- Chemotherapy.
- Radiation therapy.
- **Brachytherapy.** This is the use of radioactive "seeds." They are put into the breast at the site where the tumor was removed.
- Hormonal therapy.
- Stem cell or bone marrow transplant.
- Clinical trials.

Signs & Symptoms

- Solid tumors.
  - *Lipomas.* These are fatty tumors that can grow very large. They are usually benign.
  - *Fibroadenomas.* These lumps are round, solid, and movable. They are usually benign.
  - *Cancerous lumps.* Often, these are firm to hard masses that do not move when felt. They are often an irregular shape.

- Cysts. These are fluid filled sacs. They are painful and feel lumpy or tender. Cysts can occur near the surface of the skin of the breast. They can also be deep within the breast. This second type may need to be tested with a biopsy to make sure the cyst is benign. Cysts can be very small and diffuse as in fibrocystic breast disease.

- Nipple-duct tumors. These occur within the part of the nipple that milk flows through. They cause a discharge from the nipple. These tumors should be removed by surgery.

In rare cases, a bloody discharge from the nipple could be a sign of cancer. Breast cancer often occurs without signs and symptoms. Early screening can help detect it.

Causes

Breast lumps are often caused by fluid filled sacs (cysts), fibroadenomas, and fibrocystic changes. Breast cancer results from malignant tumors that invade and destroy normal tissue. When these tumors break away and spread to other parts of the body, it is called metastasis. Breast cancer can spread to the lymph nodes, lungs, liver, bone, and brain.

Risk Factors
- Being a woman is the main risk factor. Yearly, about 192,000 women find out they have breast cancer. About 40,000 women die from it.

{*Note:* Men can get breast cancer, too. Yearly, about 450 men in the U.S. die from breast cancer. Men should look for and report a breast lump or other change to their doctors.}

Breast Lumps & Breast Cancer, Continued

■ Increase in age.

Current Age	Chances of Getting Breast Cancer in the Next 10 Years
20	1 in 1,837
30	1 in 234
40	1 in 70
50	1 in 40
60	1 in 28
70	1 in 26
Lifetime risk	1 in 8

Source: American Cancer Society Surveillance Research, 2007

■ Changes in BRCA1, BRCA2, and other cancer genes.

■ Personal history of breast cancer.

■ Family history of breast cancer for a woman whose mother, sister, or daughter has had it, especially at an early age.

■ One or more breast biopsies were done, especially if they showed certain changes in breast tissue.

■ Dense breast tissue (shown on mammograms).

■ High-dose radiation to the chest before age 30.

■ Never giving birth or having a first full term pregnancy after age 30. Never breast-fed a baby.

■ Menstruation started before age 12. Menopause occurred after age 55.

■ Being overweight or obese after menopause.

■ Alcohol. The more used, the higher the risk.

■ Race. Caucasian women have a greater risk than Asian, African American, Hispanic, and Native American women.

■ Eastern and Central European Jewish ancestry.

■ Hormone therapy (estrogen plus progestin) after menopause and/or recent use of birth control pills may be factors.

Ask your doctor about your risk for breast cancer. You can also call 800.4.CANCER (422.6237) or access www.cancer.gov/bcrisktool for the Breast Cancer Risk Assessment Tool.

Questions to Ask

Do you see or feel any lumps, dimpling, thickening, or puckering in a breast? Or, do you notice any changes in the size, shape, or contour of the breast? If you have been diagnosed with a benign lump, do you notice any new lumps or has a lump changed in size?

YES → See Doctor

NO ↓

Do you have any of these problems?
• Redness, swelling, and warmth in a breast.
• The skin on a breast appears pink, reddish purple, or bruised.
• Pain or constant tenderness in a breast.
• Nipples become drawn into the chest, invert totally, change shape, or become crusty from a discharge.
• Nonmilky discharge when you squeeze the nipple of either breast.

YES → See Doctor

NO ↓

Flowchart continued on next page

Treatment

For Breast Lumps

- *Mammogram.* This X-ray of the breasts can detect breast problems before they can be felt.

- *Ultrasound.* This tells whether the lump is fluid-filled (usually harmless) or solid.

- *Needle aspiration.* With this, a needle is put into the lump to remove fluid or cells.

- *Biopsy.* There are many types. A sample of breast tissue is taken and examined.

- *Ductal lavage.* Fluid is sent through a catheter to the milk ducts. Cells inside the milk ducts are collected and checked for the risk of breast cancer.

Get more information from:

HealthyLearn®
www.HealthyLearn.com
Click on MedlinePlus®

Cancer Information Service
800.4.CANCER
    (422.6237)
www.cancer.gov

Breast Lumps & Breast Cancer, Continued

Do you have a family history of breast cancer and are you concerned about breast cancer, even if you don't notice any problems? **YES** →

Self-Care / Prevention

For Cystic Breasts

- Do a breast self-exam as advised by your doctor.

- Get to and stay at a healthy body weight.

- Follow a low saturated fat diet. Eat soy foods.

- Limit or have no caffeine.

- Limit salt and sodium. This helps to prevent fluid buildup in the breasts.

- Don't smoke. Don't use nicotine gum or patches.

- Take an over-the-counter pain reliever. Take vitamin E, as advised by your doctor.

- Wear a bra that provides good support. You may want to wear it while you sleep, too.

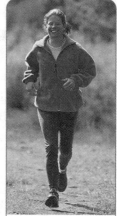

Regular exercise promotes blood flow to the breasts.

For Breast Pain and/or Swelling (without Lesions or Redness)

- For pain due to trauma or surgery: Apply cold packs for the first 48 hours. Do this for 10 to 15 minutes at a time. Do it every 2 to 4 hours. After 48 hours, apply heat. Use a hot water bottle, warm shower, etc. Do this 10 to 15 minutes at a time. Do it 4 times a day.

- For pain not due to trauma or injury apply a heating pad set on low or a hot water bottle. Do this for 30 minutes. Then apply an ice pack for 10 minutes. Repeat as needed.

- Take vitamins, as advised by your doctor.

- Take an over-the-counter medicine for pain and/or swelling, as directed.

Breast Lumps & Breast Cancer, Continued

To Reduce the Risk for Breast Cancer

- If you are at a high risk for breast cancer, ask your doctor if you should take prescribed medicine, such as raloxifene.

- Eat a variety of fruits and vegetables and whole-grain breads and cereals.

- Get to and stay at a healthy body weight.

- Get 30 or more minutes of moderate activity most days of the week. Daily is better.

- Avoid X-rays that aren't needed. Wear a lead apron when you get dental and other X-rays not of the chest.

- Limit alcohol intake to 1 drink per day, if any.

- Breast-feed your babies.

Breast Awareness & Breast Self-Exam

Breast awareness is knowing how your breasts normally look and feel and checking for changes. You can do this while you shower or get dressed. A breast self-exam (BSE) is a step-by-step method to examine your breasts. ***Beginning at age 20, ask your health care provider about the pros and cons of doing a BSE.*** If you choose to do a BSE, examine your breasts during times of the month when they are not normally tender or swollen. If you menstruate, the best time may be within 3 days after your period stops.

1. ***Lie down.*** Place a pillow under your right shoulder. Put your right hand behind your head. Move 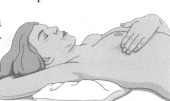 the pads of your left hand's 3 middle fingers, held flat, in small, circular motions as you start to feel your right breast tissue.

Use this circular motion in an up and down pattern as you check the entire breast area. This includes the area from your collarbone to the ribs below your breast; and from your right side (from under your arm) to the middle of your chest bone. Feel every part of this entire area with 3 different levels of pressure:

- Light – Feel the tissue closest to the skin.

- Medium – Feel a little deeper than the skin.

- Firm– Feel the tissue closest to your chest and ribs.

2. Squeeze the nipple gently. Check for a clear or bloody discharge.

3. Repeat steps 1 and 2 for the left breast using the finger pads of your right hand.

4. Stand in front of a mirror. Press your hands firmly on your hips. Look for: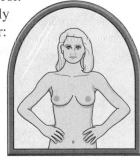

- Any changes in the size, shape, or contour of your breasts.

- Puckering, scaling, or redness of the skin.

- Nipple changes or discharge.

5. Sit or stand. Raise your arm slightly. Examine each underarm area for lumps or changes.

If you a find a lump or any change in the way your breasts normally look or feel, let your health care provider know right away. Most lumps that are found and tested are not cancer.

Cervical Cancer

The cervix is the lower, narrow part of the uterus. Cancer of the cervix is found most often in women over the age of 30. (Source: Centers for Disease Control and Prevention.) It is rare in women under age 20, but is also common in women in their 20s.

Causes

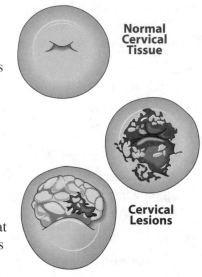

Normal Cervical Tissue

Cervical Lesions

- The main risk factor is being infected with human papillomavirus (HPV). This is passed from one person to another during sex. Only some, not all women who are infected with HPV, get cervical cancer. There are many types of HPV. Certain high risk types of HPV cause most cervical cancers. Other types increase the risk for genital warts or other conditions that are not cancer. Any woman who has ever had sex is at risk for getting HPV. The risk increases for persons who:

  - Started having sex at an early age.

  - Had or have sex with multiple partners. The more partners, the greater the risk.

  - Had or have sex with a partner who: Has HPV; began having sex at a young age; and/or has or had many sexual partners.

- Not having routine Pap tests. These tests screen for cells on the surface of the cervix that are abnormal and that can turn into cancer cells. It can take several years for this to occur, but could happen in a short period of time, too. These changing cells can be treated so they don't turn into cancer.

- Having a current or past sexually transmitted infection (STI), such as chlamydia. This increases the chance of getting HPV.

- Smoking.

- Taking drugs or having HIV/AIDS or other condition that lowers the immune system.

- Being the daughter of a mother who took a drug known as DES during pregnancy. This drug was used from about 1940 to 1970, mostly to prevent miscarriages.

Signs & Symptoms

Screening tests, such as Pap tests are important, because signs and symptoms are not often present in the early stages of the disease.

Late Stage Symptoms:

- Vaginal bleeding or spotting of blood between menstrual periods.

- Vaginal bleeding after sex, douching, or a pelvic exam.

- Vaginal bleeding that is not normal for you.

- Increased vaginal discharge.

- Pain in the pelvic area.

- Pain during sex.

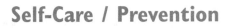

Cervical Cancer, Continued

Treatment

If found early, the cancer can be cured in most women. To find it early, have regular Pap tests and pelvic exams. (See **Health Tests & When to Have Them** on page 22.) Get tested for HPV, chlamydia, and other sexually transmitted infections (STIs), as advised by your doctor.

Treatment depends on what is found. The precancerous form of cervical cancer is called dysplasia. Mild cases of this can be monitored with more frequent Pap tests. Medical treatment can also be given. This includes laser therapy and removing part of the cervix. Surgery, radiation therapy, and/or chemotherapy are needed for cervical cancer.

If the cancer has not spread and a woman wants to become pregnant in the future, just part of the cervix is removed. If a woman does not want a future pregnancy, a hysterectomy may be chosen.

Questions to Ask

Are **late stage symptoms of cervical cancer** listed on page 308 present?

→ **YES** See Doctor

↓ **NO**

Have you not had a Pap test and pelvic exam for 3 or more years?

→ **YES** See Doctor

↓ **NO**

 Use Self-Care

See Self-Care / Prevention in next column

Self-Care / Prevention

- Three doses of HPV vaccine protect against cervical cancer and genital lesions that lead to it. The vaccines are recommended for girls aged 11 to 12 years old, but can be given from age 9 to age 26. Males aged 9 to age 26 years old may be advised by their doctors to get HPV vaccines, too.

- Have Pap tests and pelvic exams as often as your doctor advises. Ask your doctor if he or she uses a "Thin Prep Pap Test." This gives fewer false negative results and fewer unclear readings.

- Use **Safer Sex** to help prevent HPV and other STIs. (See page 252.)

- Don't douche. If you do, don't do this more than once a month.

- Don't smoke. If you smoke, quit!

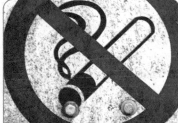

Don't smoke. Avoid secondhand smoke.

Get more information from:

HealthyLearn® • www.HealthyLearn.com
Click on MedlinePlus®

Cancer Information Service
800.4.CANCER (422.6237)
www.cancer.gov

National Cervical Cancer Coalition
800.685.5531 • www.nccc-online.org

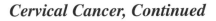

Endometriosis

The lining inside of the uterus is called the endometrium. Sometimes cells from it are found outside of the uterus. This is called endometriosis. Women in their 20s, 30s, and 40s are most likely to notice problems. Teens and women past menopause can have them, too.

Signs & Symptoms

- Pain before and during menstrual periods. The pain is usually worse than normal menstrual cramps.
- Pain during or after sex.
- Pain when you pass urine.
- Lower back pain. Painful bowel movements. Loose stools with menstrual periods.
- The pelvis feels sore or tender.
- Spotting of blood before a monthly period starts.
- Menstrual periods are longer or heavier than normal.
- Infertility.

Some females have no pain.

Causes

The exact cause is not known. It could be that some of the lining of the uterus moves backwards through the fallopian tubes into the abdominal cavity. It then attaches and grows in these places. It could also be due to problems with the immune system and/or hormones. The condition may also run in families.

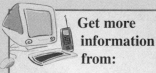

Get more information from:

HealthyLearn®
www.HealthyLearn.com
Click on MedlinePlus®

Endometriosis Association (EA)
800.992.3636
414.355.2200
www.endometriosisassn.org

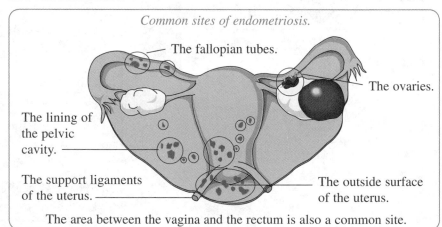

Common sites of endometriosis.

The fallopian tubes.

The ovaries.

The lining of the pelvic cavity.

The support ligaments of the uterus.

The outside surface of the uterus.

The area between the vagina and the rectum is also a common site.

Endometriosis, *Continued*

A gynecologist diagnoses endometriosis. He or she can examine the organs in the abdomen and pelvis to find out the extent of the problem. To do this, the doctor inserts a slim telescope through a very small opening made in the navel. This is done in an outpatient setting.

Treatment

Surgery Options

- One type uses a very small, lighted tube to remove or destroy areas of endometriosis. This reduces pain. It allows pregnancy to occur in some women.

- Another type removes the ovaries. The fallopian tubes and uterus can also be removed. This gets rid of the pain. A woman can't get pregnant after this is done.

Medication Therapy Options

- Pain medicines. These include ibuprofen and naproxen sodium.

- Birth control pills. These are given in a certain way to stop ovulation and menstruation for a set amount of time. They are used for very mild cases.

- Anti-estrogens. These cause a woman's body to make less estrogen.

- Progesterone. This destroys endometrial cells.

- Drugs called GnRH agonists. These stop the body from making estrogen. This causes a temporary "menopause."

Questions to Ask

Do you have a lot of pain at any of these times?
- During sex.
- With monthly menstrual periods and this has gotten worse over time.
- When you pass urine.

YES → See Doctor

NO ↓

Do you have any of these problems?
- Spotting of blood before your period starts.
- Menstrual periods are heavier or last longer than normal.

YES → Call Doctor

NO ↓

Use Self-Care

Self-Care / Prevention

Endometriosis needs medical treatment. What can you do?

- Get regular exercise.

- Eat a diet high in nutrients and low in fat, especially saturated fat. This is mostly found in coconut and palm oils, animal sources of fat, and hydrogenated vegetable fats.

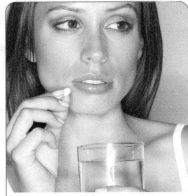
Take medicine for pain.

- Take an over-the-counter medicine for pain. Ask your doctor which one(s) he or she prefers you take.

Fibroids

Fibroids are benign tumors made mostly of muscle tissue. They are in the wall of the uterus. Sometimes they are on the cervix. They range in size from that of a pea to that of a cantaloupe or larger. With larger fibroids, the uterus can grow to the size of a pregnancy more than 20 weeks along. About 20 to 25% of women over age 35 get fibroids.

Causes

The exact cause is not known, but fibroids need estrogen to grow. They may shrink or go away after menopause.

Reasons a Woman Is More Likely to Get Fibroids

- She has not been pregnant.

- She has a close relative who also had or has fibroids.

- She is African American. The risk is 3 to 5 times higher than it is for Caucasian women.

Signs & Symptoms

When symptoms occur, they vary due to the number, size, and locations of the fibroid(s). Symptoms include:

- Swelling in the abdomen.

- Heavy menstrual bleeding. Bleeding between periods or after sex. Bleeding after menopause.

- Backache. Pain during sex. Pain with periods. Pressure on the internal organs causes the pain.

- Feeling pressure in the pelvis. Passing urine often. Pressure on the bladder causes this.

- Chronic constipation. Pressure on the rectum causes this.

- A lot of bleeding can lead to anemia.

- Infertility.

- Miscarriage. If the fibroid is inside the uterus, the placenta may not implant the way it should.

Treatment

- **"Watchful waiting."** A doctor will "watch" for any changes and suggest "waiting" for menopause. Why? Fibroids often shrink or go away after that time. A woman may choose to get treatment for the fibroids, if she has problems. These include: Too much pain; too much bleeding; an abdomen that gets too big; the need to take daily iron to prevent anemia; and other abdominal problems.

- **Medication**. One type is called GnRH agonists. These stop the body from making estrogen. This is not a cure. The fibroids return when the drug is stopped. Taking the drug shrinks the fibroids. This might allow a minor surgery (with less blood loss) to be done instead of a major one. GnRH agonists are taken for a few, but not more than six months. Why? Their side effects mimic menopause and may lead to osteoporosis. In some cases, GnRH agonists can be used longer with "Add Back Therapy." This uses low dose estrogen to make side effects milder.

Fibroids, *Continued*

- **Surgery**. There are many methods:

  - **Myomectomy**. The fibroids are removed. The uterus is not. This method may allow fibroids to grow back. The more fibroids there are to begin with, the greater the chance they will grow back.

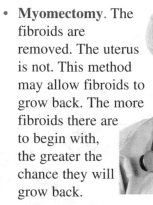

  - **Procedures to destroy the uterine lining**. These do not remove fibroids or the uterus, but stop or lighten menstrual flow from then on. The uterine lining can be destroyed using a laser, heat, or ultra cold.

  - **Uterine artery embolization**. A catheter is inserted in a large blood vessel in the groin and sent to the level of the uterine arteries. A substance is given that blocks blood flow to the uterine arteries that nourish the fibroids. This treatment shrinks the fibroids.

  - **Hysterectomy**. This surgery removes the uterus and the fibroids with it. This method is advised when the fibroid is very large or when other treatments don't stop severe bleeding. It is the only way to get rid of fibroids for sure. A women can no longer get pregnant after the surgery. This treatment is also advised if the fibroid is cancer. This occurs rarely.

Questions to Ask

Do you have severe abdominal pain? **YES** →  Get Medical Care Fast

NO ↓

Do you have any of these problems?
- Heavy menstrual bleeding. Is a pad or tampon saturated in less than an hour?
- Bleeding between periods, after sex, or after menopause.
- Paleness. Weakness. Fatigue.
- Pain during sex or with menstrual periods.
- Pain in the lower back, not due to a strain or any other problem.
- Feeling pressure on your bladder or rectum or you pass urine often.

YES → See Doctor

NO ↓

Use Self-Care

Self-Care / Prevention

- Maintain a healthy body weight. Follow a diet low in fat. The more fat you have, the more estrogen your body is likely to have. This promotes fibroid growth.

- Do regular exercise. This may reduce your body's fat and estrogen levels.

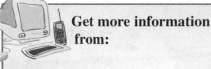

Get more information from:

HealthyLearn® • www.HealthyLearn.com
Click on MedlinePlus®

National Women's Health Information Center
800.994.9662 • www.womenshealth.gov

Menopause

Menopause occurs when menstrual periods have stopped for one whole year. It is also called "the change of life." In general, this occurs between the ages of 45 and 55. It can, though, occur as early as age 35 or as late as age 65. It can also result when both ovaries are removed by surgery.

Causes

Hormone changes that come with aging cause menopause. The body makes less estrogen and progesterone.

Signs & Symptoms

Signs and symptoms usually span 1 to 2 years. This is called peri-menopause.

Physical Signs and Symptoms

- Hot flashes.

- Irregular periods. Bleeding can occur between periods. Periods get shorter and lighter for 2 or more years. They can stop for a few months, start up again. They are more widely spaced.

- Vaginal dryness.

- Headaches. Dizziness.

- Loss of bladder tone. **Stress incontinence.** (See page 175.)

- The skin is more likely to wrinkle. Hair grows on the face, but thins at the temples.

- Muscles lose some strength and tone. Bones become more brittle. This increases the risk for **osteoporosis**. (See page 199.)

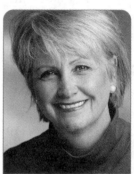

Skin and hair changes are common with menopause.

Emotional Signs and Symptoms

- Mood changes. Feeling very cranky.

- Lack of concentration. Memory problems.

- Tension. Anxiety. Depression.

- Insomnia. Hot flashes can interrupt sleep.

Treatment

Self-care may be all that is needed. Just estrogen can be prescribed. This is estrogen therapy (ET). Estrogen plus progestogen can be prescribed. This is called EPT. The term hormone therapy (HT) is used for both ET and EPT. Hormone therapy helps protect against osteoporosis, but has health risks. Each women should discuss the benefits and risks of HT and non-estrogen treatments with her doctor.

Get more information from:

HealthyLearn®
www.HealthyLearn.com
Click on MedlinePlus®

National Women's Health Information Center
800.994.9662
www.womenshealth.gov

Menopause, Continued

Questions to Ask

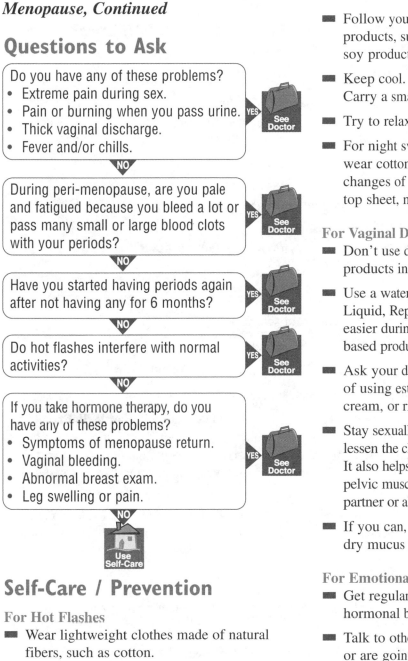

Do you have any of these problems?
- Extreme pain during sex.
- Pain or burning when you pass urine.
- Thick vaginal discharge.
- Fever and/or chills.

YES → See Doctor

NO

During peri-menopause, are you pale and fatigued because you bleed a lot or pass many small or large blood clots with your periods?

YES → See Doctor

NO

Have you started having periods again after not having any for 6 months?

YES → See Doctor

NO

Do hot flashes interfere with normal activities?

YES → See Doctor

NO

If you take hormone therapy, do you have any of these problems?
- Symptoms of menopause return.
- Vaginal bleeding.
- Abnormal breast exam.
- Leg swelling or pain.

YES → See Doctor

NO

Use Self-Care

Self-Care / Prevention

For Hot Flashes
- Wear lightweight clothes made of natural fibers, such as cotton.

- Have cool drinks, especially water, when you feel a hot flash coming on and before and after you exercise. Avoid hot drinks. Limit or avoid alcohol. Limit caffeine.

- Follow your doctor's advice for taking herbal products, such as black cohosh, as well as, soy products.

- Keep cool. Use air conditioning and/or fans. Carry a small fan with you.

- Try to relax when you get a hot flash.

- For night sweats (hot flashes during sleep), wear cotton nightwear that fits loosely. Have changes of nightwear ready. Sleep with only a top sheet, not blankets. Keep the room cool.

For Vaginal Dryness and Painful Sex
- Don't use deodorant soaps or scented products in the vaginal area.

- Use a water soluble lubricant, such as K-Y Liquid, Replens, etc. This makes penetration easier during sex. Avoid oils or petroleum-based products. They promote infection.

- Ask your doctor about the benefits and risks of using estrogen (pills, patches, vaginal cream, or rings).

- Stay sexually active. Having sex often may lessen the chance of having the vagina constrict. It also helps to maintain natural lubrication and pelvic muscle tone. Reaching orgasm with a partner or alone gives these benefits.

- If you can, avoid using antihistamines. They dry mucus membranes in the body.

For Emotional Symptoms
- Get regular exercise. This helps maintain hormonal balance.

- Talk to other women who have gone through or are going through menopause.

- Avoid stress as much as you can. Deal with it, too. (See **Manage Stress** on page 53.)

- Eat healthy. Take vitamins and minerals as advised.

315

Menstrual Bleeding Problems

Menstrual bleeding usually lasts from 2 to 7 days. It occurs about every 28 days.

Signs & Symptoms

- Spotting of blood between periods.

- Menstrual periods that occur more often than every 21 days or less often than every 35 days.

- Periods last longer than 7 days.

- Two or more times the average amount of blood is lost during a period.

- A tampon or a sanitary pad is soaked through every hour for 6 hours in a row.

Get more information from:

HealthyLearn®
www.HealthyLearn.com
Click on MedlinePlus®

National Women's Health Information Center
800.994.9662
www.womenshealth.gov

Causes

- It is normal for changes to occur at certain times. This includes: When monthly periods begin; during peri-menopause; and when some birth control methods are started, stopped, and changed.

- Light bleeding can occur for 2 to 3 days when you ovulate. This is usually normal, too.

- Starting or stopping estrogen therapy. Using an IUD for birth control.

- Weight gain or loss. Too much exercise. Anorexia nervosa.

- Vaginal irritation or infection.

- Endometriosis. Fibroids. Ovarian cysts.

- Ectopic pregnancy. Miscarriage.

- Cancer of the cervix or uterus.

- Hypothyroidism. Pituitary and adrenal gland disorders.

- Side effects of blood-thinners or corticosteroids.

- Bleeding or clotting disorders. One example is **Von Willebrand disease**. This is a genetic bleeding disorder. Often, it is not diagnosed. Bleeding is excessive with menstrual periods and after surgery, dental work, etc. Nosebleeds occur often. Bruises occur easily.

- **Polycystic ovarian syndrome (PCOS)**. This is caused by an excess of a certain hormone. It can result in irregular periods or no periods.

Treatment

- Iron supplements to treat anemia, if present. (See **Anemia** on page 212.)

- Medicines. Examples are birth control pills; GnRH agonists; Danazol (low dose); and a medicine called tranexamic acid.

- Surgery, as needed, for the cause of the problem.

Menstrual Bleeding Problems, Continued

Questions to Ask

Could you be pregnant? If so, do you have any of these problems?
- Sudden fainting.
- Abnormal vaginal bleeding. This can range from spotting that persists to bursts of bleeding.
- Severe cramping in one side of your lower abdomen.
- Sharp pains in one side of your lower abdomen, rectum, or shoulder.

YES → Get Medical Care Fast

NO ↓

With menstrual bleeding, do you have any of these problems?
- Pelvic pain is much worse than normal or causes you to double over.
- The bleeding is heavier than normal.
- You feel dizzy, faint, or lightheaded when you sit up.

YES → Get Medical Care Fast

NO ↓

Do periods return after not having one for 6 months?

YES → See Doctor

NO ↓

With irregular menstrual periods, do you have any of these problems?
- Your abdomen is tender and/or bloated.
- Pain in your pelvis or back.
- Pain during sex.
- The skin on your abdomen feels sensitive.
- Vaginal discharge with abnormal color or odor. This occurs when you are not having a period.
- Change in menstrual flow.
- Fever. Chills.

YES → See Doctor

NO ↓

Flowchart continued in next column

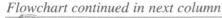 To Learn More, See Back Cover

Do you have **symptoms of hypothyroidism** or of **hyperthyroidism** listed on page 260?

YES → See Doctor

NO ↓

With irregular menstrual periods, do you have any of these problems?
- Nausea, vomiting, or pain is worse than with normal periods.
- Periods are heavier than normal or last longer than 10 days.
- After taking birth control pills for 3 months, you bleed more or you keep bleeding or spotting between periods.

YES → Call Doctor

NO ↓

 Use Self-Care

Self-Care / Prevention

- Keep track of how many days and how much you bleed to know what is normal for you.

- Change tampons and sanitary napkins as needed. Note if they are soaked through.

- Avoid stress and physical exertion that lead to increased bleeding.

- Don't have too much alcohol.

- Take ibuprofen or naproxen sodium as directed. Don't use aspirin. It can prolong bleeding. Take iron, as advised by your doctor.

- If you have an IUD, check it as advised to make sure the strings can be felt. If Depo-Provera or an IUD cause bleeding problems, change birth control methods.

- Don't have sex until treatment is done. Follow your doctor's advice.

- To prevent vaginitis from vaginal dryness, use a prescribed estrogen cream, as needed.

Menstrual Cramps

Menstrual cramps are also called painful periods. Most females have them sometime during their lives.

Signs & Symptoms

- Pain or discomfort in the lower abdomen right before or with a menstrual period. The pain can range from mild to severe.
- The pain can occur with:
  - A backache.
  - Fatigue.
  - A headache.
  - Diarrhea and/or vomiting.
- Symptoms can vary from month to month or year to year.

Causes

Menstrual cramps occur when muscles of the uterus squeeze the lining out. This is part of normal menstruation. They occur often in females who have just begun to menstruate. They may go away or be less severe after a woman reaches her mid-twenties or gives birth. Childbirth stretches the uterus.

Menstrual cramps are common in females who have just begun to menstruate.

Menstrual cramps occur much less often in women who do not ovulate. In fact, birth control pills reduce painful periods in 70 to 80% of females who take them. When the birth control pill is stopped, the same level of pain returns.

Menstrual cramps can be due to other problems, such as fibroids, endometriosis, ovarian cysts, and rarely, cancer. An intrauterine device (IUD) can also cause cramps, especially in women who haven't been pregnant. The Progestasert IUD is different. It lessens cramps and lightens menstrual flow.

Treatment

Often, self-care treats menstrual cramps. If not, a doctor can diagnose the cause and prescribe treatment.

Questions to Ask

With menstrual cramps, do you have any of these problems?
- Black stools or blood in the stools.
- The pain is extreme.
- Menstrual periods have been pain-free for years, but now occur with severe cramps.

YES → See Doctor

NO

Flowchart continued on next page

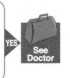

Menstrual Cramps, Continued

Have your periods been very painful since having an intrauterine device (IUD) inserted? Or, do you still have cramps after your period is over?

YES → **See Doctor**

NO ↓

With menstrual cramps, do you have any signs of infection, such as fever or foul-smelling vaginal discharge?

YES → **See Doctor**

NO ↓

Do any of these things apply?
• Bleeding with a period is heavier than normal.
• You could be newly pregnant (your period is late by one week or longer) and you have pain that feels like menstrual cramps.

YES → **Call Doctor**

NO ↓

 Use Self-Care

Self-Care / Prevention

To Relieve Menstrual Cramps

- Take an over-the-counter pain reliever, such as ibuprofen, naproxen sodium, or aspirin. Acetaminophen can help the pain, too. {*Note:* Do not give aspirin or any medication with salicylates to anyone 19 years of age or younger, due to its link with Reye's Syndrome.}

- Hold a heating pad or hot-water bottle on your abdomen or lower back.

- Take a warm bath.

- Gently massage your abdomen.

- Do mild exercises. Stretch. Do yoga. Walk. Bicycle. Exercise may improve blood flow and reduce pelvic pain.

- When you can, lie on your back. Support your knees with a pillow.

- Get plenty of rest. Limit stress as your period nears.

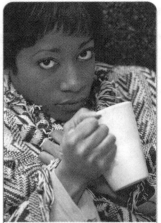

A warm cup of regular, chamomile, or mint tea can help relieve menstrual cramps.

- Consider using the birth control pill or the Progestasert IUD. These lessen menstrual cramps.

If you still feel pain after using self-care measures, call your doctor.

Get more information from:

HealthyLearn®
www.HealthyLearn.com
Click on MedlinePlus®

National Women's Health Information Center
800.994.9662
www.womenshealth.gov

Ovarian Cysts & Cancer

The ovaries are two almond-sized organs. One is found on each side of the uterus.

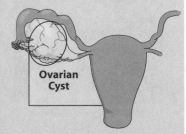

Ovarian Cyst

Growths called cysts or tumors can form in, on, or near the ovaries.

Cysts are sacs filled with fluid or semisolid matter. Ovarian cysts are common in women before menopause. Rarely, are these cysts cancer.

Tumors are solid masses. Most often, tumors in the ovary are benign. Malignant tumors are **ovarian cancer**. This type of cancer occurs most often between the ages of 50 and 75. It can occur at other ages, too.

Signs & Symptoms

For Ovarian Cysts

Ovarian cysts may cause no symptoms. When they occur, symptoms include:

- A feeling of fullness or swelling of the abdomen.
- Weight gain.
- A dull, constant ache on either or both sides of the pelvis.
- Pain during sex.
- Delayed, irregular, or painful periods.
- Growth of facial hair.
- Sharp, severe abdominal pain. Fever. Vomiting. These can be caused by a cyst that bleeds, breaks, or twists.

For Ovarian Cancer

In many cases, the cancer has spread by the time it is found. When symptoms appear, they are vague problems and are often ignored. Symptoms, even in early-stage ovarian cancer are:

- Bloating.
- Pain in the abdomen or pelvis.
- Difficulty eating or feeling full quickly.
- Urgent need to pass urine or passing urine often.

These symptoms last almost daily for more than a few weeks.

Other symptoms can include:

- Back pain. Pain with intercourse.
- Constipation. Indigestion.
- Fatigue.
- Menstrual irregularities.

Causes

For Ovarian Cysts

- Some cysts are due to changes in the normal way the ovaries work.

Ovarian Cysts & Cancer, *Continued*

- Some cysts result from cell growth. Most of these are benign, but need medical treatment. Examples are:
  - *Dermoid cysts.* These are growths filled with many types of tissue. Examples are fatty material, hair, teeth, bits of bone, and cartilage.
  - *Polycystic ovaries.* These are caused by a buildup of multiple small cysts from hormone problems. Irregular periods, body hair growth, and infertility can result.

Risk Factors for Ovarian Cysts
- Being between the ages of 20 and 35.
- Endometriosis. Pelvic inflammatory disease (PID). The eating disorder bulimia.
- Obesity.

Taking hormones does not cause ovarian cysts.

Risk Factors for Ovarian Cancer
- Not having children. Having children at an older age.
- Never taking birth control pills.
- Menopause occurred after age 55.
- Family history of ovarian, colon, breast, prostate, or lung cancer.
- Personal history of breast, uterine, colon, or rectal cancer.
- Being Caucasian.
- Increasing age.

Treatment

Growths on ovaries are diagnosed with a pelvic exam and medical tests, as needed. Ways to detect growths include yearly pelvic and rectal exams and an ultrasound. No completely reliable test exists for ovarian cancer. A CA-125 blood test can detect the progression of ovarian cancer in a woman who has it. It is not a reliable screening test.

For Ovarian Cysts
Treatment depends on:
- The size and type of cyst(s).
- The woman's desire to have children.
- The woman's health status.
- How severe symptoms are.

Some cysts resolve without any treatment in 1 to 2 months. For others, birth control pills may be tried. Hormones in them suppress the cyst. If a cyst does not respond to this treatment, surgery may be needed to remove it. If a cyst is found early, it may be removed leaving the ovary. Sometimes, the ovary needs to be removed. The uterus and/or the fallopian tube may need to be removed, as well.

For Ovarian Cancer
The sooner the cancer is found and treated, the better the chance for recovery. Treatment includes:
- Surgery. The ovaries, uterus, and fallopian tubes are removed. If the cancer has spread, the surgeon removes as much of the cancer as possible.
- Chemotherapy.
- Radiation therapy.
- Clinical trials.

Ovarian Cysts & Cancer, Continued

Questions to Ask

Do you have very severe abdominal pain, a fever, and vomiting?

YES → Get Medical Care Fast

NO ↓

Do you have **signs and symptoms for ovarian cancer** or **signs and symptoms for ovarian cysts** listed on page 320?

YES → See Doctor

NO ↓

Use Self-Care

Self-Care / Prevention

For Ovarian Cysts

- Limit caffeine.

- Have regular pelvic exams, as advised by your doctor.

- Take an over-the-counter medicine for pain as directed.

For Ovarian Cancer

- Medical care, not self-care, is needed. Follow your doctor's advice.

- Have regular pelvic exams, as advised by your doctor.

- Ask your doctor for advice if you have a family history of ovarian cancer, especially in your mother, sister, or daughter.

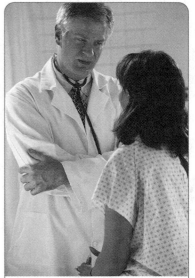

Have regular pelvic exams as advised by your doctor.

Get more information from:

HealthyLearn®
www.HealthyLearn.com
Click on MedlinePlus®

Cancer Information
Service
800.4.CANCER
    (422.6237)
www.cancer.gov

National Women's
Health Information
Center
800.994.9662
www.womenshealth.gov

Pelvic Inflammatory Disease (PID)

Pelvic inflammatory disease (PID) is an infection that goes up through the uterus to the fallopian tubes. Both females and males carry the organisms

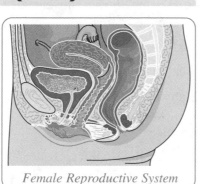

Female Reproductive System

that cause PID. These can be passed on to someone else who could then develop PID. This occurs even when no symptoms are noticed.

Signs & Symptoms

Symptoms of Acute PID

- Pain in the abdomen or back. The pain can be severe.
- Vaginal discharge with a foul odor.
- Pain during sex.
- The abdomen is tender and/or bloated.
- Menstrual cramps are very painful.
- High fever.

Symptoms of Chronic PID

- Pain in the abdomen or back is less severe. This often occurs midway in the menstrual cycle or during a pelvic exam.
- Skin on the abdomen is sensitive.
- Vaginal discharge. Change in menstrual flow.
- Nausea.
- Low-grade fever.

Causes

- Sexually transmitted infections (STIs), such as gonorrhea and chlamydia. The organisms that cause these spread to the internal reproductive organs. Many times, PID is caused by more than one of these organisms.

- Bacteria normally found in the intestines can get into the pelvic cavity. Times this can happen:
  - After sex, especially having vaginal intercourse right after having anal sex.
  - With high risk sexual practices that increase the risk of infection. Examples are having many sex partners or having sex with a person who has many partners.
  - After an intrauterine device (IUD) is put in or adjusted.

- Having had PID in the past.

- Recently having vaginitis.

Questions to Ask

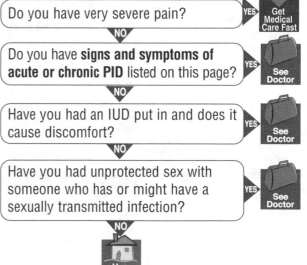

Do you have very severe pain? **YES** → Get Medical Care Fast

NO

Do you have **signs and symptoms of acute or chronic PID** listed on this page? **YES** → See Doctor

NO

Have you had an IUD put in and does it cause discomfort? **YES** → See Doctor

NO

Have you had unprotected sex with someone who has or might have a sexually transmitted infection? **YES** → See Doctor

NO

Use Self-Care

See Self-Care / Prevention on next page

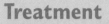

Pelvic Inflammatory Disease (PID), Continued

Treatment

Antibiotics treat diagnosed PID. Treatment for an infected sex partner is also needed. This prevents getting the infection again.

When PID is not treated, the infection can spread to other parts of the body. If it spreads to the blood, it may threaten life.

Scarring from the infection can damage a woman's reproductive organs. It can cause infertility. Also, a woman who has had PID is at increased risk for:

- A tubal pregnancy.

- Premature labor and birth.

Self-Care / Prevention

- Wipe from front to back after a bowel movement. This helps to keep bacteria from getting into the vagina.

- When you menstruate, change tampons and/or pads often.

- Don't have vaginal sex right after anal sex.

- Don't have sex with anyone who has not been treated for a current case of PID or an STI. Don't have sex with anyone who has partners that haven't been treated.

- Use barrier birth control methods with spermicides. These reduce the risk of getting PID from an infected partner. Use a male or female condom, the cervical cap, or a diaphragm. Use one of these, even if you use other forms of birth control, such as the pill.

- Don't use an IUD if you are at risk for STIs.

- If you use an IUD, have your doctor remove it if you get pregnant and then miscarry. If it is left in, your risk of PID goes up.

- Don't smoke. Smoking 10 or more cigarettes a day puts you at a higher risk for PID.

- Don't use douches. These can spread bacteria further up the vagina.

- After childbirth, wait until you stop bleeding to have sex. After a D & C, abortion, or miscarriage, wait 1 week to have sex. Use a latex or polyurethane condom for 2 weeks after having an IUD put in.

- If you are at risk for PID, get tested for chlamydia and gonorrhea every 6 months.

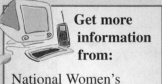

Get more information from:

National Women's Health Information Center
800.994.9662
www.womenshealth.gov

Plan for a Healthy Pregnancy

To help your pregnancy get off to a good start, take these steps before you get pregnant:

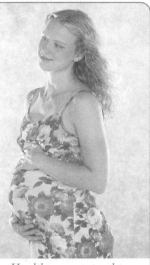

Healthy moms tend to have healthy babies.

- Get a medical checkup. Discuss your medical history and your family medical history with your doctor.

- Do you have a chronic medical problem, such as asthma, diabetes, or high blood pressure? If so, ask your doctor if changes need to be made in your treatment plan.

- Find out what medicines you can take. Ask which ones you should not take. Tell or show your doctor all prescribed and over-the-counter medicines, vitamins, herbal products, etc. that you take. Ask if you need to change any of these while you try to get pregnant.

- Take 400 to 800 micrograms (this is the same as .4 to .8 milligrams) of folic acid every day. This B vitamin can help prevent serious birth defects of the brain and spine. Make sure you take folic acid for at least one month before you get pregnant. Women who have had a baby with a serious problem of the brain or spine should take the amount of folic acid their doctors advise.

- Discuss current and past birth control methods. Ask what you should use until you decide to get pregnant.

- If you or your partner has a family history of sickle-cell disease, Tay-Sachs disease, etc., get genetic counseling. Do this, too, if you are older than age 35 or if your partner is age 60 or older.

- Do you smoke? Do you take street drugs? If so, now is the time to quit. Get help if you need it.

- Stop or limit alcohol use. This will make it easier to go without it when you are pregnant.

- Get vaccines, as advised by your doctor.

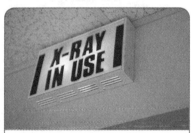

Avoid exposure to X-rays.

- Eat healthy foods. This includes:
  - Fruits and vegetables.
  - Whole-grain breads and cereals.
  - Low-fat dairy foods and other calcium-rich foods.

- Do regular exercise.

- If you are overweight, lose weight before you get pregnant.

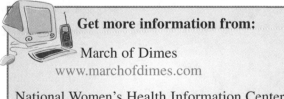

Get more information from:

March of Dimes
www.marchofdimes.com

National Women's Health Information Center
800.994.9662
www.womenshealth.gov

Premenstrual Syndrome (PMS)

Four out of ten women who menstruate have premenstrual syndrome (PMS).

Causes

The exact causes of PMS are not known. A female's response to normal monthly changes in estrogen, progesterone, and testosterone appear to be involved. So do changes in the level of serotonin, a brain chemical.

With PMS, symptoms must occur within 2 weeks before the menstrual period and go away shortly after the period begins. A symptom-free period occurs between days 4 and 12 of the menstrual cycle.

True PMS usually stops with menopause.

Signs & Symptoms

As many as 150 symptoms are linked to PMS. The most common ones are:

- Abdominal bloating. Weight gain.

- Anxiety. Depression.

- Breast tenderness.

- Fatigue.

- Feelings of hostility and anger.

- Food cravings, especially for chocolate, sweet, and/or salty foods.

- Headache.

- Feeling cranky. Mood swings.

- Tension.

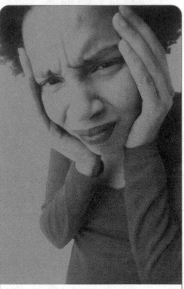

Headache and feeling tense are common symptoms of PMS.

For some women, symptoms are slight and may last only a few days before a period starts. For others, they can be severe and last the entire 2 weeks before every period. Also, other problems, such as depression, may be worse with PMS. This is called "menstrual magnification."

PMS can be confused with depression. See your doctor for a proper diagnosis.

Treatment

- Self-care measures. (See **Self-Care / Prevention** on page 327.)

- Medications. These include:
  - A water pill called spironolactone.
  - An SSRI antidepressant, such as fluoxentine or sertraline, to be taken 1 or 2 weeks before the menstrual period.
  - An anti-anxiety medicine.
  - Birth control pills.

Premenstrual Syndrome (PMS), Continued

Questions to Ask

Do symptoms of PMS, such as anxiety, depression, or anger, cause you to want to harm yourself or someone else?

 YES → Get Medical Care Fast

NO ↓

Do PMS symptoms cause you to feel out of control and unable to function?

 YES → See Doctor

NO ↓

Do you still have PMS symptoms after your period starts? Or, has self-care not brought relief?

 YES → Call Doctor

NO ↓

 Use Self-Care

Self-Care / Prevention

- Get emotional support.

- Do aerobic exercises. Swim. Walk. Bicycle.

- Eat carbohydrate-rich foods. Examples are whole grain breads and cereals, fruits, and vegetables.

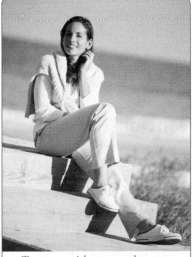

Try to avoid stress when you have PMS symptoms.

- Have good sources of calcium, such as skim milk, nonfat yogurt, collard greens, and kale. Choose cereals and juices that have added calcium. Get good sources of magnesium, too. These include spinach, other green, leafy vegetables, and whole grain cereals.

- The vitamin and minerals listed below seem to help some females with PMS. Ask your doctor if you should take any of them and in what amounts.

  • Calcium.

  • Magnesium.

  • Vitamin E.

- Learn to relax. Try deep breathing. Meditate. Do yoga. Take warm baths. Get a massage.

- Rest. Take naps if you need to.

- Limit or avoid caffeine, alcohol, and cigarettes 2 weeks before your period is due.

- Limit salt, fat, and sugar.

- If you need to satisfy a food craving, do so with a small amount. For example, if you crave chocolate, have a small chocolate bar or add chocolate syrup to skim milk. If you crave salt, eat a small bag of pretzels.

Get more information from:

HealthyLearn®
www.HealthyLearn.com
Click on MedlinePlus®

National Women's Health Information Center
800.994.9662 • www.womenshealth.gov

Toxic Shock Syndrome

Toxic shock syndrome (TSS) is a form of blood poisoning. It rarely occurs, but can be fatal.

Signs & Symptoms

Symptoms come on fast and are often severe.

- High sudden fever.

- Flat, red, sunburn-like rash on the trunk of the body that spreads. The skin on the palms of the hands and soles of the feet peels. Redness of the lips, eyes, and tongue may also occur.

- Muscle aches. Extreme fatigue and weakness.

- Vomiting. Abdominal pain. Diarrhea.

- Rapid pulse.

- Sore throat.

- Dizziness. Fainting. Confusion.

- Drop in blood pressure. **Shock.** (See page 401.)

Treatment

Toxic shock syndrome needs emergency medical care.

Causes

Toxic shock syndrome is caused when certain bacteria release toxins in the blood. Most often, TSS affects women who use super absorbent tampons. These trap and allow bacteria to grow. It can also result from wounds or an infection in the throat, lungs, skin, or bone.

Questions to Ask

Do you have **signs and symptoms of toxic shock syndrome** listed on this page?

YES → Get Medical Care Fast

NO ↓

Do you have any of these signs and symptoms?
- Vomiting, then abdominal pain, and profuse, watery diarrhea.
- Muscle aches, headaches, sore throat, and pink eye with a clear discharge.
- High fever without a skin rash, but with any other symptom listed in this question.

YES → See Doctor

NO ↓

Does a wound have increased redness, swelling, and/or pain? Does pus or other fluid drain from the wound?

YES → See Doctor

NO ↓

Use Self-Care

Self-Care / Prevention

To Help Prevent TSS

- Practice good hygiene.

- Keep wounds clean. See your doctor for signs of an infection (increased redness, swelling, and/or pain; pus; and/or fever).

- Change tampons and sanitary pads every 4 to 6 hours or more often. When you can, use sanitary napkins instead of tampons. Alternate tampons with sanitary pads or mini-pads during a menstrual period. Lubricate the tampon applicator with a water-soluble (nongreasy) lubricant, like K-Y Jelly, before you insert it.

- Don't use tampons if you've had TSS in the past.

Vaginal Infections

Vaginal infections are the most common reason females in the U.S. see their doctors. Vaginal infections cause **vaginitis**. This is swelling of the vagina.

Common vaginal infections are **bacterial vaginosis (BV)**, **vaginal yeast infections**, and **sexually transmitted infections (STIs)**. (See pages 248 to 253 for information on **STIs**.

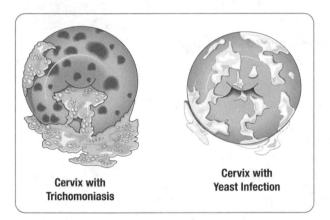

Cervix with Trichomoniasis

Cervix with Yeast Infection

Signs & Symptoms

For Bacterial Vaginosis (BV)

Nearly half of females with this infection have no symptoms. When present, symptoms include:
- A thin, gray, or milky white vaginal discharge. This has a fishy odor. The odor is noticed more after sex.
- Mild vaginal irritation or burning.

For Vaginal Yeast Infections

These are also called Monilia, *Candida*, and fungal infections. Signs and symptoms range from mild to severe. They include:
- Thick, white vaginal discharge. This looks like cottage cheese. It may smell like yeast.
- Itching, irritation, and redness around the vagina.
- Burning and/or pain when passing urine or with sex.

Causes

For Bacterial Vaginosis (BV)

The exact cause is not known. It occurs when a certain bacteria outnumber normal bacteria in the vagina.

For Vaginal Yeast Infections

These result from the overgrowth of the fungus *Candida*. This is normally present in harmless amounts in the vagina, digestive tract, and mouth.

Risk Factors for Vaginal Yeast Infections
- Hormone changes that come with pregnancy or monthly periods. Taking hormones or birth control pills.
- Antibiotic use, especially "broad spectrum" ones. Corticosteroid medicine use.
- High blood sugar. This can occur when diabetes is not controlled.
- Using douches. Using feminine hygiene sprays.
- Using hot tubs or jacuzzis often.
- Sex that irritates the vagina a lot.

Chronic vaginal yeast infections can be one of the first signs of diabetes, STIs, and HIV.

Vaginal Infections, Continued

Treatment

Different vaginal infections have the same symptoms. This makes it hard to tell one from another. A doctor may need to diagnose the cause. A sample of vaginal fluid is taken and tested. Often, this takes less than 3 minutes.

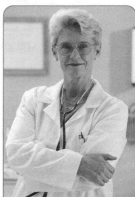

A doctor will prescribe the right treatment for a vaginal infection.

For Bacterial Vaginosis
- Prescribed antibiotic creams, gels, or pills are needed. The male sex partner(s) may also need treatment.

- Not using products that mask vaginal odor, such as feminine hygiene sprays.

- Over-the-counter (OTC) medications, such as ones for vaginal yeast infections, *do not* treat BV.

For Vaginal Yeast Infections
- Prescribed or OTC antifungal vaginal creams or suppositories. These get rid of the *Candida* overgrowth.

- Oral medicines, such as Diflucan, may be prescribed.

See pages 248 to 253 for treatment for **STIs**.

Questions to Ask

Do you have **signs and symptoms of bacterial vaginosis** listed on page 329? **YES** See Doctor

NO

Does your skin and/or the whites of your eyes look yellow after you took a prescribed, oral antifungal medicine? **YES** See Doctor

NO

Flowchart continued on next page

Vaginal Infections, Continued

With **symptoms of a vaginal yeast infection** listed on page 329, do you have any of these conditions?

- This is the first time for these symptoms.
- An infection was treated, but came back within 2 months.
- Diabetes.
- Symptoms don't improve after using self-care measures for 3 days.
- Symptoms worsen or continue 1 week or longer after using self-care.

YES ▸

See Doctor

NO ▾

Use Self-Care

Self-Care / Prevention

- Take medications as prescribed.

- For a repeat vaginal yeast infection, use an over-the-counter (OTC) antifungal vaginal medication, such as Monistat. Use it as directed.

{*Note:* Stop using any OTC product for a vaginal yeast infection at least 24 hours before a vaginal exam.}

- Ask your pharmacist about an OTC cream for itching and burning. This does not treat the infection, but may help with symptoms during treatment.

- Bathe or shower often. Clean the inside folds of the vulva. Dry the vaginal area well.

- Wipe from front to back after using the toilet.

- Don't use bath oils, bubble baths, feminine hygiene sprays, or perfumed or deodorant soaps.

- If your vagina is dry, use a water soluble lubricant, such as K-Y Liquid, when you have sex.

- Wear all-cotton underwear. Don't wear garments that are tight in the crotch. Change underwear and workout clothes right away after you sweat.

- Don't sit around in a wet bathing suit. Shower after you swim in a pool. This helps remove the chlorine from your skin. Dry the vaginal area well.

- Eat well. Include foods, such as yogurt, that have live cultures of "lactobacillus acidophilus." Or, take an OTC product that has this.

- Limit sugar. Limit foods with sugar.

- Let your doctor know if you tend to get yeast infections when you take an antibiotic. You may be told to also use a vaginal antifungal product.

- If you still menstruate, use unscented tampons or sanitary pads. Change them often.

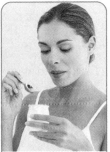

Eat yogurt with live cultures of lactobacillus acidophilus.

See also, **Self-Care / Prevention – For Genital Herpes** on page 253.

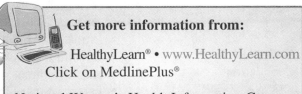

Get more information from:

HealthyLearn® • www.HealthyLearn.com
Click on MedlinePlus®

National Women's Health Information Center
800.994.9662 • www.womenshealth.gov

Chapter 19

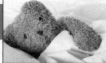

Children's Health Problems

Bed-Wetting

Passing urine during sleep is called "bed-wetting" when it occurs after age 5 or 6. Children are usually expected to have nighttime bladder control by this age. Bed-wetting is a very common problem. In the U.S., 5 to 7 million children have it.

Enuresis is a medical term for bed-wetting.

{*Note:* Bed-wetting itself, can't be prevented, but damage to a child's self-image can. Explain that bed-wetting is not his or her fault and that it will get better in time.}

Get more information from:

HealthyLearn®
www.HealthyLearn.com
Click on MedlinePlus®

National Kidney
Foundation
888.WAKE.DRY
(925.3379)
www.kidney.org

Causes

Children don't wet the bed on purpose. These are causes of bed-wetting:

- A lot of urine is made in the evening and during the night. A full bladder does not wake the child up.

- A child's small bladder does not hold urine for an entire night.

- Other conditions, such as a urinary tract infection and diabetes. (Daytime wetting and other symptoms occur with these conditions.)

- For children who have been dry at night for 6 or more months, sometimes, emotional upsets and major changes can cause bed-wetting. An example is having a new baby in the house.

- Children are more likely to wet the bed if both parents did when they were children.

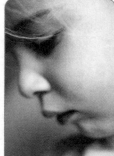

Physical or sexual abuse can cause a child to begin wetting the bed.

Treatment

Most of the time, children outgrow bed-wetting. Until then, self-care measures help with the problem. Medication can be prescribed when no other treatment works.

Questions to Ask

Does your child have these **symptoms of diabetes**?
- Drinks a lot of liquids.
- Goes to the bathroom more than normal in the day or night.
- Acts very tired.
- Eats a lot more than normal and gains weight.
- Itches around the groin.

YES → **See Doctor**

NO

Flowchart continued on next page

Bed-Wetting, *Continued*

Does your child have these **symptoms of a urinary tract infection**?

- A fever.
- Pain in the low stomach or mid back area.
- Burning when he or she passes urine.
- Bad-smelling urine.

YES **See Doctor**

NO

Is your child older than age 6 and has never been dry at night? Or, has he or she started wetting the bed again after being dry for 6 or more months?

YES **Call Doctor**

NO

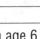 **Use Self-Care**

Self-Care / Prevention

Be patient and give your child lots of support. Children who wet the bed can't help it. Getting angry only makes the problem worse.

Until Your Child Outgrows Bed-Wetting

- Do not blame or punish your child for wetting the bed.

- Limit fluids in the evening, especially 2 hours before bedtime. Ask your child's doctor how much your child should drink. Don't give drinks with caffeine, such as colas.

- Have your child urinate in the toilet right before getting into bed.

- See that your child can easily get to the toilet during the night. Keep the path clear. Use night lights, etc. If needed, put a portable potty close to your child's bed. Assign a place the potty can be moved to for daytime, if your child wants to do this.

- Tell other members of the household that "teasing" about bed-wetting is not allowed. Respect your child's privacy and feelings.

- You may want your child to use pull-up (training) pants when he or she sleeps away from home, camps, etc. On a regular basis, encourage your child to wake up to use the toilet.

- Keep a change of pajamas, a flannel covered pad, clean sheets, dry towels, etc., near your child's bed. Show your child how to use these when he or she wets the bed. Include your child in the clean-up process.

- Have your child rehearse getting up from bed and using the toilet. Do this at bedtime. Do it during the day when your child gets the urge to urinate. Have your child lay down in his or her bed, wait a few minutes, and then get up to urinate in the toilet.

- If your child is 5 years old or older and he or she agrees to it, get a bed-wetting alarm. The child wears the alarm on his or her underwear. The first drop makes the alarm buzz. This wakes the child up. After awhile, the child learns to wake up when he or she has to urinate. Some of these alarms help prevent wet beds 85 to 90 percent of the time.

- You can get bed-wetting alarms and information from:
  - Nite Train-R Alarm: Koregon Enterprises, 800.544.4240
  - Potty Pager: Ideas for Living, 800.497.6573
  - Wet-Stop3 Alarm System: PottyMD, 877.768.8963, www.pottymd.com

Colic

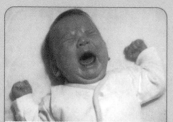

A baby with colic cries for no apparent reason, often for three or more hours a day.

Babies cry when they are hungry, sick, too hot, etc. In general, babies start to have colic when they are about three weeks old. The colic worsens at around six weeks of age and stops by 3 months of age. Colic does not harm babies, but is very hard on parents and caretakers.

Treatment

After other medical problems are ruled out, colic is treated by finding out and getting rid of colic triggers and giving comfort to the baby.

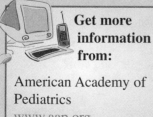

Get more information from:

American Academy of Pediatrics
www.aap.org

Signs & Symptoms

- Fussy crying occurs for no known reason. The baby is not hungry, sick, in pain, etc. The crying lasts for minutes to hours at a time.

- The baby may pull his or her knees up to the stomach.

- Colic episodes often occur in the evening.

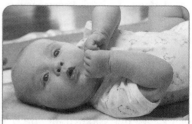

When the baby is exhausted or passes gas or stool, the crying tends to stop.

Causes

The exact cause is not known. Babies with colic are very, very sensitive to stimulation. Noises in the house bother them. Also, they may need to be cuddled more than babies without colic.

Bottle feeding too fast (less than 20 minutes) or giving too much formula can trigger colic episodes. So can foods the breast-feeding mother eats (e.g., caffeine, dairy products, and nuts).

Questions to Ask

Do any of these problems occur?
- It is hard to rouse or wake up the baby.
- The baby stares off into space.
- The baby is not normally active or acts very sick.
- The baby has been shaken.
- An infant younger than 3 months old has a temperature of 100.4°F or higher?

YES  **Get Medical Care Fast**

NO

With colic, does a baby younger than 3 months old have a temperature between 99.5°F and up to 100.4°F? Or, do you feel out of control and are you tempted to hurt the baby?

YES **See Doctor**

NO

Flowchart continued on next page

Colic, Continued

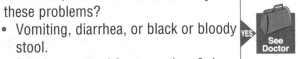

With colic, does the infant have any of these problems?
- Vomiting, diarrhea, or black or bloody stool.
- Passing no stool for more than 2 days.
- Weight loss.

YES → **See Doctor**

NO ↓

Are any of these conditions present?
- The baby with colic is younger than 2 weeks old or older then 3 months old.
- Colic episodes last more than 2 hours at a time.
- The baby with colic is taking a prescribed medicine.
- You are exhausted from the baby's crying and/or can't handle it anymore.

YES → **See Doctor**

NO ↓

Use Self-Care

Self-Care / Prevention

- Be sure the baby has enough to eat. Check with the baby's doctor about trying a new formula.

- Try different bottle nipples. Make the hole bigger if it is too small. Cut across the hole that is already there. (You will make an X-shaped hole.) Here's how to find out if the hole is too small:

  1. Put cold formula in the bottle.

  2. Turn the bottle upside down.

  3. Count the drops of formula that fall out. If the drops come out slower than 1 drop per second, the hole is too small.

- Don't allow smoking in your home.

- Do not give fruit juice (e.g., apple juice, pear juice) to infants younger than 6 months old.

- Hold the baby up for feeding. Keep holding the baby up for awhile after feeding.

- Burp the baby after each ounce of formula or every few minutes when breast-feeding.

- Use a pacifier, but never put a pacifier on a string around the baby's neck.

- Give the baby a warm bath and a massage.

- Wrap or swaddle the baby snugly in a soft blanket. Rock him or her or use a baby swing.

- Try the "colic carry." Lay the baby on his or her stomach across your arm. Put the baby's face in your hand and let the legs straddle your inner elbow. Hold the baby's back with your other hand so he or she won't fall. Walk around like this for awhile.

- Carry the baby while you vacuum. Use a baby carrier that you wear on your back or chest.

- Play soft, gentle music.

- Take your baby for a stroller or car ride.

- Run the dryer or dishwasher. Buckle your baby in a baby seat. Lean the seat against the side of the dryer or on the counter near the dishwasher. The sounds from these machines may help the baby fall asleep. Stay with your baby. Make sure the heat or steam won't hurt the baby.

- Don't give the baby antacids like Maalox or simethicone drops unless a doctor tells you to.

- Let your baby cry himself or herself to sleep if nothing else helps and your baby has been fed within 2½ hours. Do call the doctor if the baby cries for more than 2 hours without stopping.

- Get someone else to take care of your baby if you get too stressed. Get some rest.

Croup

Signs & Symptoms

Croup causes swelling around vocal cords and airways. Children usually get croup between 3 months and 5 years of age. It is a scary, but not usually dangerous condition. Croup often occurs several days after a child has mild symptoms of a cold.

- A cough that sounds like a seal's bark.
- Hoarseness.
- A harsh, crowing noise with breathing in.

Symptoms of croup can also be like symptoms of more serious problems. These include:

- **Epiglottitis**. This is a bacterial infection that can cause the back of the throat to swell up. If the throat is blocked, breathing in is very difficult. Severe respiratory distress can result. Signs of epiglottitis are:
  - Drooling.
  - Hanging the head down.
  - Sticking out the jaw to breathe.
  - Fever.
- Something can be stuck in your child's windpipe.

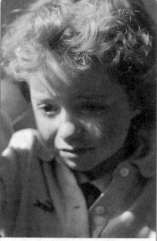

With croup, the child has a hard time breathing in.

Treatment

Self-care measures can treat symptoms. Croup usually goes away in 3 to 7 days. It is usually worse at night. Emergency care is needed for severe problems breathing.

Causes

Croup is usually caused by a certain virus. Other viruses, allergies, bacteria, and inhaled foreign objects, can mimic croup.

Questions to Ask

Does the child have any of these problems?
- Blue color around the lips or fingernails.
- Extreme shortness of breath.
- Listlessness or severe weakness.
- Coughing so much that your child can't take a breath.
- Inability to swallow or make sounds normally.

YES → Get Medical Care Fast

NO ↓

Flowchart continued on next page

Croup, *Continued*

Does the child have a hard time breathing and is he or she doing these things?
- Drooling.
- Breathing through the mouth and gasping for air.
- Sticking the chin out.

YES → **Get Medical Care Fast**

NO ↓

Without having trouble breathing, is the child doing all of the following?
- Drooling.
- Breathing through the mouth.
- Sticking the chin out.

YES → **See Doctor**

NO ↓

Does the child make a high, whistling sound like a barking seal?

YES → **See Doctor**

NO ↓

 Use Self-Care

Self-Care / Prevention

■ Don't panic. You can help your child stay calm if you stay calm. Hold your child to comfort him or her. The windpipe may open up a little if your child relaxes. Call your child's doctor or get immediate care if you are not sure what to do.

■ Go into the bathroom with your child and close the door.

   1. Turn on the hot water in the sink and shower. Let the steam fill the room.

   2. Don't put your child in the shower. Sit with your child. (Don't sit on the floor.) Read a book or play a game with your child. This will help pass the time.

   3. Open the window to let cool air in. This helps make more steam.

   4. Stay in the bathroom about 10 to 15 minutes.

■ If it is cold outside, instead of using the bathroom to make steam, put a coat, etc. on your child and take him or her outside to breathe the cold night air.

■ Use a humidifier in your child's room. Use warm, distilled water, not tap water. Clean the humidifier every day.

■ Put a humidifier on your furnace. Change the filter often.

■ Give your child a clear liquid. Warm it first. Warm liquids may help loosen the mucus. Give babies under 6 months old water or electrolyte water, such as Pedialyte, if okay with your child's doctor. Give water, apple juice, etc. to a child who is 6 months old or older.

■ Crying is a good sign. It means your child is getting better.

To Help Prevent Croup and Other Infections

■ See that your child's immunizations for diphtheria (DTaP), measles (MMR), and *H. influenzae* type b (Hib) are up-to-date. (See **Immunization Schedule** on page 23.)

■ Follow prevention measures in **Colds & Flu** on page 103.

Get more information from:

HealthyLearn® • www.HealthyLearn.com
Click on MedlinePlus®

The American Academy of Pediatrics
www.aap.org

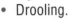

Lice are small, wingless insects about the size of a sesame seed. Lice lay up to 3 to 5 eggs a day. The eggs are called "nits." The nits hatch in 7 to 10 days. In another 7 to 10 days, a female louse matures and begins laying her own eggs.

Head lice is a common problem in children in day-care centers and schools. Head lice only affect humans. They thrive on human blood and can survive longer than 30 days. In general, head lice can't survive longer than 24 hours off their human host. Lice can also infest areas of the body other than the scalp. This is called body lice. Lice on the hair around the groin is called pubic lice.

Treatment

Over-the-counter products to get rid of lice are the preferred treatment for head lice. A prescribed medicine can treat lice and kill nits, but should be used with caution and only as directed.

Lice

Signs & Symptoms

For Head Lice

- Nits can be seen on the hair. They are small yellowish-white, oval-shaped eggs that look like dandruff. Instead of flaking off the scalp, they stick firmly to the base of a hair shaft.

- Itching of the scalp is intense.

- Small, red bumps appear on the scalp and neck.

- When hatched, head lice are clear in color, so are hard to see.

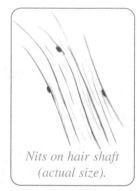

Nits on hair shaft (actual size).

Causes

Head lice does not imply poor hygiene. It is caused by the spread of the insects through direct contact of the hair or head with someone who has head lice. Sharing hats, towels, combs, helmets, etc. with an infected person can spread lice. Using pillows, head rests, etc. that an infected person used may also spread lice. Head lice don't fly or jump, so can't be spread through the air.

Questions to Ask

Does the child have any of these problems?
- Open sores are on the head from scratching.
- Lice or nits are found in the child's eyebrows, eyelashes, hair, or skin.
- Red bite marks are seen on the scalp. The child's head itches. Lymph glands in the child's neck are swollen.
- With lice, the child has a chronic illness like asthma, cancer, epilepsy, etc. Or, the child is under 2 years old.

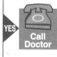

See Self-Care / Prevention on next page

Lice, Continued

Self-Care / Prevention

Check everyone in your home for lice and nits. Treat only those who have lice. Lice-killing products won't prevent lice.

- Use an over-the-counter shampoo, lotion, or cream made to get rid of lice and nits. Follow the directions on the package.

- Wear plastic or latex gloves. Don't use too much shampoo. Doing this will make the child's head too dry.

To Remove the Nits

- Shine a flashlight on the hair roots. Nits are gray and hard to see, especially in blond hair.

- Start at one spot and go row by row or even strand by strand. Use the nit comb that comes in the package. Dip the comb in vinegar first. This will help loosen the nits.

- Comb the hair from the roots to the ends. Check the comb for nits after each pass, or, break the hair up into 4 or 5 sections with hair clips. Lift about an inch of hair up and out. Put the comb against your child's head. Comb all the way to the tips of the hair. Keep going until you've done the whole head.

- Soak all combs, brushes, hair clips, and barrettes for 1 to 2 hours in the insecticidal shampoo. Or, soak them for 1 hour in soap and water, rubbing alcohol, or Lysol.

- Check for nits every 2 to 3 days for 2 to 3 weeks until all lice and nits are gone.

- A week to 10 days later, use the shampoo for lice again to kill any newly hatched nits. You don't have to remove nits after treatment is finished except for cosmetic reasons.

Other Things You Should Do

- Vacuum all mattresses, pillows, rugs, and furniture made of cloth, especially where children play. Use the long, thin attachment to suck the lice or nits out of car seats, toys, etc. Put the vacuum cleaner bags outside in the trash.

- Wash bedding and clothes right away in water 130°F or hotter. Put them in the dryer on high for 30 minutes. Heat kills the lice and nits. Dry-clean clothes and hats that you can't wash.

- Don't use bug spray on lice, furniture, stuffed animals, etc.

- As soon as you know your child has lice, call your child's school, child-care center, parents of your child's friends, etc.

- Check your children for head lice and nits once a week. Check more often if your child scratches his or her head. Look for nits behind the ears and on the back of the neck. Spread hairs apart with 2 round toothpicks to look for the nits on the hair shafts.

Things to Tell Your Child

- Don't share hats, brushes, or combs. If you must share helmets, wipe them with a damp towel and wear a baseball cap under the helmet.

- Don't lie on a pillow that another child uses.

- Wash your hair and bathe often.

Get more information from:

HealthyLearn®
www.HealthyLearn.com
Click on MedlinePlus®

National Pediculosis Association
www.headlice.org

Chapter 20

Dental & Mouth Concerns

Regular Dental Care

Take Care of Your Teeth and Gums

Dental problems affect more than your teeth and mouth. Gum (periodontal) disease and other mouth infections may increase the risk for:

- Pneumonia.

- Heart disease.

- Diabetes.

Also, an oral exam can help a dentist detect many health problems. These include diabetes, eating disorders, heart disease, osteoporosis, and a lack of vitamins.

Get more information from:

American Dental Association
www.ada.org

National Institute of Dental and Craniofacial Research (NIDR)
301.496.4261 or
www.nidr.nih.gov

Brush Your Teeth

- Do this twice a day. Brush more often, if you need to.

- Use a soft-bristled toothbrush and a toothpaste with fluoride. Brush with a gentle touch. If you have sensitive teeth, use a toothpaste made for this.

- Do a thorough job. Brush in small circles across all of the surfaces of the upper and lower teeth. Brush the outer, inner, and chewing surfaces. Brush the surfaces between the teeth.

- A child younger than 7 years old and some handicapped persons may need help to do a thorough job. A mechanical tooth brush may be helpful.

- Use a toothbrush that fits your mouth. Change your toothbrush to a new one every 3 to 4 months. Do this more often if the bristles are bent or frayed. Change it after having a throat or mouth infection, too.

- Brush your gums gently. Keep the brush perpendicular to your teeth.

- Gently brush your tongue. It can trap germs.

Floss Your Teeth

- Floss or use an interdental cleaner once a day to remove food particles and plaque from areas that your toothbrush cannot reach.

- Use a piece of floss about $1^1/_2$ feet long.

- To floss your upper teeth, hold the floss tightly between the thumb on one hand and index finger on the other. Using a gentle, sawing motion, bring the floss through the tight spaces between the teeth. Do not snap it against the gums.

Regular Dental Care, Continued

- With the floss at the gum line, curve it into a C-shape against one tooth and gently scrape the side of it with the floss. Repeat on each tooth. Use a fresh section of floss for each tooth.

- Repeat for your lower teeth, but hold the floss between both index fingers.

- Rinse your mouth after flossing.

- If it is hard for you to use dental floss, use a dental floss holder sold in drugstores.

- After flossing, rinse your mouth with water, mouthwash, or an anti-microbial mouthrinse.

It is normal for gums to be tender and bleed for the first week. If the bleeding continues, see your dentist.

Dental floss removes food particles that tooth brushing misses.

Other Tips
- Protect your teeth from damage and injury. (See **Self-Care / Prevention** for **Broken or Knocked-Out Tooth** on page 343.)

- Ask your dentist if you should use a fluoride mouth rinse, a prescribed toothpaste with fluoride, fluoride supplements, and/or a water-pik device.

- Don't lay a baby down with a bottle left in the baby's mouth if the bottle contains juice, milk, soda, etc. Water is okay, though.

Get Regular Dental Checkups
See your dentist every 6 months, at least every year, or as often as your dentist advises. Regular dental checkups are important to:
- Clean your teeth and remove plaque and tarter that buildup even after you brush and floss every day. Removing plaque and tartar helps prevent cavities, gum disease, and other problems.

- Check for cavities, gum disease, oral cancers, tooth grinding, bite problems, and other problems. When these are detected early, they are easier to treat.

- Address any areas of concern.

- Find out how to take care of your teeth and what dental care products you should use.

Also, an oral exam can help a dentist detect other health problems, such as diabetes, heart disease, eating disorders, and osteoporosis.

Diet & Dental Health Tips
- If your local water supply has fluoride, drink 6 to 10 cups of tap water every day. If not, make sure to use a fluoride toothpaste.

- Eat a well balanced diet. Limit between-meal snacks.

- Eat sticky, chewy, sugary foods with (not between) meals. Finish a meal with foods that help buffer acid formation. Examples are cheese, meat, fish, nuts, and dill pickles.

- Avoid sugar-sweetened gum and beverages. Chew a sugar-free gum instead, especially one with the artificial sweetener xylitol.

- Don't eat sweets, fruit, or starchy foods just before bedtime. Your mouth makes less saliva during the night. This allows cavity-causing bacteria to feed on food particles. Brushing your teeth doesn't effectively prevent this.

Bad Breath

Bad breath (halitosis) is a social concern. It can be a health issue, too.

Signs & Symptoms

- A bad odor from the mouth. To detect this, wipe the back of your tongue with a piece of white, sterile gauze. After 5 minutes, smell the gauze for an odor.

- An unpleasant taste is in the mouth.

- You are told you have bad breath.

Treatment

The **Self-Care/Prevention** items listed on this page treat most cases of bad breath. If not, your dentist can prescribe:

- A special toothpaste.

- A mouth rinse.

- A special brush.

- A tongue scraper.

- An antimicrobial solution.

Causes

Bacteria on the tongue, dry mouth, and strong odors of food, such as garlic and onions, are common causes of bad breath. Other causes are smoking, alcohol, ill-fitting dentures, and infections of the gums or teeth. Less often, bad breath is due to another problem, such as a sinus infection or indigestion.

Questions to Ask

With bad breath, do you have any of these problems?
- Bleeding, swelling, or pain in the mouth or throat.
- Chronic cough.
- Digestion problems. Weight loss.
- Puffy, reddened gums.

YES **See Doctor**

NO

Does bad breath continue after you use self-care for 2 weeks? **YES** **Call Doctor**

NO

Use Self-Care

Self-Care / Prevention

- Practice good oral hygiene. (See **Regular Dental Care** on page 340.)

- If you wear dentures, clean and care for them as advised by your dentist.

- Don't smoke. Limit or avoid alcohol.

- To prevent dry mouth, drink plenty of water and other liquids.

- Use a baking soda toothpaste. Brush your teeth and tongue. Do this after all meals, if you can. If not, rinse your mouth with water, chew parsley, mint leaves, celery, or carrots after meals.

- Don't rely on mouthwash or mints. They mask bad breath and help cause it, because they dry out the mouth. Try chlorophyll tablets.

- Eat at regular times. Eat nutritious foods. Limit sugary foods.

- Chew sugarless gum or suck on lemon or other citrus drops. These help make saliva. Saliva helps deal with bacteria on the teeth and washes away food particles.

Broken or Knocked-Out Tooth

Signs & Symptoms

- Loss of a tooth or part of a tooth.
- Nicked or chipped tooth or teeth.

Causes

An injury or a strain on a tooth, such as from biting on a hard object can cause a broken, knocked-out, or chipped tooth.

Treatment

When a tooth gets knocked out, go to the dentist as soon as possible. Keep the tooth moist until you get to the dentist. Follow up treatment is also needed.

Questions to Ask

Has one or more teeth been broken or knocked out?

YES → Get Medical Care Fast

(from a dentist or hospital emergency department)

NO → Use Self-Care

Self-Care / Prevention

For a Knocked-Out Tooth
- If you find the tooth, pick it up by the crown. Avoid contact with the root.
- Rinse off the rest of the tooth with clear water. Do not scrub the tooth or remove any tissue that is attached to the tooth.

- If possible (and if you're alert), gently put the tooth back in its socket or hold it under your tongue. Otherwise, put the tooth in a glass of milk, cool salt water, or a wet cloth. Don't let the tooth dry out.
- If the gum is bleeding, hold a gauze pad or a clean tissue tightly in place over the wound.
- Try to get to a dentist within 30 minutes of the accident. If the dentist is not available, go to a hospital emergency department. Take the tooth with you.

For a Broken Tooth
- To reduce swelling, apply a cold compress to the area.
- Save any broken tooth fragments. Put them in a wet cloth or milk. Take them to the dentist.

To Protect Teeth From Damage and Injury
- Don't chew on ice, pens, pencils, etc.
- Don't use your teeth to pry things open.
- If you smoke a pipe, don't bite down on the stem.
- If you grind your teeth at night, ask your dentist if you should be fitted or a bite plate.
- If you play contact sports like football or hockey, wear a protective mouthguard. Mouthguards may also be useful for non-contact sports, such as gymnastics. Discuss the need of using a mouthguard with your dentist.
- Always wear a seat belt when riding in a car.
- Don't suck on lemons or chew aspirin or vitamin C tablets. Acids in these wear away tooth enamel.

Fractured Jaw

A **fractured (or broken) jaw** is when the jaw bone breaks.

Signs & Symptoms

- Jaw and/or facial pain, swelling, or numbness.
- Not being able to open or close the mouth normally.
- Bleeding from the mouth.
- Having a hard time drinking, speaking, and swallowing.
- Drooling.
- The jaw area is bruised or discolored.
- Teeth are loose or damaged.
- The jaw area is tender to touch.

Treatment

A fractured jaw needs emergency medical care.

Causes

Most often, the cause is trauma from a blow to the face, such as from a car accident, sports injury, assault, etc. Osteoporosis can also be the cause.

Questions to Ask

Do you have any of these problems?
- The injury caused a lot of bleeding or obstructs your airway.
- Your jaw or face is tender, painful, stiff, swollen, or bruised.
- You have a very hard time or can't open your mouth widely. Or, you can't close your mouth or move the jaw at all.

YES → Get Medical Care Fast

NO → Use Self-Care

Self-Care / Prevention

First Aid Before Medical Care
- Gently align the jaws. Do not use force.
- Try not to talk. Write notes instead.
- Close your mouth and secure the jaw with a necktie, towel, or scarf tied around your head and chin. Remove this if vomiting occurs. Tie it back when vomiting stops. If you don't have anything to tie the jaw with, keep it from moving by holding the jaw gently with your hands.

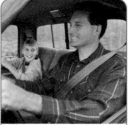

Seat belts help prevent injuries.

- Hold an ice pack on the fractured bone to reduce pain and swelling.

Self-Care after Jaw Surgery
- Follow post-operative instructions from your doctor.
- Remove elastic bands if you are choking on food or need to vomit. Go to the dentist to replace the elastic bands.

To Help Prevent a Fractured Jaw
- Wear a seat belt whenever you ride in a car, etc.
- Wear protective gear, as needed, for boxing, football, etc.

Gum (Periodontal) Disease

Signs, Symptoms & Causes

Gum (periodontal) diseases include:

Gingivitis. The gums are swollen due to bacteria from plaque and tartar on the teeth. With gingivitis, the gums are red and bleed easily.

Periodontitis. This is swelling around the tooth. It occurs when gingivitis is not treated. With periodontitis, pockets form between the gums and teeth. These expose teeth at the gum line. When left untreated, plaque grows below the gum line. Gums, bones, and connective tissue that support the teeth are destroyed. This can cause permanent teeth to separate from each other and loosen. Teeth may even need to be removed.

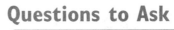

Swollen Inflamed Gums

Gingivitis

Deep Pocket

Periodontitis

Treatment

Gum disease should be treated by a periodontist or a dentist who treats this problem. Material called tartar can form, even when normal brushing and flossing are done. The dentist or dental hygienist can remove tartar on a regular basis. Treatment may also include:

- Deep cleaning (scaling and root planing).
- Medications.
- Surgical treatments. These include flap surgery and bone and tissue grafts.

Questions to Ask

Do you have any of these problems?
- Red or swollen gums that are tender or that bleed easily.
- Roots are exposed at the gum line.
- Loose permanent teeth or teeth that separate from each other.
- Pus around the gums and teeth.
- Bad breath and/or a foul taste in the mouth that doesn't go away.

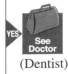
YES → See Doctor (Dentist)

NO → Use Self-Care

Self-Care / Prevention

- See your dentist as often as advised. Follow his or her advice for medication, teeth brushing and flossing and using other dental instruments.

- Don't smoke. If you smoke, quit.

- Eat a balanced diet.

- Limit sugary foods. When you eat sweets, do so with meals, not in between meals. Finish a meal with cheese. This tends to neutralize acids that form.

- Include foods with good sources of vitamin A and vitamin C daily. Vitamin A is found in cantaloupe, broccoli, spinach, winter squash, and dairy products fortified with vitamin A. Good sources of vitamin C are oranges, tomatoes, potatoes, green peppers, and broccoli.

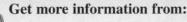

Get more information from:
HealthyLearn® • www.HealthyLearn.com
Click on MedlinePlus®

American Academy of Periodontology
312.787.5518 • www.perio.org

Mouth Sores

Treatment

Canker sores heal within 2 weeks. Self-care can help with symptoms and speed up healing. If needed, a mouthwash with tetracycline and/or an oral paste (amelxanox) can be prescribed.

Cold sores are treated with self-care measures and antiviral medications, such as acyclovir and penciclovir.

Thrush is treated with prescribed, oral antifungal medicines.

Signs, Symptoms & Causes

For Canker Sores

- Small, round, red-rimmed sores with white or gray centers are in the lining of the mouth or on the tongue, gums, or lips.

- Discomfort occurs with eating and talking.

- A burning or tingling feeling can be present.

Canker sores may be caused by any tear in the mouth's lining. This can be due to an uneven tooth, rough tooth brushing, dental work, a burn from a hot drink or food, etc. A lack of vitamins and minerals, emotional stress, and having a history of canker sores can trigger them. The sores usually resolve in 4 to 14 days.

For Cold Sores

- A tingling feeling is on or near the lips for 2 days before one or more sores appear.

- Small, red blisters filled with clear fluid rupture and weep. Scabs form.

Cold sore on lower lip.[+]

Cold sores (fever blisters) are caused by the herpes simplex virus (HSV), either HSV-1 (this is most often the cause) or HSV-2 (the usual cause of genital herpes). This virus lies dormant in the body and can return. A fever, a cold, stress, cold or windy weather, and strong sun exposure are triggers for outbreaks.

Cold sores are contagious, especially when the blisters rupture and weep.

For Thrush

- The tongue looks red. The insides of the mouth have creamy white patches. A white coating can be seen inside the mouth and the throat.

- If the throat is affected, it hurts to swallow.

Thrush is caused by a fungal infection. Often it occurs after the recent use of antibiotics or corticosteroids.

[+] This skin rash photo is courtesy of the Public Health Image Library (PHIL) of the Centers for Disease Control and Prevention.

Mouth Sores, Continued

Questions to Ask

Does a child have redness or sores in the mouth that make it hard for him or her to eat and does the child have a fever that needs immediate care for his or her age. (See **Fever** on page 226)?

 YES Get Medical Care Fast

NO

With sores or redness with white patches in the mouth, are any of these conditions present?
- HIV/AIDS.
- The person is on chemotherapy.
- Recent organ transplant.
- Diabetes.
- The person has been taking corticosteroids.

YES See Doctor

NO

With a cold sore, do you have any of these problems?
- Eye pain or the eye feels irritated.
- Severe headache.
- A fever and general achy feeling.
- Blisters in the genital area.
- The cold sore makes it hard to swallow, talk, or eat.

YES See Doctor

NO

Do you have **signs and symptoms of thrush** listed on page 346?

YES See Doctor

NO

Do cold sores last longer than 2 weeks, appear more than 4 times a year, or occur after starting a new medicine?

YES See Doctor

NO

Flowchart continued in next column

After a mouth injury or tongue or lip piercing, are any of these signs present?
- Increasing pain, redness, swelling, or tenderness around the wound or piercing site.
- Swollen glands in the neck or jaw area.
- Pus drains from the wound site.
- Temperature of 100°F (37.8°C) or higher.
- Overall ill feeling.

YES See Doctor

NO

Do mouth sores not respond to prescribed treatment or self-care?

YES Call Doctor

NO

 Use Self-Care

Self-Care / Prevention

To Treat Canker Sores

- Mix ½ teaspoon salt in 1 cup of warm water. Rinse the mouth with an ounce of this mixture 4 times a day. Don't swallow the water.

- Put ice on the canker sore. Suck on a frozen popsicle.

- Avoid spicy foods and acidic drinks like citrus juices.

- Use over-the-counter products, like Anbesol, Blistex, and aloe vera gel.

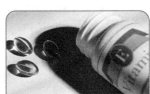
Put the gel from a vitamin E capsule on the sore several times a day.

- Swish Mylanta or milk of magnesia around the mouth to coat the sore. Then spit the medicine out.

- Take an over-the-counter pain medicine as directed.

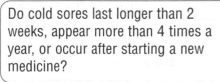

Mouth Sores, Continued

Oral Cancer Warning Signs

- Red and/or white patches inside the mouth or on the lip.

- A sore on the lip or in the mouth that won't heal.

- A lump in the neck.

- Bleeding in the mouth.

- A hard time swallowing or it feels like something is caught in the throat.

- Loose teeth or a hard time wearing dentures.

See a doctor or dentist if you have any of these signs for 2 weeks or longer. Any of these signs may be caused by oral cancer or by other, less serious problems. Don't wait for something to hurt. Pain is not usually an early symptom of oral cancer.

To Help Prevent Canker Sores

- Avoid things that injure or irritate the mouth, such as hot drinks and sharp objects.

- Use a toothbrush with soft bristles. Use a toothpaste without sodium lauryl sulfate. Don't brush too hard.

- Take vitamins and minerals, as advised by your doctor.

To Treat Cold Sores

- Apply antiviral medication, if prescribed. Or, use an over-the-counter treatment (e.g., Abreva antiviral cream, Campho-Phenique, Blistex) on the affected area at the first sign of a cold sore. You can also gently dab aloe vera or petroleum jelly on the sore.

Use a cotton swab to apply aloe vera, etc. to the affected area.

- Apply ice to the sore. Suck on a frozen popsicle.

- Take an over-the-counter medicine for pain as directed.

- Deal with stress. (See **Manage Stress** on page 53.)

- Avoid sour, spicy, or acidic foods. These may irritate the sores.

- Take vitamin C and/or zinc supplements, as advised by your doctor.

- Apply cool compresses when the sores have crusted over.

To Avoid Getting or Spreading Cold Sores

- Use medicines, as prescribed by your doctor.

- Don't share drinking glasses, towels, or cooking utensils.

- Avoid direct skin contact with the sores.

- Don't touch cold sores with your fingers. If you do touch the cold sores, do not touch your eyes. This could cause a serious eye infection.

- Try to figure out and then avoid things that trigger cold sores.

- When you are in the sun, wear a hat and use a sunblock with a sun-protective factor (SPF) of 15 or more on the lips.

- Use a lip balm on cold or windy days.

Temporomandibular Joint (TMJ) Syndrome

Temporomandibular joint (TMJ) syndrome occurs when the muscles, joints, and ligaments of the jaw move out of alignment.

Signs & Symptoms

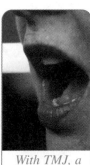

- Pain is felt in or around an ear. Pain in the jaw spreads to the face or the neck and shoulders. Pain is felt when you open and close your mouth or you can't fully open the mouth.

- Headaches. Toothaches.

With TMJ, a "clicking" noise occurs when opening the mouth or biting.

Causes

- Clenching or grinding the teeth (bruxism).

- Poor posture or sleeping in a way that misaligns the jaw or creates tension in the neck.

- Stress in life when it results in muscle tension in the neck and shoulder.

- Incorrect or uneven bite or injury to the jaw.

Treatment

- Wearing a mouthguard or bite plate.

- Physical therapy.

- Medicine to reduce swelling. One type is given through a shot in the jaw joint. Muscle relaxants for a short period of time.

- Counseling if the TMJ is caused by stress.

- Surgery is a last resort.

Questions to Ask

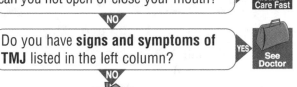

Does severe pain cause trouble eating? Or, can you not open or close your mouth? **YES** Get Medical Care Fast

NO

Do you have **signs and symptoms of TMJ** listed in the left column? **YES** See Doctor

NO

Use Self-Care

Self-Care / Prevention

Self-care measures may reduce the need for medical treatment.

- Massage the jaw area several times a day, first with your mouth open, then with it closed.

- Wear a mouth protector or mouth device, as prescribed by your doctor or dentist.

- Take medication, as prescribed.

- Don't chew gum or eat foods that are hard to chew.

- Try not to open your jaw too wide when you yawn and when you bite into foods, such as an apple, triple-decker sandwich, etc.

- To help reduce muscle spasms that can cause pain, apply moist heat to the jaw area. Use a washcloth soaked in warm water.

- If stress is a factor, use relaxation exercises.

- Take steps to reduce the risk of jaw injuries.

- Maintain a good posture.

Get more information from:

National Institute of Dental and Craniofacial Research (NIDCR)

www.nidcr.nih.gov

Causes

- A food particle, such as a popcorn hull, gets stuck between the gum and a tooth.

- Tooth grinding (bruxism). This can wear down teeth and cause cracks in them.

- A cavity or infection is beneath or around the gum of a tooth.

- **Tooth abscess**. This is swelling and/or infection in the bone and/or the tooth's canals.

- **Gum (periodontal) disease**. (See page 345.)

- Impacted teeth. Teeth may not fully erupt or can grow at odd angles.

- Temporary pain from recent dental work.

- **TMJ**. (See page 349.)

- An injury to a tooth.

- A symptom of a **sinus infection**. (See page 90.)

- A symptom of **angina**. (See page 232.) A **heart attack**. (See page 387.)

Toothaches

Signs & Symptoms

- Pain in or around a tooth that throbs or occurs with a fever and/or general ill feeling. Tooth pain occurs after you eat or drink or have something hot, cold, or sweet.

- Gums are red, swollen, and/or bleed.

- Earache and/or swollen glands on one side of the face or neck.

Treatment

Emergency care is needed for a heart attack. A dentist or doctor can diagnose and prescribe proper treatment for other problems.

Questions to Ask

With tooth pain, do you have any of these problems?
- Gnawing pain in the lower teeth or neck.
- Chest discomfort beneath the breast bone.
- Pain that travels to or is felt in the arm or neck.

YES → Get Medical Care Fast

NO

Do you have any **signs or symptoms of toothaches** listed above? **YES** → See Doctor (Dentist)

NO

Use Self-Care

Self-Care / Prevention

To Treat Tooth Pain Until You See the Dentist

- Gargle with warm salt water every hour. Hold an ice pack on the jaw. Don't drink hot or cold liquids. Avoid sweets, soft drinks, and hot or spicy foods. It may be best not to eat at all until you see your dentist.

- Gently floss around the tooth to remove food particles that could be between the teeth.

- Take an over-the-counter pain reliever. Don't place a crushed aspirin on the tooth, though. Aspirin burns the gums and destroys tooth enamel.

- For a cavity, pack it with a piece of sterile cotton soaked in oil of cloves. You can get this at a drug store.

Emergencies & First Aid

The focus of this section is to help you learn:
- When a problem needs emergency medical care.
- What to do before getting emergency care.
- When and how to give first aid.

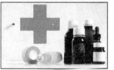

**Chapter 21
Emergency
Procedures**

Chapter 21 gives brief guidelines for CPR and first aid for choking. These **do not** take the place of formal training for these life-saving measures.

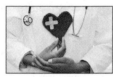

**Chapter 22
Emergency
Conditions /
First Aid**

Chapter 22 helps you decide what to do for medical emergencies and what first aid measures to give for many health conditions.

Recognizing Emergencies

What Is a Medical Emergency?
A medical emergency means death or serious harm could result without prompt care. Warning signs of a medical emergency include:
- Any **heart attack warning sign** listed on page 387.
- Any **stroke warning sign** listed on page 407.
- A hard time breathing or shortness of breath. Not being able to say 4 or 5 words between breaths.
- Fainting. Loss of consciousness.
- Change in mental status, such as unusual behavior or confusion.
- Sudden, severe pain anywhere in the body.
- Bleeding that won't stop.
- Vomiting that is severe or that persists.
- Coughing up or vomiting blood.
- Suicide attempts or gestures. Making plans for suicide. Repeated thoughts of suicide.

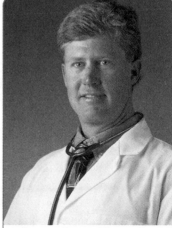

Ask your doctor if you should get emergency care for symptoms other than the ones listed here.

Being Ready for Medical Emergencies

- Learn basic first-aid skills. Take courses in CPR and first aid. These give hands-on practice in giving first aid and CPR the right way. Find out about them from your local Red Cross, police and/or fire department, etc.

- Find out what services your health plan covers and what steps you have to take to get emergency costs paid for.

- Carry the following information with you at all times:
  - Your name, address, phone number, and the person to contact if you need emergency care.
  - Your health insurance information.
  - Important medical information. This could be on a medical alert tag, on a wallet card, or on the back of your driver's license. Have a list of medications, their dosages, and things you are allergic to.
  - Emergency telephone numbers. (Post these near phones, too.)

- Read Chapter 21 (pages 353-357) and Chapter 22 (pages 358-407) to learn what to do for conditions that need emergency medical care and/or first aid.

First-Aid Kit

Keep first-aid supplies handy, but out of children's reach. Carry a first-aid kit in the car (or boat, wrapped in a waterproof container), as well as in the house. Campers, bikers, hikers, and persons who spend time in remote areas should take a first-aid kit with them. Once a year, check supplies for expiration dates. Restock items when they are used up or when expiration dates have passed.

First-Aid Supplies & Medicines
Acetaminophen, aspirin, ibuprofen, etc.
Adhesive bandages of different sizes.
Antibiotic ointment.
Antidiarrheal medicine.
Antihistamine tablets or syrup.
Antiseptic ointment or wipes.
Calibrated medicine spoon & dropper (for kids).
Cold pack.
Cotton-tipped swabs.
Elastic wrap and closures.
Flashlight and extra batteries.
Hydrocortisone ointment.
Safety pins.
Scissors.
Sterile gauze pads, a roll of gauze, and tape.
Sterile nonstick dressings.
Sunscreen (SPF of 15 or higher).
Tweezers.

Add Extra Items for a Car or Boat
Clean, folded sheet. Blanket.
Large flashlight. Extra batteries. Flares. Rope.
Plastic bottle of water, tightly capped.
Protective clothing and footwear.

{*Note:* See also **Be Prepared for Disasters & Threats** on pages 61 to 64.}

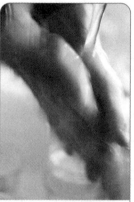

Chapter 21

Emergency Procedures

First Aid Precautions

First Aid Safety Steps

1. LOOK around. Is it safe to help? If not, call **9-1-1**, have someone else call, or seek medical help. If it is safe to help, stay calm and go to step 2.

2. CHECK for a response.
   - Gently tap the person. Ask, "Are you okay?" Ask loudly. Call the person by name if you know it.
   - If the person responds or moves, attend to his or her problem, as needed. If the person is injured or the problem is serious, call for emergency medical care. Give first aid as needed, until medical help arrives.
   - If the person does not respond or move, begin **CPR**. (See pages 354 and 355.)

3. PROTECT yourself from hepatitis B virus and HIV, the virus that causes AIDS. You can get these from an infected person's blood or other body fluids if they enter your body. These organisms can enter through cuts or breaks in your skin or through the lining of your mouth, nose, and eyes. When you give first aid or do CPR, take these steps, especially if you don't know the person:
   - Use plastic wrap or a plastic bag that you can throw away whenever you touch another person's body fluids, blood, or other objects that may be soiled with his or her blood. If possible, have the person apply pressure to the wound with his or her own hand.

   - Cover the person's open wounds with dressings, extra gauze, or water proof material.

   - Using a mouth-to-mouth barrier device when you give rescue breaths may or may not protect you from picking up an infection. If you are not willing to give mouth-to-mouth rescue breaths during **CPR**, do **Hands-Only CPR**. (See page 354.)

Wash your hands with soap and water right after you give first aid.

   - Report every incident in which you are exposed to another person's blood or other body fluids to your doctor, local health department, or EMS personnel. Do this within 1 to 2 hours.

4. FIND out if the person has certain medical needs.
   - Ask if he or she has prescribed medicine, such as nitroglycerin, to take for a heart condition. Ask where he or she keeps the medicine. Find out how much to give. Ask the person or read the directions on the medicine's label, if there is one.

   - Ask the person if you can give the medicine to him or her.

   - Look for a medical alert tag to find out about health problems the person has.

   - Find out if the person is allergic to any medicine.

CPR

CPR is **cardiopulmonary resuscitation**.

For Adults – Hands Only
Do this in 2 steps:

1. **Call 9-1-1** or get someone else to call!

2. Push hard and push fast in the center of the chest. Give 100 compressions a minute. (See step 7 on this page.) Keep this up until an **automated external defibrillator (AED)** is used or EMS takes over.

Any bystander can use this for *adults only* who suddenly collapse in places outside-the-hospital setting. **Hands-Only CPR** *should not* be used for:

• *All* infants and children.

• Adults who have collapsed due to near-drowning, a drug overdose, or breathing problems.

• Adults who are already unconscious and not breathing normally when found.

Find out more about CPR and training and updates for it from:
American Heart Association
877.AHA.4CPR (242.4277)
www.americanheart.org/cpr

See a Hands-Only™ CPR video at http://handsonlycpr.org

Conventional CPR For Adults and Children Over 8 Years Old

1. Shout for help! **Call or have someone else call 9-1-1** and get an AED, if one is nearby.

2. Follow the 9-1-1 dispatcher's instructions.

3. Until the AED can be used or until medical help arrives, do CPR.

4. Open the airway. With one hand, tilt the person's head back. With 2 fingers of your other hand, lift the person's chin up. See **A**. If the airway is still blocked, tilt the person's head gently and slowly until the airway is open.

5. Within 10 seconds, check for breathing. Look to see if the chest and abdomen rise and fall. Listen for breath sounds exhaled from the person's mouth and nose. If the person is breathing, keep the airway open. Look for other problems.

6. If the person is not breathing, take a normal (not deep) breath and give 1 "**Rescue Breath**." Pinch the nose shut. Forming a tight seal, place your mouth over the person's open mouth. See **B**. See if the chest rises. If it doesn't, do head tilt and chin lift again. See **A**. Give the 2nd full breath for 1 second. Look to see if the chest rises. {*Note:* If you do not want to or can't give mouth-to-mouth rescue breaths, do compression-only-CPR. Go to step 7.

7. Begin "**Chest Compressions**":

   • Kneel at the person's side near the chest. Place the heel of one hand ½ inch above the "V" where the ribs join the breastbone. Place the other hand on top of the one already in place. See **C**.

   • Lean over the person and press straight down on the chest using only the heels of your hands. Keep your arms straight. Depress the middle of the chest between the nipples about 1½ to 2 inches. **Push hard and push fast!** Give about 100 compressions a minute. Relax pressure completely after each compression.

8. Give cycles of 30 chest compressions and 2 rescue breaths, without a break, until: The person moves; an AED is used; or medical help takes over.

CPR For Children Ages 1 to 8 Years Old

1. Shout for help! If you are alone, do CPR first. (Do 5 cycles of 30 chest compressions and 2 breaths. See Steps 5 and 6 below.) Then **call 9-1-1**, get an AED, and return to the child. If the child is small and does not appear to have a serious injury, carry the child to a telephone and **call 9-1-1!** If you are not alone, one person should start CPR. Another person should **Call 9-1-1** and get an AED.

2. Put the child on his or her back.

3. Open the child's airway, as for an adult. See Ⓐ on page 354. If the airway is still blocked, tilt the child's head gently and slowly until the airway is open.

4. Within 10 seconds, check for breathing, as for an adult in Step 5 on page 354. If the child is breathing, keep the airway open. Look for and give first aid for other problems, as needed. If the child appears to have no serious injury, put the child in the **Recovery Position**. (See page 357.)

5. If the child is not breathing, take a normal (not deep) breath and give 1 "**Rescue Breath**." Forming a tight seal, cover an infant's open mouth and nose with your mouth. See Ⓓ. For a small child, pinch the nose closed, as for an adult. See Ⓑ on page 354. Give 1 full breath for 1 second. See if the chest rises. Give the 2ⁿᵈ full breath for 1 second. Look to see if the chest rises. If it doesn't, do head tilt and chin lift again. See Ⓐ on page 354.

Ⓓ

6. Begin "**Chest Compressions**":
   • Lean over the child. Keeping your arms straight, press straight down on the chest using the heel(s) of 1 or both hands. Don't press on the child's ribs or the lowest part of the breastbone.

• Depress the middle of the chest between the nipples about $\frac{1}{3}$ to $\frac{1}{2}$ the depth of the chest.

• **Push hard and push fast.** Give about 100 compressions a minute. Relax pressure completely after each compression.

7. Give cycles of 30 chest compressions and 2 rescue breaths, without a break. Do this 5 times. (This should take about 2 minutes.) Keep doing 30 chest compressions and 2 rescue breaths until the child starts to move, until an AED is used, or until medical help takes over. Always open the airway before giving rescue breaths.

{***Note:*** Chest compressions alone are better than doing nothing, but it is best to do both rescue breathing and chest compressions in children. Why? Airway problems are the main cause of cardiac arrest in infants and children.}

For Babies Up to 1 Year Old

1. Shout for help! If you are alone, do CPR first. Then **call 9-1-1!** If the child does not appear to have a serious injury, carry the child to a telephone and **call 9-1-1**. If you are not alone, one person should start CPR. Another person should **Call 9-1-1!**

2. Use the tips of your middle and ring finger to compress the baby's chest. Slip the other hand under the baby's back for support. See Ⓔ. Depress the breastbone $\frac{1}{2}$ to 1 inch at a rate of 100 times a minute.

Ⓔ

3. Give 1 breath after every 5ᵗʰ chest compression.

4. Give CPR, as needed, until medical help arrives and takes over.

First Aid for Choking

First Aid for Choking

The **Heimlich maneuver** can be used to clear an object blocking the airway in conscious adults and children ages 1 to 8. It lifts the diaphragm and forces air from the lungs to push the object that blocks the airway up and out.

For Persons Over 8 Years Old

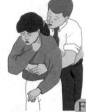

1. Ask, "Are you choking?" The person may use the choking sign. Do not interfere if he or she can speak, cough, or breathe.

2. If not able to speak, cough, or breathe, reach around the person's waist from behind. Make a fist. Place it above the navel, but below the rib cage. Grasp your fist with your other hand. Press your fist into person's abdomen and give 5 quick, upward thrusts. See F.

3. Repeat upward thrusts until the object is forced out or the person becomes unconscious. If the object is removed with success, the person should see a doctor as soon as possible.

4. If the person becomes unconscious, shout for help! **Call 9-1-1!** Tilt the head back and lift the chin to open and check the airway. {*Note:* If you suspect the person has a head, neck, or spine injury, do not move him or her. Pull the lower jaw forward to open the airway.} Give 2 slow rescue breaths. If this doesn't help, tilt the head further back (if no head, neck, or spine injury). Give 2 rescue breaths again. If the person does not respond or move, give 15 chest compressions. See G. Repeat rescue breaths and chest compressions. Each time you open the airway to give rescue breaths, check the person's mouth for the object and remove it if you can. Do CPR as needed, until the object blocking the airway is forced out or until medical help takes over.

5. Even when the object is removed with success, the person should see a doctor as soon as possible.

For Children Ages 1 to 8

1. For a conscious child, give abdominal thrusts as for adults. Don't be too forceful.

2. For an unconscious child, give first aid for choking as for an adult.

For Babies Up to 1 Year Old

1. Do not interfere if the baby coughs strongly, cries, or breathes okay.

First Aid for Choking, Continued

2. If the baby is conscious, hold the baby's head (face down) in one hand. Straddle the baby over your forearm. Rest your forearm on your leg for support. Keep the baby's head lower than the rest of his or her body.

3. With the heel of your free hand, hit the baby on the back between the shoulder blades 5 times. See **H**. Use quick, forceful motions. Repeat this procedure 3 to 4 times. If the object still blocks the airway, go to step 4.

4. Turn the baby over (face up). Cradle the baby on your forearm. Support the head with one hand. Keep the baby's head lower than the rest of his or her body. Rest your arm on your leg for support. Place 2 fingers ¹/₂ inch below and in between the nipples on the baby's chest. Give 5 quick downward thrusts. Depress the sternum ¹/₂ to 1 inch with each thrust.

5. Repeat steps 3 and 4 until the object is removed or the baby is unconscious.

6. If the baby is unconscious, shout for help. Have someone **call 9-1-1!** If no one calls **9-1-1**, give first aid for 1 minute, stop to call **9-1-1**, then resume rescue efforts.

7. Put the baby on his or her back. Tilt the head back and lift the jaw. Give 2 slow rescue breaths. If this doesn't help, give 2 rescue breaths again. Give up to 5 back blows; then up to 5 chest thrusts. If the object is expelled, stop.

8. Check for and remove the object in the airway, if visible. Repeat steps 7 and 8 as needed.

9. Don't give up! Give first aid until medical help takes over or until the object is removed. Even if it is, get medical care right away.

Recovery Position

The recovery position may need to be used in many conditions that need first aid, such as unconsciousness. It should not be used when a person: Is not breathing; has a head, neck, or spine injury; or has a serious injury.

To Put a Person in the Recovery Position

1. Kneel at his or her side.

2. Turn the person's face toward you. Tilt the head back to open the airway. Check the mouth if the person is unconscious and remove false teeth or any foreign matter.

3. Place the person's arm nearest you by his or her side and tuck it under the person's buttock.

4. Lay the person's other arm across his or her chest. Cross the person's leg that is farthest from you over the one nearest you at his or her ankles.

5. Support the person's head with one hand and grasp his or her clothing at the hip farthest from you. Have him or her rest against your knees. See **I**.

6. Bend the person's upper arm and leg until each forms a right angle to the body. Pull the other arm out from under his or her body. Ease it out toward the back from the shoulder down. Position it parallel to the person's back. See **J**.

7. Make sure the person's head is tilted back to keep the airway open.

To Learn More, See Back Cover

Chapter 22

Emergency Conditions / First Aid

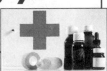

Bites & Stings

For Bites

Signs & Symptoms

- Swelling. Redness. Pain. Itching.

- Bleeding.

- Tissue loss, if the wound is severe.

- Skin rash. With **Lyme disease**, a red bull's eye rash with a white center around the bite occurs. Fatigue, fever, and joint pain may also occur.

- **Lockjaw.** This is a painful, persistent stiffness of the jaw due to a toxin. Tetanus shots can prevent this. (See **Immunization Schedule** on page 23.)

- Allergic reaction, such as with insect bites. (See **Signs & Symptoms** of **Allergies** on page 208.)

Causes

- Dog, cat, and human bites are the most common animal bites in the U.S.

- Black widow and brown recluse spider bites can cause severe reactions.

- Deer tick bites can cause **Lyme disease**, a bacterial infection.

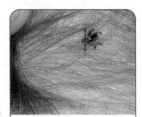

Deer tick on scalp

- Less common, but more dangerous, are bites from skunks, raccoons, bats, and other animals that live in the wild. These animals can have **rabies**. This is a serious viral infection. It can be fatal. Most house pets are vaccinated for rabies. It's unlikely they carry the virus.

- Mosquito bites can cause **West Nile virus** if the mosquito is infected with it.

- Snake bites can be fatal if the bite is from a poisonous snake (e.g., rattlesnakes, cotton mouths, copperheads, and coral snakes).

- Shark bites are a potential problem when swimming in shark-infested waters.

Treatment

Self-care can be used for dog and cat bites that cause scratches on the skin and for insect bites that do not cause a severe allergic reaction. All human bites that break the skin should be checked by a doctor due to the high risk for infection.

A series of rabies shots can prevent the spread of rabies to humans. The shots should begin soon after a bite from an infected animal.

Antivenom can be given for poisonous snake bites at emergency medical facilities. It should be given within 4 hours of the bite.

Bites & Stings, Continued

For Stings

Signs & Symptoms

- Quick, sharp pain.
- Swelling, itching, and redness at the sting site. These can occur beyond the sting site.
- Raised bump (with or without pus).
- **Signs of a severe allergic reaction**. (See page 208.)

Causes

- Insect stings. (See page 128 and 129.)
- Marine animals that sting include jellyfish, Portuguese Man-of-War, and sea nettles.

Treatment

Self-care treats mild reactions to stings. A severe allergic reaction needs immediate care. Symptoms of a severe allergic reaction usually happen soon after or within an hour of the sting.

Persons with a severe allergic reaction to a sting in the past should carry an emergency kit, prescribed by a doctor. A medical alert tag should be worn to let others know of the allergy. Persons who have had severe reactions to bee or wasp stings should ask their doctors about allergy shots.

Questions to Ask

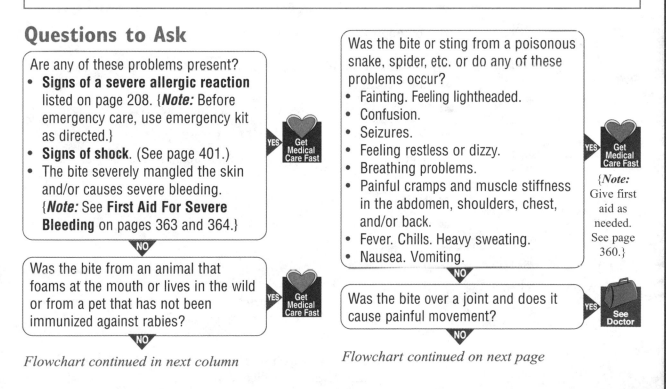

Are any of these problems present?
- **Signs of a severe allergic reaction** listed on page 208. {**Note:** Before emergency care, use emergency kit as directed.}
- **Signs of shock**. (See page 401.)
- The bite severely mangled the skin and/or causes severe bleeding. {**Note:** See **First Aid For Severe Bleeding** on pages 363 and 364.}

YES → Get Medical Care Fast

NO

Was the bite from an animal that foams at the mouth or lives in the wild or from a pet that has not been immunized against rabies?

YES → Get Medical Care Fast

NO

Was the bite or sting from a poisonous snake, spider, etc. or do any of these problems occur?
- Fainting. Feeling lightheaded.
- Confusion.
- Seizures.
- Feeling restless or dizzy.
- Breathing problems.
- Painful cramps and muscle stiffness in the abdomen, shoulders, chest, and/or back.
- Fever. Chills. Heavy sweating.
- Nausea. Vomiting.

YES → Get Medical Care Fast

{**Note:** Give first aid as needed. See page 360.}

NO

Was the bite over a joint and does it cause painful movement?

YES → See Doctor

NO

Flowchart continued in next column

Flowchart continued on next page

To Learn More, See Back Cover

Bites & Stings, Continued

> Do you have a fever, pus, or increased swelling and/or redness 24 or more hours after the animal bite? **YES** → See Doctor

NO ↓ Use Self-Care

Self-Care / First Aid

For Non-Poisonous Snake Bites

- Gently wash the site with soap and water.

- Treat the bite as a minor wound. (See **For Minor Cuts and Scrapes** on page 403.)

- If you notice signs of an infection, call your doctor.

For Poisonous Spider Bites Until Emergency Care Arrives

- Perform rescue breathing, if needed. (See **"Rescue Breath"** on page 354.)

- If you can, keep the bitten area lower than the level of the heart.

- Calm the person and keep him or her warm.

- Gently clean the site of the bite with soap and water or rubbing alcohol.

- Put an ice pack over the bite site for pain relief.

- If you can, catch the spider in a closed container to show what kind it is.

For Poisonous Snake Bites Before Medical Care

- Carefully move the person away from the snake. Calm the person. Have him or her rest. Moving about can help spread the venom.

- Gently wash the bite area with soap and water. Keep the limb of the bite site level with the heart (or just below this). Apply a splint to the limb of the bite site to keep it from moving.

- Being careful, note, if you can, the shape of the snakes eyes, pupils, and head, the colors it is, and if it has rattles.

- Don't try to kill the snake, cut the fang mark, or suck out the venom.

- Don't apply a tourniquet, a bandage, or ice to the bite.

For Poisonous Spider and Scorpion Bites Before Medical Care

- Do rescue breathing, if needed.

- If you can, keep the bitten area lower than the level of the heart.

- Calm the victim and keep him or her warm.

- Gently clean the site of the bite with soap and water or rubbing alcohol.

- Put an ice pack over the bite site to relieve pain.

- If you can, catch the spider in a closed container to show the doctor.

- Get emergency care!

For Human Bites Before Medical Care

- Wash the wound area with soap and water for at least 5 minutes. Don't scrub hard. Rinse with running water or with an antiseptic solution, such as Betadine.

- Cover the wound area with sterile gauze. Tape only the ends of the gauze in place. Then get medical care.

Bites & Stings, Continued

For Deer Tick Bites

- Remove any ticks found on the skin. Use tweezers to grasp the tick(s) as close to the skin as you can. Firmly, but gently, begin rotating the head part in a counterclockwise manner until the whole headpiece comes out. Or, pull gently and carefully in a steady upward motion at the point where the tick's mouthpart enters the skin. Try not to crush the tick. The secretions released may spread disease.

- After you remove the ticks, wash the wound area and your hands with soap and water. Apply rubbing alcohol to help disinfect the area.

- Use an ice pack over the bite area to relieve pain.

- Save one tick in a closed jar with rubbing alcohol to show the doctor.

For Dog and Cat Bites

- Wash the bite area right away with soap and warm water for 5 minutes. If the bite is deep, flush the wound with water for 10 minutes. Dry the wound with a clean towel. Then get medical care.

- If the wound is swollen, apply ice wrapped in a towel for 10 minutes.

- Get a tetanus shot, if needed.

- If the bite hurts, take an over-the-counter (OTC) medicine for pain.

- Report the incident to the animal control department. If a pet's immunizations are not current, arrange with the animal control department for the pet to be observed for the next 10 days to check for rabies.

- Observe the wound for a few days. Look for signs of infection. Often, cat bite wounds need an antibiotic.

For a Stingray Bite

- Remove the person from the water.

- Apply a local pressure bandage for a wound that bleeds a lot.

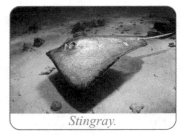

Stingray.

- Immerse the wound area in hot water for 30 to 90 minutes. Make sure the water is not hot enough to burn the skin.

- Scrub the wound area well with soap and water.

- Unless the wound is a slight one in only one limb, get medical help right away.

For Stings from Jellyfish or Sea Nettles, etc.

- Remove the person from the water. Don't touch the sting area with bare hands.

- Rinse the sting area with salt (not fresh) water right away. Don't put ice on the skin. If you can, put vinegar or rubbing alcohol on the area several times for 30 or more minutes until the pain is relieved.

- Apply dry or moist heat to the sting area until the pain subsides. You can mix one part ammonia with 3 parts salt water and apply this to the sting area.

- Wear gloves when you remove stingers. Use a towel to wipe the stingers or the tentacles off. Use tweezers to lift large tentacles. Don't scrape or rub them.

- To relieve itching, apply OTC calamine lotion or 1% hydrocortisone cream to the affected area as directed on the label.

- Contact your doctor for any **signs of infection**. (See page 120.)

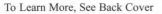

Bleeding

Signs & Symptoms

Most adults can donate a pint of blood without harmful side effects, but losing a quart of blood, quickly, can lead to shock and even death. In a child, losing a pint (or less depending on the child's size) can put the child in extreme danger.

For External Bleeding

- A skin wound.
- Dark red blood gushes or flows from veins.
- Bright red blood spurts from arteries.
- Blood oozes from capillaries. The bleeding usually clots off by itself.

For Internal Bleeding

- Vomiting or coughing up true, red blood. This includes blood-tinged sputum.
- A bruise on the skin of the chest or abdomen, especially if it is in a place where no blow was struck.
- Fractured ribs.
- Dizziness. Fainting. Weakness.
- Lethargy. Excessive sleepiness. Mental status changes. These can occur with trauma to the head, even if it is mild.
- Fast pulse. Cold, moist skin.
- Stools contain bright red blood or are black (not due to taking iron).

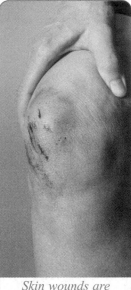

Skin wounds are common causes of bleeding.

Treatment

When bleeding occurs, the goal is to find the source, stop or lessen the bleeding, and help the body cope with the loss of blood.

- For severe bleeding, treatment includes first aid measures and emergency medical care.
- For minor bleeding, treatment depends on the cause and other medical conditions present.
- Bleeding disorders need to be treated by a doctor.

Causes

For External Bleeding

- Abrasions (scraped skin). Lacerations (cut skin with jagged edges). Punctures. (See **Skin Injuries / Wounds** on page 402.)
- Knife, gunshot, or other wounds can graze or penetrate the skin. These can damage internal blood vessels and body organs.
- Injury wounds.

Bleeding, Continued

For Internal Bleeding

- A bruise. This is bleeding from and damage to tissues beneath the skin.

- Damage to blood vessels and/or internal structures. This includes a blunt injury that does not break the skin, a bleeding ulcer, and an aneurysm.

- Bleeding disorders.

Taking blood-thinning drugs can result in both internal and external bleeding.

Questions to Ask

Are any of these problems present?
- A body part has been amputated.
- Bleeding from a wound is severe.
- Blood spurts from the wound and it is not controlled with direct pressure.
- **Signs of shock**. (See page 401.)

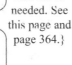 YES

{Note: Give first aid as needed. See this page and page 364.}

↓ NO

Are any of these problems present?
- Bleeding comes from a deep wound (it appears to go down to the muscle or bone) and/or a bone is exposed.
- The skin on or around the wound site hangs open.
- A deformity is at the injury site.
- Bleeding from what appears to be a minor wound continues after 20 minutes of applied pressure.

 YES

{Note: Give first aid as needed. See this page and page 364.}

↓ NO

Are any **signs of internal bleeding** listed on page 362 present? (**Note:** These may take days after an injury to occur.)

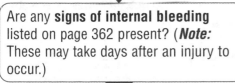 YES

↓ NO

Flowchart continued in next column

Does a person with a bleeding disorder or who takes blood-thinning medicine have a hard time controlling bleeding?

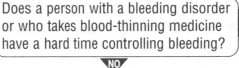 YES — Get Medical Care Fast

↓ NO

Does a person with a bleeding disorder or who takes blood-thinning medicine have a minor wound?

 YES — See Doctor

↓ NO

Are any of these problems present?
- Frequent nosebleeds.
- Small red dots or clusters of small, pinpoint-sized red specks under the skin.
- Easy bruising.
- Excessive bleeding from cuts.
- In females, excessive or prolonged menstrual bleeding or vaginal bleeding after menopause.
- Blood in the urine or stools.

YES — See Doctor

↓ NO

 Use Self-Care

Self-Care / First Aid

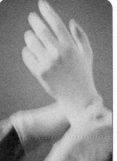

Wear waterproof gloves or use another waterproof material when you give first aid for bleeding.

For Severe Bleeding

- Without delay, apply direct pressure to the wound using a sterile dressing or clean cloths. {**Note:** If the cut is large and the edges of it gape open, pinch the edges of the wound while you apply pressure.}

- **Call 9-1-1** or take the person to nearest hospital emergency department.

Bleeding, Continued

Pressure Points

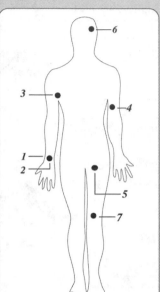

1. *Wrists: palm surface, thumb side.*

2. *Wrists: palm surface, pinky side.*

3. *Under armpits.*

4. *Inside of arms, halfway between the elbows and armpits.*

5. *Groin, about halfway between hips and genitals.*

6. *Temples.*

7. *Behind knees.*

- Do not remove an object that is stuck in a wound. Pack it in place with padding. Put tape around the padding so it doesn't move.

- If bleeding continues before getting medical help, put extra cloths, etc. on top of existing ones. Keep putting pressure on the wound until bleeding stops or until medical help takes over.

- The most important thing to do is to apply direct pressure on the bleeding site. Some health experts advise to do these things, too, if needed:
  - Elevate the wounded area higher than heart level while applying pressure. Do this if no bone is broken.

  - Apply pressure to a "pressure point" if bleeding still continues after 15 to 20 minutes of direct pressure. Use the pressure point closest to the bleeding site that is between the wound and the heart. (See **Pressure Points** at left.)

- Don't apply a tourniquet except to save a life.

- While giving first aid for bleeding, keep looking for **signs of shock**. (See page 401.)

For an Amputation

- Control bleeding. See **First Aid for Severe Bleeding** on page 363 and on this page.

- Wrap the severed part in a clean, dry (not wet) cloth or sterile gauze. Place the wrapped part in a plastic bag or other waterproof container. Put these on a bed of ice. Do not submerge the severed part in cold water or ice.

For Bleeding from the Scalp

- Use a ring pad to apply pressure around the edges of the wound, not on the wound. Make a ring pad (shaped like a doughnut) with a bandage of narrow, long strips of cloth. Start with one end of the narrow bandage and wrap it around all four fingers on one hand until you form a loop. Leave a long strip of the bandage material to weave in and around the loop so it doesn't unravel.

{See also **Self-Care / First Aid** in **Skin Injuries / Wounds** on page 403.}

Broken Bones / Dislocations

For Broken Bones

Signs & Symptoms

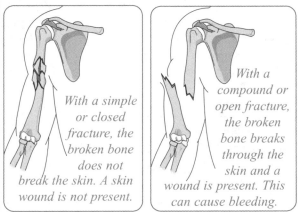

With a simple or closed fracture, the broken bone does not break the skin. A skin wound is not present.

With a compound or open fracture, the broken bone breaks through the skin and a wound is present. This can cause bleeding.

Symptoms of broken bones are pain, swelling, bruising, and loss of function or feeling. The injured area looks crooked, misshaped, or deformed.

Below the injured site, numbness and tingling can occur. The skin can be pale, blue, purple, or gray. It feels colder than the skin on the uninjured limb.

Causes

- Injuries from falls and accidents.
- **Osteoporosis.** (See page 199).
- Too much or repeated stress on a bone.

Treatment

The bone may need to be reset. A splint or cast may need to be worn. {*Note:* Broken fingers, toes, and ribs don't need a cast.} Muscles and joints near the fracture site need to be exercised.

For Dislocations

Signs & Symptoms

A dislocation is a separation of the end of a bone and the joint it meets. The bone is displaced from its proper position. A dislocated joint is swollen, misshaped, very painful, and discolored.

Dislocations can cause damage to the membrane lining the joint, tears to nearby muscles and ligaments, and nerve damage.

The shoulders are especially prone to dislocation injuries. The elbow is a common site in toddlers. Fingers, hips, ankles, elbows, jaws, and even the spine can be dislocated. A dislocated vertebrae in the spine often damages the spinal cord and can paralyze body parts lower than the injury site.

Causes

- Injuries from contact sports or falls. Over stretching bones that touch in joints.
- Joints weakened by previous injury.
- Suddenly jerking a toddler's hand or arm. Force applied in the wrong direction can snap the ball of the upper arm bone out of the shoulder socket.

Treatment

Medical care is needed to put a dislocated bone back into its socket. With this, the dislocated joint should function within 24 to 48 hours. Limited activity for 4 to 6 weeks allows enough time for the injury to heal.

Broken Bones / Dislocations, Continued

Questions to Ask

Do any of these problems occur?
- A severe injury to the head, neck, and/or back.
- Severe bleeding and a bone pushes through the skin.
- A very hard time breathing.
- An elderly person has fallen and can't move or get up.
- Severe abdominal pain after trauma to the abdomen or back.

NO

*{**Note:** Give first aid for the problem as needed. See page 367.}*

Are any of these problems present?
- Bleeding cannot be controlled with 10 minutes of direct pressure.
- Sweating. Dizziness. Thirst or an ashen skin color.
- Sudden shortness of breath follows an injury.
- A bone is broken in the hip, pelvis, or thigh and the person can't move or get up.
- The skin under the fracture is cold and blue. Or, a pulse can't be felt below the fracture site.
- Numbness or severe pain occurs below any other injured area.
- After an injury to the neck or back, a limb feels numb, weak or tingles.
- A bone breaks through the skin or bulges just under the skin.
- A limb or fracture site looks deformed.

NO

*{**Note:** Give first aid for the problem as needed. See page 367.}*

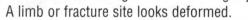

Get more information from:

HealthyLearn®
www.HealthyLearn.com
Click on MedlinePlus®

National Institute of Arthritis and Musculoskeletal and Skin Diseases (NIAMS)
www.niams.nih.gov

Are any of these problems present?
- The person can't move the limb, bear weight on it, or extend and flex it.
- Pain is severe.
- Pain, swelling, and discolored skin occur within 30 minutes of the injury.
- Pain and swelling get worse after 2 hours of using cold packs on the injured site and elevating it.

NO

Flowchart continued on next page

Broken Bones / Dislocations, Continued

Are any of these problems present?
- An injury to the face does not allow the jaw to open and close.
- A lot of bruising appears around the injury. Or, the area around an eye is swollen and discolored.
- It is hard to move the joint closest to the injury.

YES → **Get Medical Care Fast**

NO ↓

Does the area discolor more in the first 24 hours after the injury? Or, do pain and swelling not improve or respond to Self-Care/First Aid?

YES → **See Doctor**

NO ↓

 Use Self-Care

Self-Care / First Aid

For Broken Bones Before Getting Medical Care
{*Note:* If a head, neck, or spine injury is suspected, see **Head / Neck / Spine Injuries** on page 384.)

For an Open Fracture
- Monitor for **signs of shock**. (See page 401.)
- Control bleeding with direct pressure. Do not press on or move a bone that sticks out. Do not reset the bone.
- Immobilize the wound with a splint. Use a firm material, such as a folded newspaper or broom handle. Secure the splint above and below the injury or tie the injured part to an uninjured part. Use shoe laces, belts, etc. to hold the splint in place. Do not tie too tightly. Check the area below the splint to make sure that the skin is warm and pink in color. If not, loosen the ties.

For Fractures to Limbs
- To make an arm splint, put padding between the arm and the body. If an elbow is not involved, place the arm across the chest and wrap a cloth around the entire body. If the elbow is involved, place the arm straight or slightly bent against the body. Wrap the cloth around the body and arm.
- Make a sling with a triangular piece of cloth. Place the largest part under the arm and tie the ends at the neck.
- Make a splint for a leg or tie the injured leg to the other leg. Place padding in between the legs. Do not tie the splint too tightly. This could interfere with blood flow.
- Use cold packs on the injured site. **Do not use ice next to the skin. This can cause frostbite.**
- For pain, take an over-the-counter pain reliever as directed. Don't use aspirin if you have bleeding.

For Dislocations
Dislocations need medical care. The longer they are out, the harder it is to get them back in.
- If a head, neck, or back injury is suspected, see **Head / Neck / Spine Injuries** on page 384.
- Immobilize the injured area above and below the injured joint.
- Don't try to straighten a bone or joint that is misshaped. Don't try to put a joint back in its socket.
- Apply cold packs to relieve pain and swelling.
- Follow your doctor's instructions.
- Take an over-the-counter medicine for pain as directed.

To Learn More, See Back Cover

Burns

Causes

Burns can result from dry heat (fire), moist heat (steam, hot liquids), electricity, chemicals, or from radiation, including sunlight. The longer the skin is exposed to the burn source, the worse the burn can be.

Treatment

Third-degree burns always need emergency care. A second-degree burn needs immediate care if it is on the face, hands, feet, genitals, a joint, or if the burn affects a large area. **Self-Care/First Aid** treats most first-degree burns and second-degree burns.

Signs & Symptoms

First-degree burns affect only the outer skin layer. The skin area appears dry, red, and mildly swollen. First-degree burns are painful and sensitive to touch. They should feel better in 1 to 2 days. They heal in about a week.

Second-degree burns affect the skin's outer and lower layers. The skin is painful, swollen, red, and has blisters. The skin also has a weepy, watery surface.

Third-degree burns affect the outer and deeper skin layers and organs below the skin. The skin appears black-and-white and charred. It swells. Tissue under the skin is often exposed. Third-degree burns may have less pain than first-degree or second-degree burns. Why? No pain is felt where nerve endings are destroyed. Pain may be felt around the margin of the burn, though.

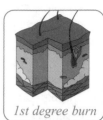

1st degree burn

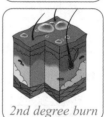

2nd degree burn

3rd degree burn

Questions to Ask

With or following a burn, do any of these problems exist?
- Loss of or decreasing level of consciousness. (See **Fainting & Unconsciousness** on page 378.)
- Breathing problems, chest pain, fast or irregular pulse.
- The person was in an enclosed room with exposure to a large amount of smoke from a fire.

YES ▸ Get Medical Care Fast

NO

Does the burn affect outer and deeper skin layers and do any of these signs occur?
- The skin looks charred or black and white and dry.
- Skin layers separate. This may look like burned pages of a paper book.
- The burned area covers more than the size of the person's palm.
- Pain is not felt.

YES ▸ Get Medical Care Fast

{*Note:* See "First Aid For Severe Burns Before Emergency Care" on page 369.}

NO

Flowchart continued on next page

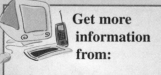

Get more information from:

National Safety Council
www.nsc.org

Burns, Continued

Does the burn appear red with swelling, blisters, and pain at the time of the burn? If so, do any of these problems occur?

- The burn is on an infant or child and it covers more than an area the size of the palm of the child's hand.
- The burn is on an adult and the area affected is larger than 10 square inches or is more than two times the size of an adult's palm.
- The burn is on the face, hands, feet, genital area, or on any joint.

YES → Get Medical Care Fast

{*Note:* Give first aid for burns as needed. See next column.}

NO ↓

Does a chemical burn affect a large area of the body? Or, does it affect the hands, feet, face, eyes, or genital area?

YES → Get Medical Care Fast

{*Note:* Give first aid for burns as needed. See next column.}

NO ↓

Do any of these problems occur?

- A sunburn affects a large area of the body. It is very painful. The skin appears red, dry, and shiny. Shivering or chills also occur.
- A burn affects a person who is diabetic, elderly, or who has a lowered immune status from illness, taking medicine, etc.
- A burn causes uncontrolled pain despite using **Self-Care/First Aid**.
- The burn has not improved in 48 hours.

YES → See Doctor

NO ↓

Use Self-Care

See Self-Care / First Aid in next column

Self-Care / First Aid

For Severe Burns Before Emergency Care

- Remove the person from the source of heat. For electrical burns, see **Electric Shock** on page 373. **Call 9-1-1!** Keep the person's airway open. Treat for **Shock**. (See page 401.)

- Remove hot or burned clothes that come off easily, not if they are stuck to the skin.

- Cover the burns loosely with clean cloths. Use direct pressure to control bleeding. Don't rub.

- Stay with the person until medical care arrives.

- If lye or a dry chemical gets on the skin, brush off the powder. Then flush with clean water for at least 20 minutes or until EMS arrives. Remove glasses, but not contacts, before treating the eyes.

For First-Degree and Second-Degree Burns (that are less than 3" in diameter)

- Use cold water or cloths soaked in cold water on burned areas for 15 minutes or until the pain subsides. **Do not use ice at all. Doing this could result in frostbite.**

- Cover the area loosely with a dry cloth, such as sterile gauze. Hold it in place by taping only the edges of the gauze. Change the dressing the next day and every 2 days after that.

- Don't use ointments. Aloe vera can be applied over closed skin 3 to 4 times a day. For a more severe burn less than 3" x 2", use Second Skin Moisture Pads, etc.

- Don't break blisters. If they break on their own, apply an antibacterial spray or ointment or treatment prescribed by your doctor. Keep the area loosely covered with a sterile dressing.

- Prop the burned area higher than the rest of the body, if you can.

To Learn More, See Back Cover

Choking

With **choking**, the airway is partly or completely blocked. When it is completely blocked, the brain doesn't get oxygen. Without oxygen, the brain can begin to die in 4 to 6 minutes.

Signs & Symptoms

When a person's airway is completely blocked, he or she:
- Can't talk.
- Can't breathe.
- Can't cough.
- May turn blue.

When a person's airway is partly blocked, he or she:
- Wheezes.
- Coughs.
- Has fast and/or labored breathing.
- Has chest pain when breathing in.

Causes

- Food goes down the windpipe. Small objects get stuck in the throat and airway.
- Fluids, such as mucus or liquids, are swallowed the wrong way and block the airway.
- Snoring. Choking can occur when the tongue blocks the airway.

Treatment

Emergency action is needed for a person who cannot breathe, speak, or cough forcefully. The Heimlich maneuver can expel an object that blocks the airway. It is used for a person who is conscious. Emergency medical care is needed for a person who loses consciousness. Rescue breaths and chest compressions are needed before medical help arrives. Even if the object is expelled, the person should see a doctor or go to a hospital emergency department.

Questions to Ask

Is the person unconscious? Or, is the person choking and not breathing? {**Note:** While waiting for emergency medical care, give or have someone give **First Aid for Choking** on page 356.}

NO

Does the person have any of these problems?
- A hard time swallowing. Fast and/or labored breathing.
- Persistent cough with a hard time breathing.
- Severe wheezing that doesn't go away.
- Drooling a lot. The person can't swallow saliva.
- Constant or unrelieved gagging.
- The feeling that something is stuck in the esophagus or throat.

NO

Flowchart continued on next page

Choking, Continued

After a choking incident, does the person have wheezing, a cough that doesn't go away, chest pain when breathing in, and/or a fever?

YES → Get Medical Care Fast

NO → Use Self-Care

Self-Care / First Aid

For **first aid for choking for a conscious and an unconscious person**, see page 356.

First Aid for Choking When Able to Breathe and Speak (or an infant or child can cry)

- Cough to clear the airway.

- Take a slow, deep breath to get a lot of air into the lungs.

- Give a deep, forceful cough. Breathe in deeply enough to be able to cough out 2 or 3 times in a row before taking a second breath.

- Don't slap a person on the back. Doing this can drive the object down deeper.

- Have the person sit or stand. Bending forward may cause the object to fall against the vocal cords. Get emergency care right away!

Prevention

- Chew all foods well before swallowing. Eat at a slow pace.

- Limit alcoholic drinks before you eat. This lessens the chance of swallowing large pieces of food.

- If you wear dentures, make sure they fit well. Since your mouth sensation is lessened, you are at a higher risk of choking. Eat slower. Chew food more thoroughly.

- Try not to laugh and eat at the same time. Laughing can draw food into the windpipe.

- Don't run or play sports with objects in the mouth.

- For children under 5 years old, cut hot dogs, sausages, seedless grapes, and caramels into small pieces before you give these to them. And don't give them nuts; popcorn; foods with pits, (e.g., cherries); gum (especially bubble gum); hard candy, throat lozenges, and cough drops.

- Don't let your child chew or suck on rubber balloons or pieces of them.

- Keep small, solid objects, such as paper clips, away from children 3 years old and younger. Make sure, too, that they don't get toys that have small parts, such as eyes on stuffed animals, game pieces, dice, etc. A young child should not play with any object smaller than his or her closed fist.

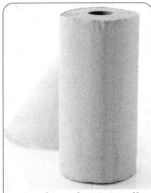

Anything that is small enough to fit through the center of a paper towel roll is a choking hazard for babies and small children.

- Put childproof latches on cupboards that have harmful items.

- Store all medicines and vitamins out of children's reach and in containers with childproof lids. Keep these items in locked cabinets, if needed.

- Remove plastic labels and decals from baby walkers and other kiddy furniture before children can peel them off.

Dehydration

Dehydration is when the body loses too much water and needed minerals (electrolytes).

Signs & Symptoms

For Severe Dehydration

- Severe thirst (sometimes).

- Sunken and dry eyes. Tearless eyes. (Infants may not show this sign.)

- Dry mouth, tongue, and lips.

- No urine or a low amount of urine that is dark yellow.

- Sunken fontanelle (the soft spot on an infant's head).

- Headache. Feeling lightheaded, especially when getting up quickly.

- Dry skin that doesn't spring back when pinched.

- Feeling dizzy. Confusion. Severe weakness.

- Increase in breathing and heart rate.

Causes

- The body does not get enough fluids for it's needs.

- Too much water or other body fluids and electrolytes, such as sodium and potassium, are lost. This can result from: Repeated episodes of diarrhea and/or vomiting; heavy sweating; heat exhaustion; or heat stroke.

Treatment

Fluids and electrolytes must be replaced. If this can't be done by mouth, they are given through an IV solution.

Questions to Ask

Do any of these problems occur?
- **Signs of severe dehydration** listed at left.
- A child or person has been left in a hot car or other hot, enclosed place and has any of the signs listed at left.
- After being in hot conditions, 2 or more **signs of heat exhaustion** listed on page 389 occur.

Self-Care / First Aid

- If vomiting isn't present, adults and children over age 12 should drink about 2 cups of fluid per hour. Fluids of choice are: Sports drinks; flat cola; clear sodas; broths; popsicles; and gelatin.

- If you have high blood pressure, heart disease, kidney disease, diabetes, or a history of stroke, you should find out what fluids your doctor prefers you take when you need to replace lost fluids.

- For children under 2 years old, consult your child's doctor about the amount and type of fluid to give. Ask your child's doctor about using over-the-counter products that give fluid and electrolytes. Examples are Pedialyte and Infalyte.

- For children over 2 years old, give up to $1\frac{1}{2}$ quarts of fluid per day.

Electric Shock

Electric shock occurs when an electric current flows through the body. The human body is made up of 60% to 70% water. This makes it a good conductor of electricity. Burns, damage to internal organs, heart rhythm problems, and death, can result from electric shock.

Signs & Symptoms

- Shocking sensations. Numbness or tingling. A change in vision, speech, or in any sensation.

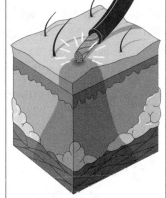

Electric Shock can cause tissue damage under the skin's surface.

- Burns or open wounds. These occur where the electricity enters and exits the body.

- Muscle spasms or contractions.

- Sudden immobility or fractures. A body part may look deformed.

- Interrupted breathing. Irregular heartbeats or chest pain.

- Seizures.

- Unconsciousness.

A small child who bites or sucks on an electric cord can have a facial injury or distinct burn around the rim of the mouth.

Causes

- Touching a high-voltage (more than 1,000 volts) source, such as high-tension wires that fall during a storm. Touching someone who is still touching a live current. Touching a low-voltage (less than 1,000 volts) current source, such as an electric socket or worn cord.

- Mixing water and electricity.

- Being struck by lightning. A bolt of lightning carries as many as 30 million volts.

Questions to Ask

Do any of these problems occur?
- The person is still in contact with the electric source or was in contact with a high-voltage wire.
- The person was struck by lightning.
- The person is not breathing.

YES → Get Medical Care Fast

{Note: Give first aid for the problem as needed. See page 374.}

NO ↓

Has an electric shock gone through the body in such a way that it might have passed through the center of the chest? Or, are any **signs and symptoms of electric shock** listed in the left column present?

YES → Get Medical Care Fast

NO ↓

After having an electric shock, are any of these problems present?
- Cough with phlegm. Fever. Headache.
- Wounds are not healing.
- Tetanus shots are not up-to-date.

YES → See Doctor

NO ↓

 Use Self-Care

See Self-Care / First Aid on next page

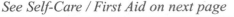

Electric Shock, Continued

Treatment

Contact with electricity from a high-voltage wire or being struck by lightning needs emergency medical care. Contact with electricity from a low-voltage current needs emergency medical care if any signs or symptoms listed on page 373 are present. A person who does not have any symptoms should still see a doctor to check for possible internal injuries.

To Avoid Being Harmed by Lightning

- Heed weather warnings.

- Take shelter in a building, if you can.

- Stay in your car (if it is not a convertible) rather than out in the open.

- If you are caught outside, avoid tall trees, open water, metal objects, and high ground. Crawl into a low-lying place or curl up on the ground, head to knees with your head touching the ground.

Self-Care / First Aid

Beware! Do not put yourself in danger to give first aid. Do not touch the person until power is shut off.

- If the source is a high-voltage wire or lightning, **call 9-1-1!**

- It is safe to touch a person struck by lightning.

- If the source is a low-voltage current, remove the fuse or switch off the circuit breaker to the electrical outlet.

- If you can't shut off the source, with dry feet and hands, use a board, wooden stick, rope, etc. to get the person away from the source.

- If it is safe for you to touch the person, check for a response. (See Step 2 on page 353.) Give **CPR**, as needed. (See pages 354 to 355).

  - Unless it is absolutely necessary, don't move the person. He or she could have a traumatic injury, especially to the head or neck.

  - Check for burns. Cover burned areas with dry, sterile dressings.

  - Give first aid for **Shock** (see page 401), if needed.

Prevention

- Stay clear of fallen wires. Inform the police, electric company, etc.

- Install ground-fault circuit-interrupters (GFCIs) in wall outlets of bathrooms, kitchens, etc. With GFCIs, when an electrical appliance falls into water, the current is instantly cut off.

- Don't turn electrical switches on or off or touch an electric appliance while your hands are wet, while standing in water, or when sitting in a bathtub.

- Replace worn cords and wiring.

- Cover all electric sockets with plastic safety caps.

Heed warnings to avoid electrical hazards.

- Before you do electrical repairs, remove the fuse from the fuse box or switch off the circuit breaker. Don't just turn off the appliance or light switch.

Eye Injuries & Irritation

Signs & Symptoms

Signs and symptoms depend on the cause. Common symptoms are:

- Pain and/or swelling in or around the eye(s).
- The eyes burn, are dry, and/or itch.

Causes

For Eye Injuries
Causes include:

- A physical blow to the eye.
- Harsh chemicals.
- A foreign body is stuck in the eye.

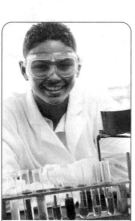

For Eye Irritation
Causes include:

- Particles in the eye.
- Too much sun exposure.
- Low humidity.
- Strong wind.
- Scratches from contact lenses.

Eye goggles help protect the eyes from harsh chemicals.

Other causes are allergies, infections, and conditions that make the eyes dry. With aging, the eyes can get irritated more easily because they make less tears.

Treatment

Mild eye irritations and injuries can be treated with self-care. More serious problems need medical care.

Questions to Ask

Do any of these problems occur?
- A foreign body is stuck in the eye.
- One or both eyes were exposed to acid, alkali, or any harmful chemicals.

YES → Get Medical Care Fast

{Note: Give first aid for the problem as needed. See page 376.}

NO ↓

Did super glue get in the eye(s)? *{Note: Before emergency care, do not try to pry the eye(s) open. Rinse the eyes with warm tap water for 20 to 30 minutes.}*

YES → Get Medical Care Fast

NO ↓

Do any of these problems occur?
- A severe blow to the eye with or without a broken bone of the face.
- Vision loss, blurred vision, double vision, or blood in the pupil after an eye injury.
- A cut to the eye or eyelid.
- **Signs of a severe allergic reaction** (see page 208) after a bite or sting to the eye. *{Note: Before immediate care, use emergency kit as directed.}*

YES → Get Medical Care Fast

{Note: Give first aid for the problem as needed. See page 377.}

NO ↓

Do you have eye pain or visual changes after exposure to a welder's flame or other ultraviolet source?

YES → Get Medical Care Fast

NO ↓

Do you have a contact lens in an eye and can't find it or remove it or does it cause eye pain?

YES → Get Medical Care Fast

NO ↓

Flowchart continued on next page

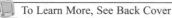 To Learn More, See Back Cover

Eye Injuries & Irritation, Continued

Is eye pain present? — **YES** — See Doctor

NO / Use Self-Care

Self-Care / First Aid

For a Foreign Body Sticking Into the Eye

- Do not remove the object.

- Don't press on, touch, or rub the eye.

- Cover the injured eye with a clean object, such as a paper cup that will shield, but not touch the eye or the foreign object. Use tape to hold the cup in place without putting pressure on the eye or the foreign object.

- Gently cover the uninjured eye with a clean bandage and tape, too. This helps to keep the injured eye still. Get Immediate Care!

For Harmful Chemicals in the Eye(s)

- Flush the eye(s) with water immediately!

- Hold the injured eye open with your thumb and forefinger. At the faucet or with a pitcher or other clean container, flush the eye with a lot of water. Start at the inside corner and pour downward to the outside corner. This lets the water drain away from the body and keeps it from getting in the other eye.

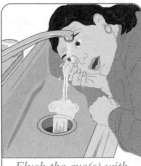

Flush the eye(s) with water immediately!

- Keep pouring the water for 10 to 30 or more minutes. Flush the eye with water until you get medical help.

- If both eyes are injured, pour water over both eyes at the same time. Or, flush one eye at a time with water. Switch back and forth quickly to treat both eyes. Or, place the face in a sink or container filled with water. Tell the person to move his or her eyelids up and down and remove the face from the water to take breaths. Use this method if chemicals get in your eyes and you are alone.

- Loosely bandage the eye with sterile cloth and tape. Don't touch the eye. Get Medical Care Right Away!

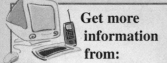

Get more information from:

HealthyLearn®
www.HealthyLearn.com
Click on MedlinePlus®

Prevent Blindness America
800.331.2020
www.preventblindness.org

Eye Injuries & Irritation, Continued

For a Bruise from a Minor Injury that Surrounds the Eye, But Does Not Damage the Eye Itself

- Put a cold compress over the injured area right away. Do this for 15 minutes, every hour, for 48 hours.

- Take an over-the-counter medicine for the pain and swelling.

- After 48 hours, put a warm compress over the injured area.

- Seek medical care if these measures do not help.

To Remove a Foreign Particle On the White of the Eye or Inside the Eyelids

- Do not remove an object stuck in the eye, a metal chip, or a foreign body over the colored part of the eye. (See **For a Foreign Body Sticking Into the Eye** on page 376.)

- Wash your hands.

- If the foreign object is under the upper lid, look down and pull the upper lid away from the eyeball by gently grabbing the eyelashes. Press a cotton-tipped swab down on the skin surface of the upper eyelid and pull it up and toward the brow. The upper lid will invert.

- Twist a piece of tissue. Moisten the tip with tap water (not saliva). Gently try to touch the speck with the tip. Carefully pass the tissue over the speck which should cling to the tip.

- Do not rub the eye or use tweezers or anything sharp to remove a foreign object.

- Gently wash the eye with cool water.

For Dry, Irritated Eyes

With your doctor's okay, use over-the-counter artificial tear drops, such as Ocu-Lube. Refrigerate the solution, if needed. Wash your hands before using.

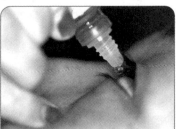

When you use eye drops, follow the label's directions.

For an Insect Bite Without a Severe Allergic Reaction

- Wash the eye(s) with warm water.

- Take an antihistamine if okay with your doctor.

Prevention

- Wear safety glasses when your eyes are exposed to sawdust, etc. Wear sunglasses that block UV rays.

- When using harsh chemicals, wear rubber gloves and protective glasses. Don't rub your eyes if you've touched harsh chemicals. Turn your head away from chemical vapors.

- To help prevent dry eyes, use a humidifier. Limit exposure to smoke, dust, and wind. Don't drink alcohol.

- Use artificial tear drops with your doctor's okay.

- Don't stare directly at the sun, especially during a solar eclipse.

- Don't use eye makeup when an allergy or chemical irritant bothers your eye(s).

- Don't allow a child to stick his or her head out of the window of a moving car, etc. Sand, insects, and other flying objects can strike the eye and irritate or damage the cornea.

- Don't let children play with or near sparklers, bottle rockets, and other fireworks.

Fainting & Unconsciousness

Signs & Symptoms

Fainting is a brief loss of consciousness. It can last from seconds to 30 minutes. Just before fainting, a person may feel a sense of dread, feel dizzy, see spots, and have nausea.

If a person falls and can't remember the fall itself, he or she has fainted.

An **unconscious** person is hard to rouse and can't be made aware of his or her surroundings. The person is unable to move on his or her own.

Treatment

Treatment depends on the cause.

Causes

Fainting is due to a sudden drop in blood flow or glucose supply to the brain. This causes a temporary drop in blood pressure and pulse rate. Medical reasons for this include:

- Low blood sugar (hypoglycemia). This can occur in diabetics, in early pregnancy, in persons on severe diets, etc.

- Anemia. Eating disorders.

- Conditions which cause rapid loss of blood.

- Abnormal heart rhythm. Heart attack. Stroke.

- Head injury. Heat stroke. Heat exhaustion.

Other things that can lead to feeling faint or fainting include:

- A sudden change in body position like standing up too fast. This is called **postural hypotension**.

- A side effect of some medicines. Drinking too much alcohol.

- Anxiety or sudden emotional stress or fright.

- Being in hot, humid weather or in a stuffy room. Standing a long time in one place.

- Extreme pain.

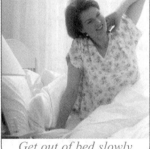

Get out of bed slowly.

Questions to Ask

Do any of these problems occur?
- The person is not breathing. {***Note:*** Give **Rescue Breaths**, and **CPR**, as needed. See pages 354 to 355.}
- The person is unconscious or is having a hard time breathing.
- Any **heart attack warning sign**. (See page 387.)
- **Signs of dehydration**. (See page 372.)
- **Signs of shock**. (See page 401.)
- The person who fainted had sudden, severe back pain.

YES Get Medical Care Fast

NO

Flowchart continued on next page

Fainting & Unconsciousness, Continued

Did fainting occur with any of these conditions?
- A recent head injury.
- **Severe bleeding.** (*Note:* Give first aid for this. See pages 363 and 364.)
- Severe pain in the abdomen or pelvis.
- Blood in the stools or urine. Black, tarlike, or maroon colored stools.
- Being over 40 years old and this is the first time for fainting.
- A known heart problem. A fast or irregular heartbeat.
- Diabetes and the person does not respond to a glucagon injection or rubbing a sugar source, such as cake frosting paste, inside the mouth.
- Being a young person and the fainting took place during a sports activity.
- Slow, noisy, or unusual breathing.
- Seizure symptoms, such as twitching or jerking, in a person not known to have epilepsy.

Self-Care / First Aid

For Unconsciousness
- Check for a response. (See Step 2 on page 353.) **Call 9-1-1!** Give **Rescue Breaths** and **CPR,** (see pages 354 to 355), or treat for **Shock** (see page 401), as needed.

- Check for a medical alert tag or information. Call the emergency number if there is one. Follow instructions given.

- Don't give the person anything to eat or drink, not even water.

For Fainting
- Catch the person before he or she falls.

- Lie the person down with the head below heart level. Raise the legs 8 to 12 inches to promote blood flow to the brain. If the person can't lie down, have him or her sit down, bend forward, and put the head between the knees.

- Loosen any tight clothing.

- Don't slap or shake a person. Don't give anything to eat or drink.

- Check for a medical alert tag. Respond as needed.

To Reduce the Risk of Fainting
- Follow your doctor's advice to treat any medical problem which may lead to fainting. Take medicines as prescribed. Let the doctor know about any side effects.

- Get up slowly from bed or from a chair.

- Avoid turning your head suddenly.

- Wear loose-fitting clothing around the neck.

- Don't exercise too much when it is hot and humid. Drink a lot of fluids when you exercise.

- Avoid stuffy rooms and hot, humid places. When you can't do this, use a fan.

- If you drink alcohol, do so in moderation.

For a Low Blood Sugar Reaction
- Have a sugar source, such as: One half cup of fruit juice or regular (not diet) soda; 6 to 7 regular (not sugar free) hard candies; 3 glucose tablets; or 6 to 8 ounces of milk.

- If you don't feel better after 15 minutes, take the same amount of sugar source again. If you don't feel better after the second dose, call your doctor.

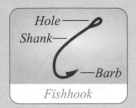

Hole
Shank
—Barb

Fishhook

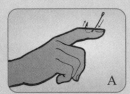

A

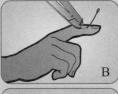

B

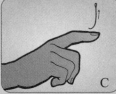

C

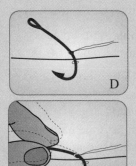

D

E

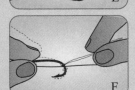

F

Fishhook Removal

Signs & Symptoms

A fishhook can nick or cut the skin, get stuck in the skin near its surface, or get deeply embedded in the skin.

Treatment

First aid treats most fishhook accidents.

Questions to Ask

Is a fishhook stuck in an eye?   YES → **Get Medical Care Fast**

NO ↓

Is the fishhook still in the skin, do **signs of an infection** (see page 120) occur, or are tetanus shots not up-to-date?   YES → **See Doctor**

NO ↓

 Use Self-Care

Self-Care / First Aid

For a Fishhook Deeply Embedded in the Skin

■ Put ice or cold water on the wound area to numb it. Push on the shaft of the hook until the barb protrudes. A   With wire cutters, snip the hook at either the shank or the barb. B   Pull the hook out. C

■ Wash the wound area well with soap and water. Treat for **a puncture wound** (see page 403).

For a Fishhook Stuck Near the Surface of the Skin

■ Put ice or cold water on the wound area.

■ Take a piece of fishing line. Loop one end and tie it to the hook near the surface of the skin. D   Grasp the shaft end of the hook with one hand and press down about $1/8^{th}$ inch to disengage the barb. E

■ Keep pressing the hook down and jerk the fishing line in a motion parallel to the skin's surface to make the shaft of the hook lead the barb out of the skin. F   Treat for **a puncture wound**. (See page 403.)

{*Note:* For nicks or surface cuts to the skin, treat for a **cut**. (See page 403.)

Frostbite & Hypothermia

Frostbite freezes the skin. It can damage tissue below the skin, too. Most often, frostbite affects the toes, fingers, earlobes, chin, and tip of the nose.

Hypothermia is when body temperature drops below 96°F. The body loses more heat than it can make. This usually occurs from staying in a cold place for a long time.

For Frostbite and Frostnip

Signs & Symptoms

- Cold, numb skin swells and feels hard and solid.

- Loss of function. Absence of pain.

- Skin color changes from white to red to purple. Blisters occur.

- Slurred speech.

- Confusion.

Frostnip is a less serious problem. The skin turns white or pale and feels cold, but the skin does not feel hard and solid.

Causes

When temperatures drop below freezing, frostbite and frostnip can occur. Both can set in very slowly or very quickly. This will depend on how long the skin is exposed to the cold and how cold and windy it is.

For Hypothermia

Signs & Symptoms

With *mild hypothermia*, symptoms include: Shivering; slurred speech; memory lapses; and the abdomen and back feel cold.

With *moderate hypothermia*, shivering stops, but the skin feels ice cold and looks blue. The person may act confused, drowsy, very cranky, and/or stuporous. Muscles may be rigid and stiff. Pulse rate and breathing slow down.

With *severe hypothermia*, the person has dilated pupils, no response to pain, and loses consciousness. The person appears to be dead. Death occurs in half or more of persons with severe hypothermia.

Causes

- Exposure to cold temperatures (wet or dry). Many factors increase the risk. Examples are: Wet clothing or lying on a cold surface; circulation problems; diabetes; and old age. The elderly are more prone to hypothermia if they live in a poorly heated home and do not dress warm enough.

- Immersion. This can be from 6 hours or less of exposure to cold water immersion. It can also be from water immersion or exposure on land to cold, wet weather near freezing for up to 24 hours.

- **Shock.** (See page 401.)

Frostbite & Hypothermia, Continued

Treatment

Self-care measures can treat frostnip. Prompt emergency medical care is needed for frostbite to keep the area affected from getting infected and to prevent the loss of a limb. Hypothermia needs emergency medical care.

Wind Chill Temperature
As the wind increases, the body is cooled at a faster rate. This causes the skin temperature to drop. Wind chill temperature combines outdoor air temperature and wind speed to give a temperature of what it "feels like" on the skin. The National Weather Service has a "Wind Chill Chart" that shows temperatures, wind speeds, and exposure times that cause frostbite. To get this, access www.nws.noaa.gov/om/windchill.

Questions to Ask

Do any of these problems occur?
- No breathing. {*Note:* Give **Rescue Breaths** or **CPR**, as needed. See pages 354 to 355.}
- Pale or blue colored skin, lips, and/or nailbeds.
- Loss of or decreasing level of consciousness. Fainting.
- Body temperature is less than 95°F.
- Rigid and stiff muscles.
- Mental confusion. Feeling drowsy.
- Slow pulse. Problems breathing.
- Stumbling. Lack of coordination.
- **Signs and symptoms of frostbite**. (See page 381.)

NO

With a low body temperature, did the person have a recent infection and now has **signs of sepsis** (lethargy, chills, vomiting, looks sick, and delirium)?

NO

Have any of these persons had prolonged exposure to the cold?
- Elderly persons.
- Persons with a history of alcoholism or drug abuse.
- Persons whose immune systems are depressed due to disease and/or medication.

NO

After being warmed, does the person continue to shiver? Or, does his or her body temperature not return to normal after 4 hours of warming?

NO

{*Note:* Continue to look for symptoms. The damage from exposure to the cold may not be noted for 72 hours.}

See Self-Care / First Aid on next page

Frostbite & Hypothermia, Continued

Self-Care / First Aid

First Aid for Frostbite and Hypothermia Before Emergency Care

- Gently move the person to a warm place and **Call 9-1-1!**

- Check for a response. (See Step 2 on page 353.) Give **Rescue Breaths** (see page 354) or **CPR** (see pages 354 to 355), as needed.

- Loosen or remove wet and/or tight clothing. Remove jewelry.

- Don't rub the area with snow or soak it in cold water.

- Warm the affected area by soaking it in a tub of warm water (101°F to 104°F) and an antiseptic solution, such as Betadine.

- Stop when the affected area becomes red, not when sensation returns. This should take about 45 minutes. If done too fast, thawing can be painful and blisters may develop.

- If warm water is not available, cover the person with blankets, coats, etc., or place the frostbitten body part in a warm body area, such as an armpit or on the abdomen (human heat) or use a blow dryer, if available.

- Keep exposed areas elevated, but protected.

- Don't rub or massage a frostbitten area.

- Protect the exposed area from the cold. It is more sensitive to re-injury.

- Don't break blisters.

First Aid for Frostnip

- Warm the affected area. This can be done a number of ways:

  - Place cold fingers in armpits.

  - Place cold feet onto another person's warm stomach.

  - Put the affected area in warm water (101°F to 102°F).

After warming the area, the skin may be red and tingling. If it is not treated, frostnip can lead to frostbite.

- Protect the exposed area from the cold. It is more sensitive to re-injury.

Prevention

To Prevent Frostbite and Outdoor Hypothermia

- Stay indoors, as much as possible, when it is very cold and windy.

- Wear clothing made of wool or polypropylene. These fabrics stay warm even when wet. Layer clothing. Wear 2 or 3 pairs of socks instead of 1 heavy pair. Wear roomy shoes. Do not wear items that constrict the hands, wrists, or feet.

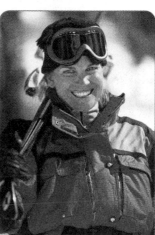

Wear outerwear that is windproof and waterproof.

- Wear a hat that keeps your head and ears warm. A major source of heat loss is through the head.

Head / Neck / Spine Injuries

Treatment

If you suspect a head, neck, or back injury, you must keep the head, neck, and back perfectly still until emergency medical care arrives. Any movement of the head, neck, or back could result in paralysis or death.

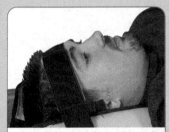

Keep the head, neck, and back perfectly still.

Signs & Symptoms

For a Severe Injury

- The scalp, neck, or back bleeds.
- It looks like the head, neck, or back is in an odd position.
- Pain is felt in the back, neck, and/or head. The pain can be severe.
- Stiff neck.
- Abdominal pain. Vomiting.
- Blood or fluid comes from the mouth, nose, or an ear.
- Loss of vision. Blurred or double vision. Pupils of uneven size.
- Inability to move any part of the body. Weakness in an arm or leg. Walking is difficult.
- New feelings of numbness occur in the legs, arms, shoulders, or any other part of the body.
- New loss of bladder or bowel control occurs.
- Confusion. Drowsiness. Personality changes.
- Convulsions.
- Loss of consciousness.

Watch for signs and symptoms for the first 24 hours after the injury. Symptoms may not occur for as long as several weeks, though. Problems can occur even if no injury is seen on the outside.

For a Whiplash Injury

- Neck pain and stiffness.
- Having a hard time raising the head off of a pillow.

Causes

Anything that puts too much pressure or force on the head, neck, or back can result in injury. Common causes are falls, accidents, and hard blows. A concussion occurs when the brain is shaken. A contusion occurs when the brain is bruised.

Head / Neck / Spine Injuries, Continued

Questions to Ask

Does the person have one or more **signs and symptoms for a severe injury** listed on page 384? {***Note:*** See **First Aid for a Severe Injury** on this page.}

YES → Get Medical Care Fast

NO ↓

Was a recent injury to the head, neck, and/or back not treated with emergency or medical care and are any of these problems present?
- Loss of consciousness, even briefly.
- Confusion.
- Vomiting.
- Severe pain.
- Numbness, tingling, or weakness in the face, arms, or legs.
- Loss of bladder control.
- A headache has lasted longer than 2 days and gets worse with time.
- Unusual feeling or sensations.
- Large or increased area of swelling despite the use of ice.

YES → Get Medical Care Fast

NO ↓

After a head, neck, or back injury, do any of these problems occur?
- Pain from a head, neck, or back injury lasts longer than 1 week or goes away and returns.
- Signs of infection (e.g., redness, fever, pus, drainage, etc.) occur at the site of the wound.
- A whiplash injury is suspected.

YES → See Doctor

NO ↓

 Use Self-Care

See Self-Care / First Aid in next column

Self-Care / First Aid

First Aid for a Severe Injury
- Do not move the person unless his or her life is in danger. If so, log roll the person, place tape across the forehead, and secure the person to a board to keep the head, neck, and back areas from moving at all. A

- **Call 9-1-1!**

- **CHECK for a response.** (See Step 2 on page 353.) If giving rescue breaths, do not tilt the head backward. Pull the lower jaw open instead. B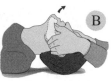

To Immobilize the Head, Neck, and/or Back
- Tell the person to lie still and not move his or her head, neck, back, etc.

- Log roll as listed above or place rolled towels, etc. on both sides of the neck and/or body. Tie in place, but don't interfere with the person's breathing. If necessary, use both of your hands, one on each side of the person's head to keep the head from moving.

- Monitor for **Bleeding** (see page 362) and **Shock** (see page 401). Keep the person warm with blankets, coats, etc.

Move Someone You Suspect Has Injured His or Her Neck in a Diving or Other Water Accident
Before emergency care arrives:
- Protect the neck and/or spine from bending or twisting. Place your hands on both sides of the neck. Keep it in place until help arrives.

- If the person is still in the water, help the person float until a rigid board can be slipped under the head and body, at least as far down as the buttocks.

Head / Neck / Spine Injuries, Continued

First Aid For Traffic Accidents

- If the person was in a motorcycle accident, do not remove the helmet. **Call 9-1-1** to do this.

- Don't move the person. He or she may have a spinal injury. **Call 9-1-1** to do this.

First Aid for Bleeding from the Scalp

- To control bleeding, put pressure around the edges of the wound. Make a ring pad (shaped like a doughnut) out of long strips of cloth to apply pressure around the edges of the wound. If this doesn't control bleeding, put direct pressure on the wound. Don't poke your hand into the person's brain, though.

- Don't wash the wound or apply an antiseptic or any other fluid to it.

- If blood or pink-colored fluid is coming from the ear, nose, or mouth, let it drain. Do not try to stop its flow.

- If no board is available, get several people to take the person out of the water. Support the head and body as one unit. Make sure the head does not rotate or bend in any way.

First Aid for Minor Head Injuries

- Put an ice pack or bag of frozen vegetables in a cloth. Apply this to the injured area. Doing this helps reduce swelling and bruising. Change it every 15 to 20 minutes for 1 to 2 hours. Do not put ice directly on the skin. Cover an open, small cut with gauze and first-aid tape or an adhesive bandage.

- Once you know there is no serious head injury, do normal activities again. Avoid strenuous ones.

- Take an over-the-counter medicine for pain as directed.

- Don't drink alcohol or take any other sedatives or sleeping pills.

- During the next 24 hours, monitor the person. While asleep, wake the person every 2 hours to check alertness. Ask something the person should know, such as a pet's name, an address, etc. If the person can't be roused or respond normally, get immediate medical care.

If You Suspect a Whiplash Injury

- See your doctor, as soon as you can, to find out the extent of injury. If your arm or hand is numb, tell your doctor.

- For the first 24 hours, apply ice packs to the injured area for up to 20 minutes every hour.

- After 24 hours, use ice packs or heat, whichever works best, to relieve the pain. There are many ways to apply heat. Take a hot shower for 20 minutes a few times a day. Use a hot-water bottle, heating pad (set on low), or heat lamp directed to the neck for 10 minutes, several times a day. (Use caution not to burn the skin.)

- Wrap a folded towel around the neck to help hold the head in one position during the night.

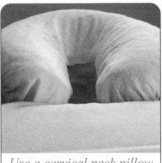

Use a cervical neck pillow or a small rolled towel behind your neck instead of a regular pillow.

Heart Attack

A **heart attack** happens when the heart does not get enough blood supply for a period of time. Part or all of the heart muscle dies.

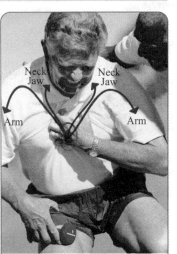

Common places heart attack pain is felt.

Signs & Symptoms

A heart attack may have warning signs. (See box below). It can occur without signs, too. This is called a "silent" heart attack.

Causes

- The most common cause is one or more blood clots that block an artery in the heart. Often, a blood clot forms in an artery already narrowed by plaque.

- Having a heart attack in the past increases the risk for another one.

- Spasms occur in the large coronary artery. This can be triggered by: Heavy physical exertion, such as shoveling snow; exposure to cold; severe emotional stress; and having a heavy meal. These triggers are more likely to affect persons who are not active.

- Cocaine or amphetamine abuse can cause a sudden heart attack. This can happen in persons with no signs of heart disease.

Heart Attack Warning Signs

Common Warning Signs

- Feeling of pain (may spread to or be felt in the arm, neck, tooth, jaw, or back), tightness, burning, squeezing, or heaviness in the chest. This lasts more than a few minutes or goes away and comes back.

- Chest discomfort with:
  - Fainting
  - Feeling lightheaded.
  - Nausea.
  - Shortness of breath.
  - Sweating.

Other Warning Signs

- Unusual chest, abdominal, or stomach pain.

- Dizziness; nausea; trouble breathing; jaw or arm pain without chest pain.

- Fast or uneven heartbeat or pulse.

- Sweating for no reason, pale, gray, or clammy skin.

Signs More Likely in Women Than Men

- An uneasy feeling in the chest with: Unexplained or extreme anxiety; unusual fatigue or weakness; fluttering heartbeats; or severe indigestion that doesn't go away with an antacid.

{*Note:* If any of these signs occur, **call 9-1-1**. Then, give **"First Aid for a Heart Attack Before Emergency Care"** listed on page 388.}

To Learn More, See Back Cover

Heart Attack, Continued

Treatment

A heart attack is a medical emergency! Treatment works best when it is given within 1 to 2 hours after symptoms start. Treatment includes:

- Medicine(s) to keep blood from clotting.

- "Clot busters" to dissolve blood clots in heart arteries.

- Tests to diagnose the status of the heart and arteries.

- Angioplasty, stents, or bypass surgery, if needed.

Prevention

- Follow prevention measures in **Heart Disease** on page 234.

- Take medications, as prescribed.

- Don't shovel snow or carry heavy objects, especially if you are not physically fit.

- Don't use amphetamines and/or cocaine.

Questions to Ask

Do any of these problems occur?
- Any **heart attack warning sign** listed on page 387.
- For a person with angina, chest pain does not respond to prescribed medicine or go away in 10 to 15 minutes.

YES → Get Medical Care Fast

NO → Use Self-Care

{*Note:* **Call 9-1-1** without delay! Then, give first aid listed below as needed.}

Self-Care / First Aid

- Call **9-1-1** or your local rescue squad right away! Call when warning signs start. Don't wait to see if the pain goes away.

First Aid for a Heart Attack Before Emergency Care
- **CHECK for a response**. (See Step 2 on page 353.) Do **CPR** (see pages 354 to 355), as needed.

- If the person uses and has nitroglycerin, place one tablet under the tongue. Give as many as 3 tablets in 10 minutes.

- Give the person a regular (325 mg.) aspirin or 4 children's chewable aspirins (81 mg. each) to chew on. Give the aspirin *after* calling **9-1-1**. Ask the **9-1-1** dispatcher if aspirin should be taken.

{*Note:* Don't use aspirin if the person is allergic to it or has a condition that makes using it risky.}

- If you can't call **9-1-1**, drive the person to the hospital right away. If you are having heart attack signs, don't drive yourself unless you have no other choice.

- Loosen clothing around the neck, chest, and waist. Don't let the person lie down, especially if he or she has breathing problems. A half-sitting position is better. Put the legs up. Bend them at the knees. Put a pillow or rolled towel under the knees. Support the back.

- Reassure the person that you have called for medical help and will stay with him or her until it arrives.

- After a heart attack, follow the doctor's treatment plan.

Heat Exhaustion & Heat Stroke

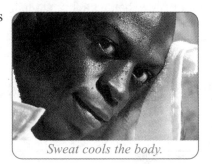

Sweat cools the body.

Sweat evaporates from the skin to cool the body. If this personal cooling system does not work right or fails to work, heat exhaustion or a heat stroke can occur.

Heat exhaustion is a warning that the body is getting too hot. With a **heat stroke**, body organs start to overheat. They will stop working if they get hot enough. If it is not treated, a heat stroke can result in death.

Signs & Symptoms

For a Heat Stroke
These signs and symptoms can occur suddenly with little warning:
- Very high temperature (104°F or higher).
- Hot, dry, red skin. No sweating.
- Deep breathing and fast pulse. Then shallow breathing and weak pulse.
- Confusion. Hallucinations.
- Convulsions.
- Loss of consciousness.

For Heat Exhaustion
- Normal, low, or only slightly elevated body temperature.
- Cool, clammy, pale skin. Sweating.
- Dry mouth. Thirst.
- Fatigue. Weakness. Feeling dizzy.
- Headache.
- Nausea. Vomiting can occur.
- Muscle cramps.
- Weak or rapid pulse.

Causes

Anything that keeps the body's natural cooling system from working right can lead to heat exhaustion and heat stroke. This includes:
- Extreme heat and humidity.
- Being in places without fans or air conditioners during hot, humid weather.
- Not being able to get to public air-conditioned places. Waiting for a bus or other type of public transportation in hot, humid weather.
- Overdressing.
- Changes in the skin due to aging.
- Poor circulation. Heart, lung, and/or kidney disease.
- Not being able to sweat due to medicines, such as water pills and some used for mental illnesses.
- Alcohol or drug use.
- Any illness that causes weakness, fever, vomiting, or diarrhea.

Heat Exhaustion & Heat Stroke, Continued

Treatment

A heat stroke is a medical emergency.

Heat exhaustion may respond to self-care measures. If not, medical care is needed.

Questions to Ask

Is any **sign of a heat stroke** listed on page 389 present? {***Note:* Call 9-1-1** without delay. Then give first aid listed below and on the top of page 391 as needed.}

YES → Get Medical Care Fast

NO ↓

Are these **signs of heat exhaustion** present?
- Dryness on the inside of the mouth.
- Fatigue. Weakness. Listlessness.
- Muscle cramps.
- Feeling lightheaded or faint.

YES → Get Medical Care Fast

NO ↓

With hot conditions, do you sweat a lot <u>and</u> have a headache and nausea?

YES → See Doctor

NO ↓

Use Self-Care

Self-Care / First Aid

First Aid for a Heat Stroke
- **Call 9-1-1!**

Before Emergency Care Arrives
- Move the person to a cool place indoors or under a shady tree. Place the feet higher than the head to avoid shock.

- Remove clothing. Either wrap the person in a cold, wet sheet; sponge the person with towels or sheets that are soaked in cold water; or spray the person with cool water. Fan the person.

- Put ice packs or cold compresses on the neck, under the armpits, and on the groin area.

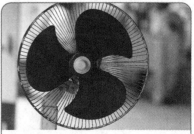

If using an electric fan, keep the person with wet items away from the fan to avoid electric shock.

Heat Exhaustion & Heat Stroke, Continued

- Once the person's temperature gets to 101°F, place him or her in the **Recovery Position**. (See page 357.) Do not lower the temperature further.

- Don't give fever reducing medicine.

- Don't use rubbing alcohol.

First Aid for Heat Exhaustion

- Move to a cool place indoors or in the shade. Lie down.

- Loosen clothing.

- Drink fluids, such as cool or cold water. Add ½ teaspoon of salt to 1 quart of water. Sip this. Or, drink sport drinks, such as Gatorade, etc.

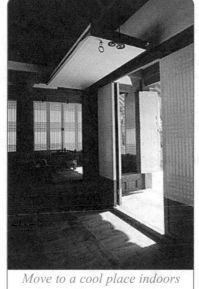

Move to a cool place indoors or in the shade.

- Have salty foods, such as saltine crackers, if you tolerate them.

- Massage and stretch cramped muscles.

Prevention

- Drink lots of liquids, especially if your urine is dark yellow. Drink water, sport drinks, such as Gatorade, etc.

- Do not stay in or leave anyone in a closed, parked car during hot weather.

- Don't have drinks with alcohol or caffeine.

- Use caution when you are in the sun. At the first sign of heat exhaustion, get out of the sun. If you can, avoid midday heat. Do not do vigorous activity during the hottest part of the day (11:00 a.m. to 4:00 p.m.).

- Wear light, loose-fitting clothing, such as cotton, so sweat can evaporate. Wear a wide-brimmed hat with vents. Use an umbrella for shade.

- If you feel very hot, try to cool off. Open a window. Use a fan. Go to an air-conditioned place.

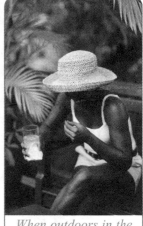

When outdoors in the sun, drink fluids and wear a hat.

- Check with your doctor about sun exposure if you take:

  - Water pills.

  - Mood-altering medicines.

  - Some antibiotics, such as tetracycline.

Hyperventilation

Hyperventilation is breathing too deeply and faster than normal. This causes too much carbon dioxide to be exhaled. As a result, levels of carbon dioxide in the blood and brain tissue drop.

Signs & Symptoms

- Your heart pounds.
- It feels like you can't get enough air.
- You feel tingling and numbness in the arms, legs, and around the mouth.
- You feel a sense of doom.
- You may pass out.

Symptoms usually last 20 to 30 minutes, but seem to last hours. Though scary, hyperventilation is not usually dangerous.

Causes

- Anxiety is the most common cause. (See **Anxiety** on page 269.)
- **Panic attacks.** (See page 269.)
- Central nervous system problems.

Treatment

Self-care may be enough to treat hyperventilation. If it persists or occurs with other symptoms, seek medical care.

Questions to Ask

Do you breathe rapidly and have any of these problems?
- Any **heart attack warning sign**. (See page 387.)
- Bluish or purple color around your lips, fingernails, or skin.
- Asthma, emphysema, or a serious lung or heart problem.
- A seizure. (See **Seizures** on page 399.)

YES → Get Medical Care Fast

NO

Do you hyperventilate often? Or, have you had 4 or more panic attacks over a 4-week span?

YES → See Doctor

NO → Use Self-Care

Self-Care / First Aid

- Open up a small paper bag. Loosely cover your nose and mouth with it. Breathe slowly into the bag. Rebreathe the air in the bag. Do this about 10 times. Set the bag aside. Breathe normally for a couple of minutes.
- Repeat the steps above for up to 15 minutes.
- Try to breathe slowly. Focus on taking one breath every 5 seconds.

See also **Self-Care / Prevention** for **Anxiety** on pages 271 and 272.

{*Note:* If you still hyperventilate after using **Self-Care / First Aid**, call your doctor.}

Near-Drowning

Near-drowning is when a person is in danger of drowning.

Each year, almost 8,000 people die from drowning. Seventy percent of all near-drowning victims recover; 25% die, and 5% have brain damage.

A toddler can drown in as little as 2 inches of water in a bathtub, sink, etc. Toilet bowls are unsafe, too, if a small child falls into one head-first.

Signs & Symptoms

- A person is in the water with signs of distress. He or she can't stay above water, swims unevenly, signals for help, etc.

- Blue lips or ears. The skin is cold and pale.

- Bloated abdomen. Vomiting. Choking.

- Confusion. Lethargy.

- The person does not respond or can't breathe.

Causes

- Not being able to swim. Being in water too deep and too rough for one's ability to swim.

- Water sport and other accidents. Not following water safety rules. Not wearing a life preserver, etc. Unsupervised swimming.

- Falling through ice while fishing, skating, etc.

- Injury or problems that occur while swimming, boating, etc. Examples are leg or stomach cramps, fatigue, and alcohol or drug use. A heart attack, stroke, seizure, and a marine animal bite or sting may have occurred.

Treatment

Immediate medical care is needed for near-drowning.

Questions to Ask

Is the person unconscious and not breathing? Or, does the person have blue lips and ears and is the skin cold and pale? Give **First Aid for Near-Drowning** below.

 YES — Get Medical Care Fast

NO

Does the person in the water show any of these signs?
- Waves or shouts for help.
- Swims in uneven motions.
- Can't stay above water.
{*Note:* Give **First Aid for Near-Drowning** below.}

YES — Get Medical Care Fast

NO

After a near-drowning incident, does the person have a fever, a cough, or muscle pain?

 YES — Get Medical Care Fast

NO

 Use Self-Care

Self-Care / First Aid

First Aid for Near-Drowning
- Shout for help! Send someone to call **9-1-1**!

- If it is safe and possible, try to reach the person. Use a long pole, rope, life preserver, etc. Then pull him or her to safety.

- Did the person fall through ice? Try a human chain rescue to safely reach the person, but stay as far away from cracked ice as you can.

Prevention

For Children

- Never leave an infant or child alone in any type of bathtub. Supervise young children in the bathroom.

- Never leave a child alone near water, swimming pools, etc. Lock gates to keep children from getting near swimming pools.

- Have a phone near outdoor pools, etc.

- Teach children to swim. Tell them not to swim alone and not to swim too far from shore without a lifeguard or other adult swimmer.

- Put a personal floatation device on each child when near the water or on a boat.

- Tell children to check the depth of water before diving in. It should be at least 9 feet deep.

- Do not allow children to go on untested ice.

- Take CPR and water safety courses.

Near-Drowning, Continued

- If you must swim to the person, be sure you are strong and capable enough. Take a flotation device with you. Approach the person from behind in a calm manner. Grab a piece of the person's clothing. Or, cup one hand under the person's chin.

- When getting the person out of the water, support the head and neck. (Suspect a neck injury, especially with diving or water sports.)

- **CHECK for a response**. (See Step 2 on page 353.) Give **Rescue Breaths** and **CPR** (see pages 354 to 355), as needed. If you suspect a spinal injury, use jaw thrust instead of chin-lift for rescue breaths.

- Once out of the water, keep checking the person for a response. Give first aid, as needed.

- Put the person in the **Recovery Position**. (See page 357.) Immobilize the person as much as possible. If the person is vomiting, clear his or her mouth of it.

- Remove cold, wet clothes. Cover the person with a blanket, etc.

Prevention

For Adults

- Learn to swim. Never swim alone at the beach or in a swimming pool. A lifeguard or other adult swimmer should be nearby in case you suffer a leg cramp or other problem.

- Wear a personal floatation device when you are on a boat, when you fish, etc.

- Check the depth of the water before diving in. It should be at least 9 feet deep. Never dive into an above-ground pool.

- Do not use a hot tub or jacuzzi if you've had any alcoholic drinks. You could fall asleep, slip under the surface, and drown.

- Take CPR and water safety courses.

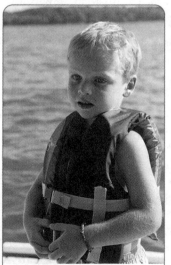

Children should wear a personal floatation device.

Objects in the Ear or Nose

A foreign object stuck in an ear or the nose needs to be removed. If not, an infection could result. Damage to structures in the nose or ear could also occur.

Signs & Symptoms

A child may be able to tell if an object was put in a nostril or an ear and didn't come out. If not, signs and symptoms can help identify this problem.

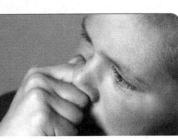

Young children like to put things in their mouths, ears, and nose.

For an Object Stuck in an Ear
- Feeling of fullness in the ear.
- Ear pain or discomfort.
- Hearing loss and/or feeling dizzy.
- Foul odor from the ear and/or drainage from the ear.
- Bleeding from an ear.

For an Object Stuck in the Nose
- Constant nasal discharge from one nostril.
- Foul odor. Pus or blood drains from a nostril.
- Pain, swelling, and/or tenderness.

Causes

- An object or substance is placed in the ear or nose on purpose and won't come out.
- Objects get stuck in the nose or ear by injury or by accident.
- An insect flies or crawls into an ear.

Questions to Ask

Do any of these problems occur?
- A sharp object is stuck in a nostril or ear.
- An object stuck in a nostril or ear causes severe pain or a lot of bleeding.
- Removing an object from a nostril caused a severe nosebleed.
- A button-size battery is stuck in a nostril or ear.

YES → Get Medical Care Fast

NO ↓

Do any of these problems occur?
- Hearing loss or feeling dizzy.
- Signs of an infection, such as fever, pain, swelling, foul odor, pus drainage, etc.
- An insect cannot safely be removed from an ear.
- After several tries, an object cannot be removed from a nostril or an ear.

YES → See Doctor

NO ↓

 Use Self-Care

See Self-Care / First Aid on next page

Objects in the Ear or Nose, Continued

Treatment

Medical care is needed for foreign objects that can't be removed with self-care. After an object is removed, an antibiotic may be needed if an infection is present. Small, button-sized batteries need to be removed to prevent burns.

Self-Care / First Aid

To Remove an Insect from an Ear

■ Kill the insect before you try to remove it. To do this, tilt the person's head to put the ear with the insect in an upward position. Pour warm (not hot) mineral, olive, or baby oil into the ear. As you pour the oil, straighten the ear canal. In a child, pull the earlobe gently backward and downward; backward and upward in an adult.

■ The goal is to suffocate the insect and cause it to float out.

To Remove Objects Other Than Insects

■ Don't use oil.

■ Tilt the head toward the side with the foreign object. Gently shake the head toward the floor to try to get the object out. **Do not shake a baby.** Gently pull the ear up and back.

■ Don't use a sharp tool, cotton swab, etc., to try to locate and remove the object. This risks pushing the object farther into the ear. Doing this could damage the middle ear.

■ Remove the object with blunt tweezers if it is easily seen and can be grasped and pulled out.

To Remove Objects in the Nose

■ Don't use a sharp tool, cotton swab, etc., to try to locate and remove the object.

■ Breathe through the mouth until the object is removed.

■ Apply gentle pressure to close the other nostril and gently try to blow the object out.

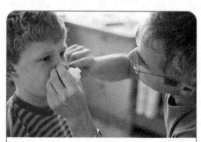

To reduce swelling, spray a nasal decongestant in the nostril with the foreign object.

■ Remove the object with blunt tweezers, if it is easily seen and can be grasped and pulled out.

Poisoning

Poisons are harmful substances that are swallowed, inhaled, or that come in contact with the skin. Each year about 10 million poisonings occur; 80% of them are in children under five years old.

Signs & Symptoms

Signs and symptoms depend on the substance. They include a skin rash, upset stomach, and more severe problems. Some poisons can cause death.

Causes

Things Not Meant to Be Swallowed or Inhaled

- Household cleaners, such as bleach, drain cleaners, ammonia, and lye.
- Insecticides. Rat poison.
- Gasoline. Antifreeze. Oil. Lighter fluid. Paint thinner.
- Lead.
- Airplane glue. Formaldehyde.
- Rubbing alcohol. Iodine. Hair dye. Mouthwash. Mothballs.
- Some indoor and outdoor plants.
- Carbon monoxide. This has no color, odor, or taste.

Things That Are Poisonous in Harmful Amounts

- Alcohol. Drugs. Over-the-counter and prescribed medicines.
- Medicinal herbs.
- Vitamins and minerals. Iron in these can be deadly to a small child.

See also **Food Poisoning** on page 158 and **Bites & Stings** on page 358.

Questions to Ask

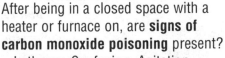

Is the person unconscious, having convulsions, or not breathing? {*Note:* See **First Aid For Unconsciousness** on page 379; **First Aid For Seizures with Convulsion** on page 400; and **Rescue Breathing** on page 354.}

YES ▶ Get Medical Care Fast

NO

After being in a closed space with a heater or furnace on, are **signs of carbon monoxide poisoning** present?
- Lethargy. Confusion. Agitation.
- Sudden shortness of breath.
- Severe headache. Abdominal pain.
- Seizure.
- Chest pain or irregular heartbeat.
- **Signs of shock**. (See page 401.)

YES ▶ Get Medical Care Fast

NO

Do any of these problems occur?
- Pulse rate is 140 or more beats per minute or 40 or fewer beats per minute.
- Shortness of breath. Breathing 10 or fewer breaths per minute. Time lapses of more than 8 seconds between breaths.
- Any change in mental status.
- Hallucinations.

YES ▶ Get Medical Care Fast

{*Note:* First, call Poison Control Center at 800.222.1222.}

NO

Has any substance been swallowed, inhaled, or absorbed by the skin that has "Harmful or fatal if swallowed" or a skull-and-crossbones sign on the label? Or, did the person take a substance that could be poisonous.

YES ▶ Get Medical Care Fast

{*Note:* First, call Poison Control Center at 800.222.1222.}

NO

Use Self-Care

See Self-Care / First Aid on next page

397

Poisoning, Continued

Treatment

Treatment depends on the poison and its effects.

Information to give the Poison Control Center, emergency department, etc.:

- The name of the substance taken.

- The amount and when it was taken.

- A list of ingredients on the label.

- Age, gender, and weight of the person who took the poison. How the person is feeling and reacting. Any medical problems the person has.

Get more information from:

National Poison Control Center
800.222.1222
www.poisonprevention.org

Home Safety Council®
www.homesafetycouncil.org

Self-Care / First Aid

For Swallowed Poisons

1. If the person is unconscious, shout for help. **Call 9-1-1!**

2. For a conscious person, call the Poison Control Center (800.222.1222). Follow instructions. Do not give Syrup of Ipecac to induce vomiting unless the Poison Control Center tells you to. {*Note:* The American Academy of Pediatrics recommends that parents *don't* give Syrup of Ipecac to children.}

3. Lay the person on his or her left side to keep the windpipe clear, especially if the person vomited. Keep a sample of the vomit and the poison container.

For Inhaled Poisons

1. Protect yourself. Move the person to fresh air (outdoors if you can). Try not to breathe the fumes yourself.

2. Follow steps 1 and 2 above for **Swallowed Poisons**. Get medical care.

For Chemical Poisons on Skin

1. Protect yourself. Flood the skin with water for 5 or more minutes. Remove clothing that was in contact with the person.

2. Gently wash the skin with soap and water. Rinse well. Get medical care.

Prevention

- Buy household products, vitamins, and medicines in child-resistant packaging. Keep these and all poisons out of children's reach.

- Put child-resistant latches on cabinet doors. Follow instructions for use and storage of pesticides, household cleaners, and other poisons.

- Keep products in original containers. Don't transfer them to soft drink bottles, plastic jugs, etc.

- Teach children not to take medicine and vitamins unless an adult gives it to them. Don't call these "candy" in front of a child.

- Wear protective clothing, masks, etc., when using chemicals that could cause harm if inhaled or absorbed by the skin.

- Install carbon monoxide detectors in your home and garage.

Seizures

A **seizure** is a sudden "episode" caused by an electrical problem in the brain. With a seizure, a person has change in awareness, body movements, or sensation.

Signs & Symptoms

There are many types of seizures. Common types are:

- **A Generalized Tonic Clonic Seizure.** This is also called a **grand mal seizure**. A **convulsion** occurs with this type. Signs of a convulsion include:
  - Brief loss of consciousness. Falling down.
  - The arms and legs stiffen, jerk, and twitch.
  - This type usually lasts 1 to 2 minutes. When it ends, the person's muscles relax. He or she may lose bladder control, be confused, have a headache, and fall asleep. This is the type most people think of with the word "seizure."

- **An Absence Seizure.** This is also called a **petit mal seizure**. A convulsion does not occur with this type. Signs of an absence seizure include:
  - Blank stares. It looks like the person is daydreaming or not paying attention.
  - Lip smacking. Repeated blinking, chewing or hand movements.
  - This type of seizure usually lasts only a few seconds, but can occur many times a day. When the seizure ends, the person is not confused, but is not aware that the seizure occurred.
  - Absence seizures are common in children and can result in learning problems.

- **A Fever (Febrile) Seizure.** This type is brought on by a high fever in infants and small children. High fevers cause most seizures in children aged 6 months to 5 years. Signs are ones of a convulsion listed in the left column. Most febrile seizures last 1 to 2 minutes, but can last longer. Seeing a child have a febrile seizure causes alarm. In general, these seizures are harmless.

Causes

Causes include **epilepsy** (a brain disorder), infections that cause a high fever, heat stroke, and electric shock. Head injury, stroke, and toxic substances can also cause a seizure. Sometimes the cause of a seizure is not known.

Treatment

Seizure disorders are treated with medication. Other medical treatments may be needed.

Questions to Ask

Did the seizure occur with or after any of the following?
- The person stopped breathing. {**Note:** Give **Rescue Breaths**. See page 354.}
- A head or other serious injury. {**Note:** See **Head / Neck / Spine Injuries** on page 384.}
- **Signs and symptoms of a heat stroke**. (See page 389.)
- **Electric shock**. (See page 373.)
- **Poisoning**. (See page 397.)
- **Symptoms of meningitis**. (See page 101.)
- An illness with symptoms of lethargy and confusion, flu, or chicken pox.

YES ▶ Get Medical Care Fast

NO ▼

Flowchart continued on next page

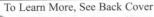

Seizures, Continued

Febrile Seizure Prevention
For a child who has had a febrile seizure in the past, give acetaminophen or ibuprofen at the first sign of a fever. Give the right kind and dose for his or her weight. Insert suppositories that lower fevers, instead, if prescribed by the child's doctor.

{*Note:* Don't give aspirin to anyone less than 19 years old.}

- Dress the child in light, loose clothes.

- Apply washcloths rinsed in lukewarm (not cold) water to your child's forehead and neck. Sponge the child's arms, legs, and trunk with lukewarm water. **Don't use cold water, ice, or rubbing alcohol.**

- Keep trying to bring the fever down until it is 101°F or less.

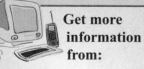

Get more information from:

National Institute of Neurological Disorders and Stroke (NINDS)
www.ninds.nih.gov

Are any of these conditions present?
- This is the first time the person had a seizure or the seizure lasts longer than 5 minutes.
- The person has a second seizure soon after the first one or has multiple seizures.
- The person has a hard time breathing.
- The person who had the seizure is pregnant or has diabetes.
- The seizure is different from the typical seizure the person has. (It may take longer to wake up after the seizure ends.)

YES → Get Medical Care Fast

NO ↓

Has the person stopped taking medicines for seizures? Or, do seizures occur more often or are they more severe?

YES → See Doctor

NO ↓

 Use Self-Care

Self-Care / First Aid

For Seizures with Convulsions
- Stay calm. Protect the person from injury. Cushion the head with a pillow, a coat, etc. Move sharp objects out of the way.

- Loosen tight clothes, especially around the neck.

- If the person vomits, clear the mouth of it.

- Do not hold the person down or throw water on the face. Don't put anything into the mouth. (A spoon in the mouth does not prevent tongue biting.)

- If the seizure in a child is due to a fever, start bringing the child's temperature down as soon as the seizure stops. Sponge the child's body with room temperature water. Do not put the child in a bathtub. Do not use ice. Do not use rubbing alcohol.

- Report how long the seizure lasts and the symptoms that occur.

- After the seizure, lay the person on his or her side. Let the person sleep. Check for a medical alert tag. Respond as needed. Do not embarrass the person.

- **Call 9-1-1** (except for a febrile seizure or a seizure in a person you know has a seizure disorder).

Shock

Shock occurs when the circulation system fails to send blood to all parts of the body. With shock, blood flow or blood volume is too low to meet

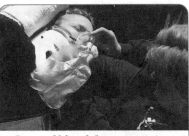

Loss of blood from any injury can cause shock.

the body's needs. Areas of the body are deprived of oxygen. The result is damage to the limbs, lungs, heart, and brain.

Signs & Symptoms

- Weakness. Trembling.
- Feeling restless. Confusion.
- Pale or blue-colored lips, skin, and/or fingernails. Cool and moist skin.
- Rapid, shallow breathing. Weak, but fast pulse.
- Nausea. Vomiting. Extreme thirst.
- Enlarged pupils.
- Loss of consciousness.

Causes

- A heart attack.
- Severe or sudden blood loss from an injury or serious illness. Bleeding can occur inside or outside the body.
- A large drop in body fluids, such as following a severe burn.

Treatment

Shock requires emergency medical care.

Questions to Ask

Are **signs and symptoms of shock** listed on this page present? {*Note:* **Call 9-1-1**! Then, give first aid listed below.}

 YES Get Medical Care Fast

 NO Use Self-Care

Self-Care / First Aid

First Aid for Shock Before Emergency Care

- **CHECK for a response**. (See Step 2 on page 353.) Give **Rescue Breaths** or **CPR** as needed. (See pages 354 to 355.)
- Lay the person flat, face-up, but do not move him or her if you suspect a head, back, or neck injury.
- Raise the person's feet about 12 inches. Use a box, etc. Do not raise the feet or move the legs if hip or leg bones are broken. Keep the person lying flat.
- If the person vomits or has trouble breathing, raise him or her to a half-sitting position (if no head, back, or neck injury). Or, turn the person on his or her side to prevent choking.
- Loosen tight clothing. Keep the person warm. Cover the person with a coat, blanket, etc.
- Monitor for a response. Repeat the steps listed above, as needed.
- Do not give any food or liquids. If the person wants water, moisten the lips.
- Reassure the person. Make him or her as comfortable as you can.

Skin Injuries / Wounds

Signs & Symptoms

Cuts slice the skin open. This causes bleeding and pain.

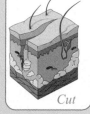

Cut

Scrapes are less serious than cuts, but more painful because more nerve endings are affected.

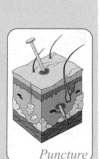

Scrape

Punctures are stab wounds. This causes pain, but may not result in bleeding.

Puncture

Bruises cause black and blue or red skin. As they heal, the skin turns yellowish-green. Pain, tenderness, and swelling also occur.

Causes

For Cuts, Scrapes & Punctures
The cause can be any object that penetrates the skin. This includes cut glass, a splinter, stepping on a nail or tack, falling on pavement, etc.

For Bruises
Common causes are falls or being hit by some force. Bruises result when broken blood vessels bleed into the tissue under the skin. Persons who take blood-thinners bruise easily.

For information on **Burns**, see pages 368 and 369.

Treatment

Treatment depends on the cause and how severe the skin injury is. Simple wounds can be treated with self-care. An antibiotic treats a bacterial infection. Medical care, such as stitches, may be needed for deep cuts or ones longer than an inch.

Questions to Ask

With an injury, do any of the following occur?
- Loss of consciousness. {***Note:*** See **Self-Care / First Aid For Unconsciousness** on page 379.}
- **Signs of shock**. (See page 401.)
- Severe bleeding or blood spurts from the wound. (Apply direct pressure on the wound site while seeking care.)
- Bleeding continues after pressure has been applied for more than 10 minutes (or after 20 minutes for a minor cut).
- A deep cut or puncture appears to go down to the muscle or bone and/or is located on the scalp or face.
- A cut is longer than an inch and is located on an area of the body that bends, (e.g., the elbow, knees, etc.).
- The skin on the edges of the cut hangs open.

NO

Flowchart continued on next page

YES Get Medical Care Fast

{***Note:*** Give first aid as needed. See **First Aid** sections in **Bleeding** on page 364 and in **Skin Injuries/ Wounds** on page 403.}

Skin Injuries / Wounds, Continued

Does any **sign of infection** occur?
- Fever and/or general ill feeling.
- Redness. Or, red streaks extend from the wound site.
- Increased swelling, pain, or tenderness at or around the wound.

YES → See Doctor

NO ↓

Was the cut or puncture from dirty objects, rusty nails, or objects in the soil? Or, did a puncture go through a shoe, especially a rubber-soled one?

YES → See Doctor

NO ↓

Do you have any of these problems?
- Bruises appear often and easily, take longer than 2 weeks to heal, or occur more than 3 times a year for no known reason.
- Vision problems occur with a bruise near the eye.

YES → See Doctor

NO ↓

Use Self-Care

Self-Care / First Aid

{*Note:* For severe bleeding, see **Self-Care / First Aid – For Severe Bleeding** on page 363.}

For Minor Cuts and Scrapes

- Clean in and around the wound thoroughly with soap and water.

- Press on the cut for up to 10 minutes to stop the bleeding. Use sterile, wet gauze or a clean cloth. Dry gauze can stick to the wound. Don't use a bandage to apply pressure.

- If still bleeding, lift the part of the body with the cut higher than the heart, if practical.

- After the bleeding has stopped and when the area is clean and dry, apply a first-aid cream.

- Put one or more bandages on the cut. The edges of the cut skin should touch, but not overlap. Use a butterfly bandage if you have one.

- Keep a scrape clean and dry. Dress it with gauze and first-aid tape. Change this every 24 hours.

For Punctures that Cause Minor Bleeding
- Let the wound bleed to cleanse itself.

- Remove the object (e.g., splinter). Use clean tweezers. Hold a lit match or flame to the ends of the tweezers to sterilize them. Let them cool and wipe the ends with sterile gauze.

- Two to 4 times a day, clean the wound area with soapy water. Dry it well and apply an antibacterial cream. Do this for several days.

For Bruises
- Apply a cold pack to the bruised area as soon as possible (within 15 minutes of the injury). Keep the cold pack on for 10 minutes at a time. Apply pressure to the cold pack. Take it off for 30 to 60 minutes. Repeat several times for 2 days.

- Rest the bruised area and raise it above the level of the heart, if practical.

- Two days after the injury, use warm compresses for 20 minutes at a time.

- Do not bandage a bruise. Try to avoid hitting the bruised area again.

Get more information from:

HealthyLearn® • www.HealthyLearn.com
Click on MedlinePlus®

National Safety Council
www.nsc.org

Sprains, Strains & Sports Injuries

Common Sports Injuries

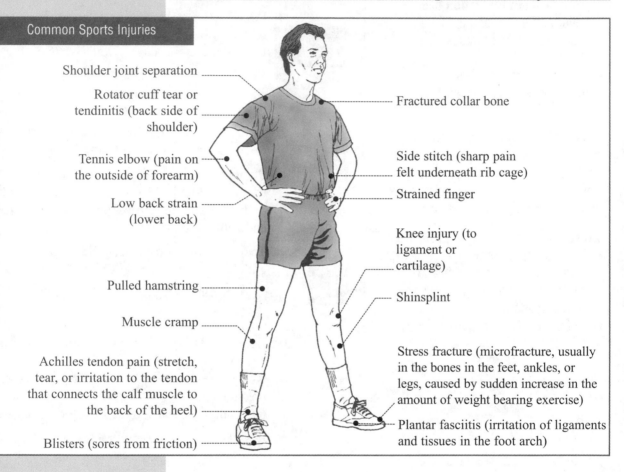

Shoulder joint separation

Rotator cuff tear or tendinitis (back side of shoulder)

Tennis elbow (pain on the outside of forearm)

Low back strain (lower back)

Pulled hamstring

Muscle cramp

Achilles tendon pain (stretch, tear, or irritation to the tendon that connects the calf muscle to the back of the heel)

Blisters (sores from friction)

Fractured collar bone

Side stitch (sharp pain felt underneath rib cage)

Strained finger

Knee injury (to ligament or cartilage)

Shinsplint

Stress fracture (microfracture, usually in the bones in the feet, ankles, or legs, caused by sudden increase in the amount of weight bearing exercise)

Plantar fasciitis (irritation of ligaments and tissues in the foot arch)

Signs & Symptoms

For Sprains

A sprain happens when you overstretch or tear a ligament. (This is fibrous tissue that connects bones.) A joint is affected, but there is no dislocation or fracture. Symptoms are rapid pain, swelling, bruising, and a warm feeling at the injured site.

For Strains

A strain is an injury to the muscles or tendons. (These are tissues that connect muscles to bones.) Symptoms are pain, tenderness, swelling, and bruising.

Sprains, Strains & Sports Injuries, Continued

For Sports Injuries

Sports injury symptoms depend on the injury. They include pain, tenderness, swelling, and bruising. Bones may be broken or dislocated. (See **Common Sports Injuries** on page 404.)

Causes

Sprains occur from an accident, injury, fall, etc. A strain occurs when you overstretch or overexert a muscle or tendon (not a ligament). This is usually due to overuse and injuries, such as sports injuries.

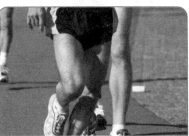

An ankle sprain can cause strain on the achilles tendon.

Questions to Ask

Do you suspect a head, neck, or spinal injury by any of these symptoms?
- Loss of consciousness.
- Paralysis. The head, neck, or back can't move.
- Inability to open and close the fingers or move the toes or any part of the arms and legs.
- Feelings of numbness in the legs, arms, shoulders, or any body part.
- It looks like the head, neck, or back is in an odd position.
- Neck pain is felt right away.

YES **Get Medical Care Fast**

{*Note:* See **First Aid** section in **Head/ Neck/ Spine Injuries** on page 385.}

NO

Flowchart continued in next column

Are any of these signs present?
- A bone sticks out or bones in the injured part make a grating sound.
- An injured body part looks bent, shortened, or misshaped.
- You can't move the injured body part or put weight on it.
- The injured area is blue, pale, or feels cool, but the same limb on the other side of the body does not.

YES **Get Medical Care Fast**

{*Note:* See **First Aid** section in **Broken Bones/ Dislocations** on page 367.}

NO

Are any of these signs present?
- You can't bend or straighten an injured limb.
- Bad pain and swelling occur or the pain gets worse.
- Pain is felt when you press along the bone near the injury.

YES **See Doctor**

NO

Does the sprain or strain not improve after using self-care for 2 days?

YES **Call Doctor**

NO

Use Self-Care

Self-Care / First Aid

- If the injury is not serious, stop what you are doing and use **R.I.C.E.** (See page 197.)

- If you sprained a finger or hand, remove rings. (If you don't and your fingers swell up, the rings may have to be cut off.)

- Take an over-the-counter medicine for pain, if needed. {*Note:* Many sports medicine providers do not recommend aspirin-like medicine at first, because it can make bleeding and bruising worse.}

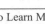

Sprains, Strains & Sports Injuries, Continued

Treatment

Treatment for sprains, strains, and sports injuries depends on the injury and on the extent of damage. Self-care may be all that is needed for mild injuries. Sports injuries and sprains may need medical treatment. Some sprains need a cast. Others may need surgery if the tissue affected is torn.

Broken bones (other than broken toes) need medical care right away.

■ Try liniments and balms. These give a cooling or warming sensation by masking the pain. They do not promote healing.

■ Once the injury begins to heal, use M.S.A.:

• *Movement.* Work toward a full range of motion as soon as possible. This will help maintain flexibility during healing and prevent any scar tissue from limiting future performance.

• *Strength.* Gradually strengthen the injured area once the swelling is controlled and a range of motion is back.

• *Alternative Activities.* Do regular exercises that do not strain the injured part. Start this a few days after the injury, even though the injured part is still healing.

Prevention

To Prevent Serious Injuries (especially during contact sports)

■ Wear the right protective gear and clothing for the sport (e.g., a helmet; shoulder, knee, and wrist pads; a mouth guard, etc.).

■ Train in the sport so you learn how to avoid injury. "Weekend athletes" are prone to injury. Follow the rules that apply to the sport.

General Prevention

■ Ease into any exercise program. Build up gradually.

■ Avoid running on hard surfaces like asphalt and concrete. Run on flat surfaces. Running uphill puts added stress on the achilles tendon.

■ Don't lock your knees. When you jump, land with your knees bent.

■ Wear shoes and socks that fit well. The widest area of your foot should match the widest area of the shoe. You should be able to wiggle your toes with the shoe on when you sit and when you stand. Wear shoes that provide shock absorption and stability.

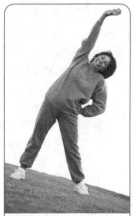

Do warm-up exercises before the activity.

Get more information from:

HealthyLearn®
www.HealthyLearn.com
Click on MedlinePlus®

National Institute of Arthritis and Musculoskeletal and Skin Diseases (NIAMS)
www.nih.gov/niams

■ Stop if you feel pain. Don't do the activity until you can do it without pain.

■ Cool down after exercise. Do the activity at a slower pace for 5 minutes.

Stroke (Brain Attack)

A **stroke** is also called a "brain attack." With a stroke, brain cells die due to a blood clot or rupture of a blood vessel in the brain. The end result is brain damage (and possible death).

In the U.S., strokes are the 3rd leading cause of death. They are the leading cause of adult disability.

Stroke Warning Signs
Sudden numbness or weakness of the face, arm, or leg, especially on one side of the body.
Sudden confusion, trouble speaking or understanding.
Sudden trouble seeing in one or both eyes.
Sudden trouble walking, dizziness, loss of balance or coordination.
Sudden severe headache with no known cause.

Causes

Most strokes are caused by a blood clot in an artery in the neck or brain. Some are caused by bleeding into or around the brain.

Risk Factors for a Stroke

- **Transient ischemic attack (TIA)**. This is a temporary lack of blood supply to the brain. With a TIA, stroke symptoms can appear for a short term and then go away. A TIA is a warning that a stroke may follow.

- **Atrial fibrillation**. This is an irregular beating of the heart.

- High blood pressure. Cigarette smoking. Diabetes. Heart disease.

Questions to Ask

Does any **stroke warning sign** occur? {*Note:* **Call 9-1-1** without delay! Then, follow first aid listed below.} — **YES** → **Get Medical Care Fast**

NO ↓

In the past, have stroke warning signs occurred briefly and then gone away? — **YES** → **See Doctor**

NO ↓

Use Self-Care

Self-Care / First Aid

First Aid before Emergency Care

- Note the time when the first sign(s) of stroke occurred. Report this time to emergency personnel. For the most common type of strokes, a clot-busting drug should to be given within 3 hours of the start of symptoms.

- Do not give the person anything to eat or drink. Do not give aspirin.

Prevention

- Take medicine(s), as prescribed, to control blood pressure, blood cholesterol, diabetes, and atrial fibrillation. Aspirin may help reduce the risk of stroke in women ages 55-79 years. Discuss this with your doctor.

- Get to and stay at a healthy weight. Get regular exercise.

- Don't smoke. If you smoke, quit. Use alcohol in moderation. Manage stress.

Get more information from:

American Stroke Association
888.4.STROKE (478.7653)
www.strokeassociation.org

Index

M

N

O